£44.00

This book is to be returned on or before
the last date stamped below.

2 6 DEC 1983		
27 APR 1984		
1 4 OCT 1998		

LIBREX —

PATHOLOGY OF OXYGEN

Pathology of Oxygen

Edited by

Anne P. Autor

Department of Pharmacology
College of Medicine
The University of Iowa
Iowa City, Iowa

1982

ACADEMIC PRESS

A Subsidiary of Harcourt Brace Jovanovich, Publishers

New York   London
Paris   San Diego   San Francisco   São Paulo   Sydney   Tokyo   Toronto

ACADEMIC PRESS, INC.
111 Fifth Avenue, New York, New York 10003

United Kingdom Edition published by
ACADEMIC PRESS, INC. (LONDON) LTD.
24/28 Oval Road, London NW1 7DX

Library of Congress Cataloging in Publication Data

Main entry under title:

Pathology of oxygen.

    Includes index.
    1. Oxygen--Toxicology. I. Autor, Anne Pomeroy.
[DNLM: 1. Oxygen--Toxicity. QV 312 P297]
RA1247.09P37   615.9'1   82-6730
ISBN 0-12-068620-1   AACR2

PRINTED IN THE UNITED STATES OF AMERICA

82 83 84 85   9 8 7 6 5 4 3 2 1

Contents

CHAPTER 1
Superoxide Dismutase in Biology and Medicine
Irwin Fridovich

CHAPTER 2
Light, Oxygen, and Toxicity
Christopher S. Foote

CHAPTER 3

The Role of Active Oxygen in Microbial Killing by Phagocytes
Bernard M. Babior

CHAPTER 4

The Stimulated Granulocyte as a Source of Toxic Oxygen Compounds in Tissue Injury
Dale E. Hammerschmidt and Harry S. Jacob

CHAPTER 5

**A Mechanism for the Antiinflammatory Activity of
Superoxide Dismutase**
*Joe M. McCord, Kenneth Wong, Steven H. Stokes,
William F. Petrone, and Denis English*

CHAPTER 6

**Effect of Intraperitoneally Administered Superoxide
Dismutase on Pulmonary Damage Resulting from Hyperoxia**
Geoffrey McLennan and Anne P. Autor

CHAPTER 7

**Macrophage-Generated Superoxide Radicals:
Inflammation and Tumor Cell Growth**
Yoshihiko Ōyanagui

CHAPTER 8

Oxygen Radicals, Hydrogen Peroxide, and Parkinson's Disease
Gerald Cohen

CHAPTER 9

Oxygen Free Radicals in Central Nervous System Ischemia and Trauma
Harry B. Demopoulos, Eugene Flamm, Myron Seligman, and Dennis D. Pietronigro

CHAPTER 10

Free Radicals and Microvascular Permeability
Rolando F. Del Maestro, Jacob Björk, and Karl E. Arfors

CHAPTER 11

Studies on a Destructive Oxidant Released in the Enzymatic Reduction of Prostaglandin G_2 and Other Hydroperoxy Acids
Frederick A. Kuehl, Jr., Edward A. Ham, Robert W. Egan, Harry W. Dougherty, Robert J. Bonney, and John L. Humes

CHAPTER 21

Superoxide Dismutase Therapy in Degenerative Joint Disease
Knud Lund-Olesen

CHAPTER 22

Evaluation of Safety of Superoxide Dismutase in the Treatment of Urological Disorders
Joseph D. Schmidt and Thomas L. Schulte

Contributors

Numbers in parentheses indicate the pages on which the authors' contributions begin.

Karl E. Arfors (157), Department of Experimental Medicine, Pharmacia AB, S-751, 04, Uppsala, Sweden

Anne P. Autor (85), Department of Pharmacology, University of Iowa, Iowa City, Iowa 52242

Bernard M. Babior (45), Department of Medicine, Blood Research Laboratory, Tufts-New England Medical Center, Boston, Massachusetts 02111

George Bartsch (327), Department of Urology, University of Innsbruck, Innsbruck A6020, Austria

Isabel B. Bize[1] (207), Radiation Research Laboratory, University of Iowa, Iowa City, Iowa 52242

Jacob Björk (157), Department of Experimental Medicine, Pharmacia AB, S-75104 Uppsala, Sweden

Robert J. Bonney (175), Department of Immunology, Merck Sharpe and Dohme, Research Laboratory, Rahway, New Jersey 07065

Garry R. Buettner (207), Department of Chemistry, Wabash College, Crawfordsville, Indiana 47933

William S. Chelack (223), Medical Biophysics Branch, Whiteshell Nuclear Research Establishment, Atomic Energy of Canada, Ltd., Pinawa, Manitoba ROE 1LO, Canada

Gerald Cohen (115), Department of Neurology, Mount Sinai School of Medicine, City University of New York, New York, New York 10029

Rolando F. Del Maestro (157), Brain Research Laboratory, Department of Clinical Neurological Sciences, Victoria Hospital, University of Western Ontario, London, Ontario N6A 4G5, Canada

[1] *Present address:* Embryology Laboratory, I.C.B., Catholic University of Chile, Casilla 114-D, Santiago, Chile.

Harry B. Demopoulos (127, 191) Department of Pathology and Neurosurgery, New York University School of Medicine, New York, New York 10016

James Doroshow[2] (245), Institute for Toxicology and Department of Biochemistry, University of Southern California, Los Angeles, California 90033

Harry W. Dougherty (175), Department of Biochemistry of Inflammation, Merck Institute for Therapeutic Research, Rahway, New Jersey 07065

Folke Edsmyr (315), Radiumhemmet, Karolinska Hospital, S-104 01, Stockholm 6, Sweden

Robert W. Egan (175), Department of Inflammation and Arthritis, Merck Institute for Therapeutic Research, Rahway, New Jersey 07065

Denis English (75), Division of Pediatric Oncology-Hematology, Vanderbilt University Medical Center, Nashville, Tennessee 37232

Lawrence J. Fischer (261), Department of Pharmacology, University of Iowa, Iowa City, Iowa 52242

Eugene Flamm (127), Department of Neurosurgery, New York University School of Medicine, New York, New York 10016

Christopher S. Foote (21), Department of Chemistry, University of California, Los Angeles, California 90024

Irwin Fridovich (1), Department of Biochemistry, Duke University Medical School, Durham, North Carolina 27710

Henry G. Friesen (223), Physiology Department, University of Manitoba, Winnipeg, Manitoba R3T 2N2, Canada

Edward A. Ham (175), Department of Inflammation and Arthritis, Merck Institute for Therapeutic Research, Rahway, New Jersey 07065

Dale E. Hammerschmidt (59), Division of Hematology, Department of Medicine, University of Minnesota Medical School, Minneapolis, Minnesota 55455

A. W. Harman (261), Department of Pharmacology, University of Iowa, Iowa City, Iowa 52242

Paul Hochstein (245), Institute for Toxicology and Department of Biochemistry, University of Southern California, Los Angeles, California 90033

James A. Hokanson (191), Department of Preventive Medicine and Community Health, University of Texas Medical Branch, Galveston, Texas 77550

John L. Humes (175), Department of Inflammation and Arthritis, Merck Institute for Therapeutic Research, Rahway, New Jersey 07065

---

[2] *Present address:* Department of Medical Oncology, City of Hope National Medical Center, Duarte, California 91010.

Harry S. Jacob (59), Division of Hematology, Department of Medicine, University of Minnesota Medical School, Minneapolis, Minnesota 55455

Kenneth Kelly (223), Immunology Department, University of Manitoba, Winnipeg, Manitoba R3E OW3, Canada

Frederick A. Kuehl, Jr. (175), Department of Biochemistry of Inflammation, Merck Institute for Therapeutic Research, Rahway, New Jersey 07065

Susan W. H. C. Leuthauser (207), Radiation Research Laboratory, University of Iowa, Iowa City, Iowa 52242

Knud Lund-Olesen (339), Ringe Hospital, 5750 Ringe, Denmark

H. Marberger (327), Department of Urology, University of Innsbruck, Innsbruck A6020, Austria

Joe M. McCord (75), Department of Biochemistry, College of Medicine, University of South Alabama, Mobile, Alabama 36688

John E. McGinness (191), Department of Physics, University of Texas Cancer Center, Houston, Texas 77030

Geoffrey McLennan[3] (85), Department of Pharmacology, University of Iowa, Iowa City, Iowa 52242

A. M. Michelson (277), Institut de Biologie Physico-Chimique, Service de Biochimie-Physique, 75005 Paris, France

Larry W. Oberley (207), Radiation Research Laboratory, University of Iowa, Iowa City, Iowa 52242

Terry D. Oberley (207), Department of Pathology, University of Wisconsin, Madison, Wisconsin 53706

Yoshihiko Ōyanagui (99), Research Laboratories, Fujisawa Pharmaceutical Co., Ltd., 1-6, 2-Chome, Kashima, Yodogawa-ku, Osaka 532, Japan

Abram Petkau (223), Medical Biophysics Branch, Whiteshell Nuclear Research Establishment, Atomic Energy of Canada, Ltd., Pinawa, Manitoba ROE 1LO, Canada

William F. Petrone (75), Department of Biochemistry, College of Medicine, University of South Alabama, Mobile, Alabama 36688

Dennis D. Pietronigro (127), Department of Neurosurgery, New York University Medical Center, New York, New York 10016

Peter H. Proctor (191), Department of Pharmacology, University of Texas Medical Branch, Galveston, Texas 77550

Joseph D. Schmidt (355), Division of Urology, Department of Surgery, University of California, San Diego, School of Medicine, La Jolla, California 92093

---

[3] *Present address:* Thoracic Medical Unit, The Royal Adelaide Hospital, Adelaide, South Australia 5000, Australia.

Thomas L. Schulte (355), Division of Urology, Department of Surgery, University of California, San Diego, La Jolla, California 92093

Myron Seligman (127), Department of Pathology and Neurosurgery, New York University School of Medicine, New York, New York 10016

John R. J. Sorenson (207), College of Pharmacy, Department of Pharmacology, University of Arkansas School for Medical Sciences, Little Rock, Arkansas 72201

Steven H. Stokes[4] (75), Department of Biochemistry, College of Medicine, University of South Alabama, Mobile, Alabama 36688

Nguyen T. Van (191), Baylor College of Medicine, Houston, Texas 77030

Roy P. Villasor (303), Oncology Service, Department of Medicine, Far Eastern University — N. Reyes Medical Foundation, Tumor Service, City Hospital of Manila, Makati, Metro Manila, Philippines 3117

Kenneth Wong (75), Department of Biochemistry, University of Alberta, Edmonton, Alberta, Canada

---

[4] *Present address:* Division of Radiation Oncology, Washington University School of Medicine, St. Louis, Missouri 63110.

Preface

Physicians have known for decades that oxygen, administered as therapeutic hyperoxia, has a well-defined toxic component. Rapid advances in basic and clinical research have now resulted in a much deeper understanding of the underlying mechanisms of the pathophysiology of oxygen. Concomitant with this enlarged understanding of mechanism has come the realization that oxygen toxicity, now known to be expressed through oxygen-derived free radicals and high energy singlet oxygen, is a much greater clinical problem than ever previously recognized.

Oxygen radical cytotoxicity plays a fundamental role in a wide spectrum of pathologic conditions; for example, edema induced by certain chemicals, inflammation originating from diseases such as arthritis and from bacterial infections, and toxic side effects of cancer chemotherapeutic agents and radiation. Oxygen radicals are now implicated in the pathogenesis of such diverse conditions as Crohn's disease, and other autoimmune diseases, organ ischemia, a variety of urologic diseases, neurologic disorders, diabetes, and cancer. Only a partial listing of pathologic conditions deriving from oxygen metabolites is possible here. The important recent advances in medical research associated with oxygen radical toxicity have occurred rapidly and have taken place in diverse and often unrelated areas.

This volume has been designed to provide clinicians and medical investigators with a working knowledge of the advances in the field of oxygen toxicity with the intention that the topics described in each chapter will be immediately useful. The book is divided into three general sections. The first section, comprising two chapters, explains the molecular and biochemical basis of our current understanding of oxygen radical toxicity as well as the means by which normal aerobic cells protect themselves from the toxic effects of oxygen radicals. The second and third sections of about equal length are concerned consecutively with *in vivo* and *in vitro* laboratory studies of oxygen toxicity in animals and with the results of clinical studies of patients. The chapters in the final clinical section describe, for the most part, evaluative studies of patients treated with the antioxidant, antiinflammatory enzyme superoxide dismutase which has been assessed for effectiveness in treating a variety of pathologic conditions associated with oxygen radical toxicity. Because of the absolute substrate specificity of this enzyme for the superoxide free radical, it has provided both an irreplaceable tool for the understanding of the cytopathology of oxygen and a very promising therapeutic agent, the use of which has a firm rational basis. Some of the chapters in the clinical section describe work in progress, some describe observations with only one or a few patients, and some are complete double-blind, placebo-controlled studies. All, however, are provocative enough to stimulate further clinical studies and trials in order to understand the etiology and to develop effective therapy for the many apparently unrelated pathologic conditions described herein.

It is hoped that this book will give physicians in practice and in clinical research, toxicologists, pharmacologists, as well as biochemists, and medicinal chemists, a working knowledge of the dramatic advances in this field, an understanding of the breadth of applicability, and an appreciation of the excitement in a rapidly advancing, important new area of experimental medicine.

This volume had its inception at a Symposium entitled *Active Oxygen and Medicine* which was held in Hawaii in 1979. Most, but not all, of the chapters in this book are based on studies presented at that meeting. The Symposium and the impetus for publishing the collected papers were made possible by the unstinting generosity of The Alexander Medical Foundation of Woodside, California. As the organizer of *Active Oxygen and Medicine,* I acknowledge with deep gratitude the particular generosity and unfailing support of Mrs. Patricia W. Hewitt who, although not formally trained in science, has a deep understanding of the need to advance the frontiers of experimental medicine. Without her interest and participation, the Symposium could never have occurred. Dr. Thomas L. Schulte, Medical Director for The Alexander Medical Foundation, gave unending support and encouragement to the planning of the Symposium and the production of this book. As a practicing urologist of many years, Dr. Schulte has a first-hand understanding of the need to develop better and more effective therapy for suffering patients. In pursuit of this goal, he has generously given the benefit of his experience, his ideas, and his support to medical investigation.

The invaluable assistance of Mr. Tomlinson I. Moseley (President of The Alexander Medical Foundation), Mrs. Roselle Howell, and Nancy B. Frank during the Symposium is acknowledged with thanks.

I thank very especially Mr. Galen Miller who assisted me not only with the planning and the running of the Symposium but also with compiling and preparing manuscripts for this book. His devoted, conscientious work and careful attention to detail throughout, made the organizing and editing tasks possible.

PARTICIPANTS*

Anne P. Autor
The Toxicology Center
Department of Pharmacology
The University of Iowa
Iowa City, Iowa 52242

Bernard M. Babior
Department of Medicine
Tufts-New England Medical Center
Boston, Massachusetts 02111

George Bartsch
Department of Urology
University of Innsbruck
Anichstrasse 35
Innsbruck A6020
Austria

William T. Brady
430 Trousdale Place
Beverly Hills, California 90211

Charles D. Brown
Texas A & M Veterinary School
College Station, Texas 77843

Gerald Cohen
Neurology Department
Mount Sinai School of Medicine
5th Avenue and 100th Street
New York, New York 10029

Richard C. Cutler
Gerontology Research Center
National Institute on Aging
Baltimore City Hospital
Baltimore, Maryland 21224

Rolando F. Del Maestro
Department of Neurosurgery
University of Western Ontario
London, Ontario
Canada N6A 5A5

Harry Demopoulos
Department of Pathology
New York University Medical Center
New York, New York 10016

Folke Edsmyr
Radiumhemmet
Karolinska Hospital
S-104 01 Stockholm 6
Sweden

Edwin W. Ellett
Texas A & M Veterinary School
College Station, Texas 77843

Christopher S. Foote
Department of Chemistry
University of California
Los Angeles, California 90024

Irwin Fridovich
Department of Biochemistry
Duke University Medical Center
Durham, North Carolina 27710

Jaime G. Gomez
Department of Neurological Surgery
Neurological Institute of Colombia
Apdo Aereo 90303
Bogota, Colombia
South America

Elwood Hansen
340 El Portal
Hillsborough, California 94010

Patricia W. Hewitt
Friendship Farms
Route 2, Box 612
Coaltown Road
East Moline, Illinois 61244

Milton M. Howell
P. O. Box 98
Hana, Hawaii 96713

Ronald H. Jones
Medical Research Institute
Florida Institute for Technology
Melbourne, Florida 32901

Frederick A. Kuehl
Department of Inflammation and Arthritis
Merck Institute for Therapeutic Research
Rahway, New Jersey 07065

Joe M. McCord
Department of Biochemistry
College of Medicine
University of South Alabama
Mobile, Alabama 36688

Eleanor J. McDonald
M.B. Anderson Clinic
2107 University Avenue
Houston, Texas 77030

John McGinness
Department of Physics
University of Texas Cancer Center
Houston, Texas 77030

* Participants in the symposium *Active Oxygen and Medicine,* which took place in Honolulu, Hawaii in 1979.

Geoffrey McLennan
Thoracic Medical Unit
The Royal Adelaide Hospital
Adelaide
South Australia 5000
Australia

S. Qasim Mehdi
Department of Nuclear Medicine
Stanford University
Stanford, California 94305

A.M. Michelson
Institut de Biologie Physico-Chimique
13 rue Pierre et Marie Curie
75005 Paris
France

Tomlinson I. Moseley
297 Park Lane
Atherton, California 94025

Larry W. Oberley
Radiation Research Laboratory
University of Iowa
Iowa City, Iowa 52242

Yoshihiko Ōyanagui
Research Laboratories
Fujisawa Pharmaceutical Co.
1-6, 2-chome Kashima
Yodogawa=ku
Osaka 532
Japan

Abram Petkau
Medical Biophysics Branch
Whiteshell Nuclear Research Establishment
Atomic Energy of Canada
Pinawa, Manitoba
Canada ROE 1L0

Dennis Pietronigro
Department of Pathology
New York University Medical Center
New York, New York 10016

Lawrence H. Piette
Cancer Center of Hawaii
University of Hawaii at Manoa
1236 Lauhala Street
Honolulu, Hawaii 96813

Charles B. Preacher
St. Luke's Hospital
1227 E. Rusholme Street
Davenport, Iowa 52803

Peter H. Proctor
Department of Pharmacology
University of Texas Medical Branch
Galveston, Texas 77550

Vernon Riley (deceased)
Pacific NW Research Foundation

1102 Columbia Street
Seattle, Washington 98104

Richard Rock
R.R. 2, Box 277
East Moline, Illinois 61244

Joseph D. Schmidt
University of California Medical Center
University Hospital
225 Dickinson Street
San Diego, California 92103

Thomas L. Schulte
218 Family Farm Drive
Woodside, California 94062

Lewis N. Sears
1414 7th Street
Moline, Illinois 52722

Sandor Shapiro
Cardeza Foundation
Jefferson Medical College
1015 Walnut Street
Philadelphia, Pennsylvania 19107

William Sheremata
Department of Neurology
University of Miami
School of Medicine
Box 520876
Miami, Florida 33152

Noriyasu Takayanagi
Research Lab.
Toyo Jozo Co., Ltd.
Ōhito-Cho
Tagata-Gun Shizuoka
Japan

David E. Turfler
336 W. Navaive
South Bend, Indiana 46616

Roy P. Villasor
Far Eastern University
Chief of Tumor Service
City Hospital of Manila
8 Antares, Bel Air IV
Makati, Metro Manila
Philippines

Brooks Walker
1280 Columbus
San Francisco, California 94133

Tetsuo Watanabe
Toyogozo Co. Ltd.
Matsuda Yeasu-doro Bldg.
1-10-7 Hacchoboro Chuo-ku
Tokyo
Japan

Ernest H. Willers
5799 Kalanianaele Hwy.
Honolulu, Hawaii 96821

Chapter 1

Superoxide Dismutase in Biology and Medicine

IRWIN FRIDOVICH

INTRODUCTION

Given the perfect clarity of hindsight, it now seems obvious that the biological reduction of molecular oxygen should be accompanied by the production of dangerously reactive free-radical intermediates. Indeed, it is predictable from the electronic structure of oxygen and the tenets of quantum mechanics. However, it was the accumulated weight of empirical data, rather than brilliant deductions from first principles, that forced this knowledge upon us. To this generation of biologists it still seems strangely frightening that free radicals of oxygen, long associated with the effects of ionizing radiation, should be normal products of aerobic metabolism; yet it is so, and our survival in the face of this endogenous flux of toxins is entirely dependent on a system of elegantly contrived defenses. Given this situation of a constant threat neutralized by an intricate defense, one can easily imagine circumstances in which the delicate balance is upset, with pathological consequences. As will become apparent in this volume, such situations do arise and it is then that exogenous superoxide dismutases may be applied to good advantage. As an introduction to such clinical material I will briefly review the biological production and scavenging of oxygen radicals.

The complete reduction of a molecule of oxygen to water requires four

1

PATHOLOGY OF OXYGEN
Copyright © 1982 by Academic Press, Inc.
All rights of reproduction in any form reserved.
ISBN 0-12-068620-1

electrons, and in a sequential univalent process several intermediates are encountered. These are the superoxide anion-radical, hydrogen peroxide, and the hydroxyl radical, and they are too reactive (1) to be well tolerated within living systems. The primary defense is provided by enzymes that catalytically scavenge the intermediates of oxygen reduction. The superoxide radical is eliminated by superoxide dismutases, which catalyze its conversion to hydrogen peroxide plus oxygen (2). Hydrogen peroxide is removed by catalases (3), which convert it to water plus oxygen, and by peroxidases (4), which reduce it to water, using a variety of reductants available to the cell. Figure 1 illustrates the univalent pathway of oxygen reduction and the catalytic scavenging of intermediates. It is clear that efficient removal of the first two intermediates of oxygen reduction, O_2^- and H_2O_2, prevents formation of the third, $HO\cdot$. This is fortunate, since the hydroxyl radical reacts avidly with many substances (5) and its specific enzymatic scavenging would be impossible.

At present, we are aware of superoxide dismutases with either iron or manganese at the active site and still others with both copper and zinc (2). There are catalases that are hemoproteins (3) and others, found in organisms incapable of heme synthesis, that may be flavoproteins (6). There are heme-containing peroxidases (4) that can utilize a wide variety of electron donors for the reduction of H_2O_2 and others that contain selenium and specifically utilize reduced glutathione as the reducing substrate (7). The biological production of hydrogen peroxide and the existence of catalases and peroxidases have been known for more than a century (3). In contrast, the corresponding production of superoxide radical and the existence of superoxide dismutases have been appreciated for approximately one decade.

SUPEROXIDE RADICAL

The superoxide radical is a minor, but not a trivial product of biological oxygen reduction. The dictates of quantum mechanics lead to a spin restriction that hinders the divalent reduction of O_2 and favors the univalent pathway (8). Oxidative enzymes have been evolved that circumvent the spin restriction and accomplish the divalent and even the tetravalent reduction of O_2^-, without the release of intermediates. Thus, most of the oxygen consumed by respiring cells is utilized by cytochrome oxidase, which reduces oxygen to water without releasing either O_2^- or H_2O_2 (9). The strategy of minimizing oxygen toxicity by avoiding the production of O_2^- and H_2O_2 has clearly been employed. Nevertheless, O_2^- is made in re-

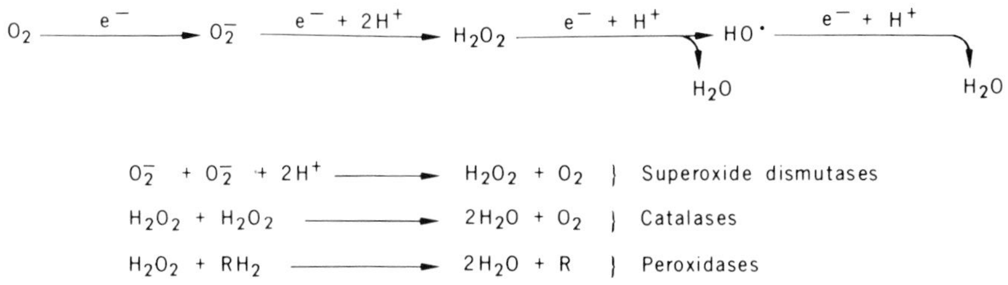

$$O_2 \xrightarrow{\ e^-\ } O_2^- \xrightarrow{\ e^- + 2H^+\ } H_2O_2 \xrightarrow{\ e^- + H^+\ } HO^\cdot \xrightarrow{\ e^- + H^+\ }$$

$$H_2O \qquad\qquad\qquad\qquad\qquad H_2O$$

$$O_2^- + O_2^- + 2H^+ \longrightarrow H_2O_2 + O_2 \quad\} \quad \text{Superoxide dismutases}$$

$$H_2O_2 + H_2O_2 \longrightarrow 2H_2O + O_2 \quad\} \quad \text{Catalases}$$

$$H_2O_2 + RH_2 \longrightarrow 2H_2O + R \quad\} \quad \text{Peroxidases}$$

Fig. 1. Univalent pathway of oxygen reduction and catalytic scavenging of intermediates.

spiring cells. We cannot easily ascertain the extent of its production *in vivo* because of the ubiquity of superoxide dismutases. However, in extracts of *Streptococcus faecalis* the superoxide dismutase activity of which was suppressed by the addition of a specific inhibiting antibody, 17% of the oxygen consumption resulted in O_2^- production (10). In whole cells the proportion of univalent oxygen reduction is probably smaller.

It may be helpful to mention reactions known to produce a substantial amount of O_2^-. The autoxidations of hydroquinones (11), leukoflavins (11,12), catecholamines (13,14), thiols (15), and tetrahydropterins (16) have all been shown to generate O_2^-. Reduced ferredoxins are also subject to spontaneous oxidation, which produces O_2^- (17). Hemoglobin and myoglobin, in their oxygenated forms, have classically been considered to be ferrooxy compounds, but there are good reasons for thinking of them as ferrisuperoxy compounds, and they do slowly liberate O_2^- as they are converted to methemoglobin and metmyoglobin (18,19). The production of methemoglobin is sufficiently substantial that erythrocytes contain a methemoglobin reductase to carry out a net reversal of the process. A number of enzymes, including xanthine oxidase, aldehyde oxidase, and dihydroorotic dehydrogenase, produce O_2^-, as do several flavin dehydrogenases (2). The superoxide radical has also been demonstrated to be an intermediate in the mechanisms of action of galactose oxidase (20), indoleamine dioxygenase (21), and 2-nitropropane dioxygenase (22), and other enzymes will undoubtedly be found to produce it. Fragments of subcellular organelles, such as mitochondria (23,24) and chloroplasts (25–27), produce O_2^-. Polymorphonuclear leukocytes, or granulocytes, have also been shown to liberate a large amount of it during the respiratory burst that accompanies active phagocytosis (28). Thus, we can confidently conclude that O_2^- is made during biological oxygen reduction, although we can neither specify the predominant responsible reaction in any particular cell nor precisely quantitate the extent of O_2^- production.

DANGERS OF SUPEROXIDE

Fluxes of O_2^-, generated enzymatically or photochemically, inactivate viruses (29), induce lipid peroxidation (30), damage membranes (31,32), and kill cells (33). There are indications that O_2^- is not itself the species that causes these effects but is the precursor of a more potent oxidant, the generation of which depends on the simultaneous presence of H_2O_2. For example, methional ($CH_3SCH_2CH_2CHO$), when exposed to an enzymatic source of both O_2^- and H_2O_2, was oxidatively attacked, resulting in the production of ethylene. Superoxide dismutase inhibited ethylene production, indicating the importance of O_2^-, and catalase did likewise, indicating the importance of H_2O_2. Since superoxide dismutase does not scavenge H_2O_2 and catalase does not scavenge O_2^-, we concluded that both O_2^- and H_2O_2 were needed (34). Haber and Weiss (35), in earlier studies of the catalytic decomposition of H_2O_2 by iron salts, had deduced a free-radical mechanism, one component reaction of which was $O_2^- + H_2O_2 \rightarrow OH^- + HO^. + O_2$. This suggested that O_2^- and H_2O_2 had cooperated in the production of $HO^.$, which then attacked methional and produced ethylene. In accord with this supposition was the observation that compounds such as ethanol and benzoate, which were known to scavenge $HO^.$ and to be unreactive toward O_2^- or H_2O_2, were capable of inhibiting ethylene production (34).

Similar observations have since been made by many workers; yet studies performed under carefully controlled conditions have demonstrated that the direct reaction of O_2^- with H_2O_2 is a slow process (36). One explanation for this apparent impasse invokes catalysis by iron compounds. Thus, O_2^- could reduce a ferric compound ($Fe^{3+} + O_2^- \rightarrow Fe^{2+} + O_2$), and the resulting ferrous compound could then reduce H_2O_2, as it does in the well-known Fenton reaction ($Fe^{2+} + H_2O_2 \rightarrow Fe^{3+} + OH^- + HO^.$). In accord with this proposal, an iron–EDTA complex was shown to catalyze the hydroxylation of tryptophan in the presence of O_2^- plus H_2O_2 (37). Whatever the actual mechanism, it is clear that O_2^- and H_2O_2 do conspire in the production of an oxidant more potent than themselves. In this light, it seems possible that the greatest danger posed by O_2^- is its interaction with H_2O_2 or with organic peroxides (38), which generates highly reactive entities that can then attack DNA, membrane lipids, and other essential cell components. A recent observation increases the likelihood that the iron-catalyzed Haber–Weiss reaction has *in vivo* significance: Lactoferrin, from human neutrophils, has been reported to catalyze the production of $HO^.$ from O_2^- plus H_2O_2 and to do so 5000 times more efficiently than iron–EDTA (38a).

COMPARATIVE ASPECTS OF
SUPEROXIDE DISMUTASES

Three distinct types of superoxide dismutase have been described. They all catalyze the same reaction and do so with comparable efficiency. The iron-containing (FeSOD) and manganese-containing (MnSOD) enzymes are characteristic of prokaryotes and are closely related, as shown by homologies in their amino acid sequences. The enzymes that contain both copper and zinc (CuZnSOD) are characteristic of eukaryotes and appear to have evolved independently, since they have no sequences homologous to those of FeSOD and MnSOD (39). The distribution of these enzymes must tell a fascinating story of evolutionary events, although it is tangled and difficult to unravel. Both FeSOD and MnSOD are found in bacteria, and recent surveys (10) showed that gram-positive bacteria most frequently contain only MnSOD, whereas gram-negative bacteria generally contain both FeSOD and MnSOD. However, some gram-positive bacteria, such as *Staphylococcus aureus,* contain FeSOD plus MnSOD, and some, such as *Bacillus cereus,* contain only FeSOD. Furthermore, there are gram-negative bacteria, such as *Alcaligenes faecalis,* that contain only FeSOD. The CuZnSOD is characteristic of the cytosol of eukaryotes, yet the symbiotic bacterium *Photobacterium leiognathi* has been shown to contain CuZnSOD in addition to FeSOD (40). Since this organism is one partner in a long-standing symbiosis (41) and is the only bacterium thus far found to contain CuZnSOD, it is tempting to speculate that it obtained this enzyme through a gene transfer from the host fish (2). Indeed, a recent computer-aided comparison of superoxide dismutases, on the basis of amino acid compositions, has revealed that the CuZnSOD in *P. leiognathi* is more closely related to the corresponding enzymes from a variety of fish than it is to the CuZnSOD's from fungi, plants, birds, or mammals (41a). This indicates that the gene for CuZnSOD in *P. leiognathi* originated in the ponyfish, a conclusion also supported by the lack of CuZnSOD in other bacteria, including closely related free-living photobacteria.

Eukaryotes generally contain both CuZnSOD and MnSOD. These are readily distinguished, even in crude extracts, since the former is inhibited by CN^- and is stable to treatment by a mixture of chloroform and ethanol, whereas the latter is resistant to CN^- but is denatured by chloroform and ethanol. Yeast (42), plants (43,44), chicken liver (45), rat liver (46), and pig heart (45) contain MnSOD in the mitochondrial matrix and CuZnSOD in the cytosol. Human and baboon liver also contain both MnSOD and CuZnSOD. Only MnSOD is found in the mitochondrial matrix, but the cytosol contains both enzymes (47). The mitochondrial MnSOD and the bacterial MnSOD have homologous amino acid sequences (39), in accord with the proposal that mitochondria evolved from an endocellular symbiosis between a prokaryote and a protoeukaryote.

MECHANISMS OF SUPEROXIDE DISMUTASES

The superoxide radical is unstable with respect to O_2 and H_2O_2, and it spontaneously "goes over" to these products by dismutation. Since O_2^- is the conjugate base of a weak acid, $HO_2^.$, the pK_a of which is 4.8, we must actually consider three dismutation reactions. These reactions and their rate constants (k_2) are (48–49b) as follows:

$$HO_2^. + HO_2^. \rightarrow H_2O_2 + O_2 \tag{1}$$
$$k_2 \simeq 8 \times 10^5 \ M^{-1} \ sec^{-1}$$

$$HO_2^. + O_2^- + H^+ \rightarrow H_2O_2 + O_2 \tag{2}$$
$$k_2 \simeq 8 \times 10^7 \ M^{-1} \ sec^{-1}$$

$$O_2^- + O_2^- + 2H^+ \rightarrow H_2O_2 + O_2 \tag{3}$$
$$k_2 < 0.3 \ M^{-1} \ sec^{-1}$$

The spontaneous dismutation is thus most rapid at pH 4.8, and the rate decreases by a factor of 10 for each unit increase in pH above 4.8. The dismutation between O_2^- and O_2^- [Eq. (3)] is probably so slow because electrostatic repulsion prevents the close approach that would allow electron transfer. Furthermore, the production of O_2^{2-} would be an event of very low probability considering both the mutual repulsion of negative charges in the collisional complex and its very high pK_a. Therefore, the simplest mechanism for catalysis of reaction (3) would involve alternate reduction and reoxidation of the catalyst during successive encounters with O_2^-. The catalyst would thereby accomplish the transfer of an electron from one O_2^- to another without the necessity for close approach of the anions, and if proton transfer accompanied electron transfer the need for the transient existence of O_2^{2-} could be avoided. This appears to be the actual mechanism of action of all of the superoxide dismutases that have been examined (50–55). This mechanism can be written as

$$E—Me^n + O_2^- \rightarrow E—Me^{n-1} + O_2 \tag{4}$$

$$E—Me^{n-1} + O_2^- + 2H^+ \rightarrow E—Me^n + H_2O_2 \tag{5}$$

where E denotes enzyme and Me metal. In the case of CuZnSOD it is the copper that participates in the catalytic cycle and oscillates from the cupric to the cuprous state, whereas the zinc appears primarily to play a structural role. In MnSOD and FeSOD the trivalent and divalent states of the metals are involved in the catalytic cycle. The superoxide dismutases are extraordinarily efficient catalysts, their rate of interaction with O_2^- being approximately $2 \times 10^9 \ M^{-1} \ \text{sec}^{-1}$. This is close to the diffusion limit and, as expected for a diffusion-limited process, the rate shows a very small temperature effect (energy of activation) and is diminished by increasing the viscosity of the solvent.

SUPEROXIDE AND OXYGEN TOXICITY

The conclusion that O_2^- is an important agent of oxygen toxicity and that superoxide dismutases provide an essential defense is supported by several types of evidence. Purely circumstantial evidence was obtained by surveying a range of microorganisms (56). In general, aerobes contained superoxide dismutase and obligate anaerobes did not. One organism, *Lactobacillus plantarum,* was aerotolerant, yet did not contain this enzyme. However, it did not respire during log phase growth and thus appeared in no need of a defense against O_2^-, since it could not reduce oxygen to O_2^- (56,57). *Lactobacillus plantarum* does respire during the late log and stationary phases of its growth cycle and can then accumulate millimolar levels of H_2O_2 in the medium. *Lactobacillus plantarum* and related lactobacilli require manganese-rich media for optimal growth and accumulate manganese until intracellular levels are in the 20–25 m*M* range. These organisms are oxygen tolerant when manganese replete but become oxygen intolerant when a manganese deficiency is imposed. Compounds such as plumbagin, which enhance intracellular production of O_2^-, are also better tolerated by manganese-replete than by manganese-deficient cells. A survey of lactobacilli and related organisms showed that species which accumulate manganese did not contain superoxide dismutase and, conversely, that organisms containing superoxide dismutase did not accumulate manganese. Finally, it was shown that manganese, at the levels found in *L. plantarum,* could efficiently scavenge O_2^-. It thus appears that Lactobacillaceae, which ordinarily live in manganese-rich materials such as decaying plants, have substituted millimolar levels of Mn(II) for the micromolar levels of superoxide dismutase found in most bacteria (57a,b).

More direct evidence was provided by the observations that exposure to oxygen of facultative organisms such as *Streptococcus faecalis, Escherichia coli,* and *Saccharomyces cerevisiae* resulted in increased intracellular accumulation of the enzyme and that elevated levels of the enzyme correlated with enhanced resistance to the lethal effect of hyperbaric oxygen. In the case of *E. coli,* which contains both FeSOD and MnSOD, the two superoxide dismutases responded very differently to oxygenation. The FeSOD was made whether or not oxygen was present, whereas the MnSOD was made only in the presence of oxygen (58). Transfer of cells from anaerobic to aerobic conditions resulted in prompt induction of the synthesis of MnSOD. Interference with the synthesis of MnSOD rendered the anaerobically grown cells susceptible to the toxicity of oxygen (58). Thus, we observed both induction of MnSOD and increased resistance to oxygen toxicity as a consequence of exposure to oxygen, and we concluded that the two are related. However, oxygenation of *E. coli* or of other cells certainly induces changes other than the synthesis of MnSOD, and one of these changes might have been responsible for the enhanced resistance to oxygen toxicity.

Several lines of evidence support the correlation between MnSOD and resistance to oxygen toxicity. When *E. coli* organisms were grown in a glucose-limited chemostat culture with constant and abundant oxygenation, increasing the rate of inflow of fresh medium increased the rates of growth and respiration. The content of MnSOD increased in proportion to the rate of respiration and correlated with resistance to the lethality of hyperbaric oxygen, even though oxygenation had remained constant during the growth of the cells (59). When the supply of nutrient was abruptly increased, the content of superoxide dismutase began to increase immediately, whereas the growth rate remained at the level characteristic of cells given the limited supply of nutrient. When the cellular content of superoxide dismutase reached the level that is characteristic of the growth rate in the presence of an unlimited supply of nutrients, the growth rate abruptly increased. It thus appeared that under these conditions the growth rate was limited by the intracellular level of superoxide dismutase. It should be noted that the cellular content of catalase and of peroxidase did not increase under these conditions.

In another experiment, *E. coli* organisms were grown in batch culture in an aerated rich medium containing glucose, amino acids, purines, pyrimidines, and vitamins (Trypticase Soy plus yeast extract). The energy needs of the cells were at first met by fermentation of the glucose. The rate of respiration was low, and the medium was acidified by the accumulation of lactic acid and other organic acids. When the glucose was exhausted, the cells began to use the amino acids and the accumulated organic acids. The rate of respiration and the pH of the medium increased. If superoxide dismutase provides a defense against O_2^- produced during respiration, then the level of this activity should have been low during the fermentative phase of growth and elevated during the shift to more aerobic metabolism. This was observed (60).

Strong evidence in support of the superoxide theory of oxygen toxicity was obtained by the use of paraquat (methyl viologen) (60,61). This compound, widely used as a herbicide, is easily reduced to a relatively stable radical, which then reacts with oxygen, generating O_2^-. Paraquat augments the production of O_2^- by chloroplasts and lung microsomes, and this is probably one reason for its lethality to both plants and animals. When paraquat is administered to *E. coli*, it subverts electron flow from the normal electron transport pathway. The result is an increase in cyanide-resistant respiration and in the rate of production of O_2^-. Under conditions of constant aeration, paraquat elicits a dramatic increase in the biosynthesis of MnSOD, whereas in the absence of oxygen it has no such effect. It is clear that O_2^-, directly or indirectly, increases the rate of synthesis of MnSOD in *E. coli*. When the level of MnSOD was elevated as a consequence of aerobic exposure to paraquat, the cells were rendered resistant to the lethal effect of hyperbaric oxygen (61). Many compounds are potentially capable of increasing intracellular O_2^- production by undergoing a redox cycle similar to that seen with paraquat. Only compounds that gain entry to the cells being used and that satisfy the specificity requirements of the diaphorases in these cells can be expected to have this effect. Plumbagin, pyocyanine, phenazine methosulfate, streptonigrin, juglone, and methylene blue were among the compounds found to be active with *E. coli* (61a,b).

Mutants with modifications in superoxide dismutase activity have provided additional indications that O_2^- is an agent of oxygen toxicity and that superoxide dismutase is an essential defense. One mutant of *E. coli*, which had a temperature-sensitive defect in its capacity to maintain normal intracellular levels of superoxide dismutase, showed a parallel temperature-sensitive defect in oxygen tolerance (62). Another mutant, selected on the basis of tolerance for hyperbaric oxygen, contained an elevated level of FeSOD (63). Several mutants, selected on the basis of intolerance for oxygen, lacked MnSOD, catalase, and peroxidase, which suggests the possibility of a genetic linkage between these enzymes. Revertants to oxygen tolerance fell into two classes. One group had regained the missing enzymatic activities, whereas the other group showed a diminished capacity to respire (64,64a).

RATIONALE

There is compelling evidence that superoxide dismutases are essential components of the biological defense against oxygen toxicity. It may nevertheless be surprising that enzymes are needed to catalyze a reaction that is quite rapid, even in the absence of catalysis. This is easily explained. At pH 7.8, in an aqueous environment, O_2^- dismutes spontaneously at a rate of 8×10^4 M^{-1} sec^{-1}. This is a large rate constant, but the reaction is second order in O_2^- and the first half-life is therefore a function of the steady-state level of O_2^-. Thus, at 1×10^{-10} M O_2^- the reaction would be slow. In contrast, the reaction between O_2^- and superoxide dismutase is first order in O_2^- and first order in enzyme, and the enzyme is present in most tissues at approximately 1×10^{-5} M. At 1×10^{-10} M O_2^- the enzyme-catalyzed dismutation would thus be 10^5-fold faster than the spontaneous reaction, even if the rate constant for the enzymatic reaction were the same as that for the spontaneous reaction. In fact, at physiological pH the rate constant for the enzymatic reaction is 10^4-fold greater than that for the spontaneous reaction. The net increase in the rate of dismutation of O_2^-, caused by intracellular levels of superoxide dismutase at a steady-state level of O_2^- of 0.1 nM, is thus 10^9-fold. The advantage provided by the enzyme would be even greater than this at the lower steady-state levels of O_2^- to be expected in a cell.

The dismutation of O_2^-, whether spontaneous or enzyme-catalyzed, produces H_2O_2, which is itself a dangerously reactive substance. However, as already described, there are catalases and peroxidases that scavenge it. The net effect of superoxide dismutase is to lower the steady-state level of O_2^- greatly, and the catalases and peroxidases do the same for H_2O_2. The likelihood that O_2^- or H_2O_2 will participate in deleterious reactions with other cell components is diminished in proportion to the decrease in their concentrations. The likelihood that O_2^- and H_2O_2 will collaborate in the production of even more reactive species, such as HO˙ or singlet oxygen, is diminished in proportion to the product of the decreases in their concentrations. These defensive enzymes are thus likely to exert a synergistic effect in protecting respiring cells against the consequences of the production of O_2^- and H_2O_2.

OXYGEN ENHANCEMENTS

Paraquat, which increases the rate of production of O_2^-, is much more toxic under aerobic than under anaerobic conditions. In effect, paraquat enhances the toxicity of oxygen, and oxygen enhances the toxicity of paraquat. Other oxygen enhancements are probably also related to the production of O_2^-. Oxygen enhances the toxicity of several antibiotics, including streptonigrin, mitomycin, daunomycin, adriamycin, and porfiromycin. In the case of streptonigrin this oxygen enhancement is clearly due to cyclic reduction and reoxidation, with the production of O_2^-. Increased levels of superoxide dismutase have been shown to protect against the enhancement of the lethality of streptonigrin by oxygen (58). The structures of the other substances that exhibit oxygen enhancements also suggest that they divert normal electron flow and increase the production of O_2^-.

Oxygen has long been known to enhance the lethality of ionizing radiation. The oxygen enhancement ratio (OER) quantitatively expresses this effect. Since ionizing radiation passing through water produces hydrogen atoms, hydrated electrons, and hydroxyl radicals, which, in the presence of dissolved oxygen, secondarily yield O_2^- and H_2O_2, it seemed that O_2^- might be a factor in this oxygen enhancement. In one attempt to implicate O_2^-, *E. coli* organisms containing a low level of superoxide dismutase, as a consequence of anaerobic growth, were compared with *E. coli* organisms containing a high level of this enzyme, as a consequence of aerobic growth. No difference was noted (65). However, there have been several reports of superoxide dismutase protecting against radiation damage to DNA (66), viruses and mammalian cells in culture (33), suspensions of bacteria (67), and even whole mice (68). In these cases superoxide dismutase was effective when added to the suspending medium or when injected into the mice. This effect of extracellular enzyme brought to mind earlier studies of "medium effects" (69) and suggested that the role of O_2^- in the oxygen enhancement of radiation lethality needed to be reexamined. Dilute suspensions of *E. coli* in buffer exhibited an OER of 2.4. The ratio was reduced to 1.5 when superoxide dismutase or catalase was added to the medium and was reduced to 1.2 when these enzymes were present simultaneously (70). Controls with heat-inactivated enzymes or other proteins showed no effect. It thus appears that, in the case of dilute suspensions of *E. coli*, O_2^- and H_2O_2 are important agents of the oxygen enhancement. The basis of the OER remains an area of controversy and more work is necessary to achieve clarification. Thus, the protective effects of superoxide dismutase and the role of extracellular events have been questioned (70a), and a reverse OER has been reported with *Micrococcus radiodurans* (70b).

SUPEROXIDE AND INFLAMMATION

The respiratory burst shown by activated granulocytes and the associated production of O_2^- have already been alluded to. Granulocytes are capable of chemotaxis, and they congregate at sites of injury or infection. Since a large fraction of the O_2^- produced during the respiratory burst es-

capes from the granulocytes, we might anticipate that a collection of activated phagocytes would damage each other as well as surrounding cells
and connective tissue. Enzymatically generated O_2^- has been shown to depolymerize hyaluronate, an agent that lends viscosity and lubricating
properties to synovial fluid (71). Moreover, the mortality of activated suspensions of granulocytes is decreased by superoxide dismutase added to
the suspending medium (72). The O_2^- produced by activated phagocytes,
presumably to facilitate killing of engulfed bacteria, could thus exacerbate
and prolong the inflammatory process. There is ordinarily very little superoxide dismutase in extracellular fluids, and the damaging effects of O_2^-
released into such fluids would go largely unopposed. In that case injected
superoxide dismutase should have an antiinflammatory effect. Such effects have been reported (73–75).

There is another and probably more significant aspect of the involvement of O_2^- in the inflammatory process. Aggregation and activation of
phagocytic cells is the central factor in inflammation. Cell aggregation
depends on the release of, and response to, chemotaxins. Neutrophils exhibit a positive chemotactic response toward a wide range of N-formyl-
methionyl peptides, such as might be expected to be released from
damaged bacterial cells. fMet-Leu-Phe is such a peptide, and it both at-
tracts and activates human neutrophils (76). An entirely different class of
chemotaxins appears to be generated as a consequence of the oxidation of
arachidonate (77), and O_2^- was seen to initiate the conversion of arachidonate to a potent chemotaxin via a Haber–Weiss process (78). The physiological significance of O_2^- in the inflammatory process is underscored by
the observation that O_2^- could convert a normal plasma component into a
neutrophil chemotaxin (79). Furthermore, the intradermal injection of a
source of continuous O_2^- production, such as xanthine oxidase plus xanthine, caused a transient massing of neutrophils. The natural history of a
normal inflammation would thus begin with the introduction of a few bacteria under the skin. Formylmethionyl peptides, diffusing from the bacteria, might attract and activate a few neutrophils. The O_2^- secreted by the
neutrophils during the respiratory burst would convert the plasma component to a powerful chemotaxin, which would, in turn, attract more neutrophils. The process would self-amplify until the bacteria were completely
eliminated, at which point the incoming neutrophils would find no activating contacts and, failing to be activated, would secrete no O_2^- so that the
process would subside for want of a source of continuous chemotaxin
production.

Superoxide dismutase, injected as long as 1 hr after X irradiation of
mice, has been shown to diminish the lethality of such irradiation (68).
Since the O_2^- generated during irradiation could not conceivably survive

in the mouse for such a period, one must suppose that irradiation sets in motion some continuing physiological process that is damaging to the animal and that involves the production of O_2^-. Granulocytes that are activated by the consequences of irradiation could provide the postulated source of continuous O_2^- production, and the postirradiation protection of mice by injected superoxide dismutase could be an expression of the antiinflammatory action of this enzyme.

We have been privileged to witness a new level of understanding of oxygen metabolism. Appreciation of the biological production of superoxide radicals and of the existence of superoxide dismutases for the efficient scavenging of these radicals gives us a new grasp of vexing problems of long standing. In this symposium the scientists and clinicians who have been probing the implications and applications of this new knowledge will have the rare opportunity to educate each other. It is certain that both groups and their separate endeavors will profit from the exchange.

REFERENCES

1. Czapski, G. (1971). Radiation chemistry of oxygenated aqueous solutions. *Annu. Rev. Phys. Chem.* **22**:171.
2. Fridovich, I. (1975). Superoxide dismutases. *Annu. Rev. Biochem.* **44**:147.
3. Rapoport, S. M., and Müller, M. (1974). Catalase and glutathione peroxidase. *In* "Cellular and Molecular Biology of Erythrocytes" (H. Yoskikawa and S. M. Rapoport, eds.), p. 167. University Park Press, Baltimore, Maryland.
4. Saunders, B. C., Holmes-Siedle, A. G., and Stark, B. P. (1964). "Peroxidase." Butterworth, London.
5. Dorfman, L. M., and Adams, G. E. (1973). "Reactivity of the Hydroxyl Radical in Aqueous Solutions," NSRDS-NBS No. 46. U.S. Dept. of Commerce, National Bureau of Standards, Washington, D. C.
6. Johnston, M. A., and Delwiche, E. A. (1965). Distribution and characteristics of the catalases of lactobacillaceae. *J. Bacteriol.* **90**:347.
7. Arias, I. M., and Jakoby, N. B., eds. (1976). Glutathione peroxidase. *In* "Glutathione: Metabolism and Function" (I. M. Arias and N. B. Jakoby, eds.), p. 115. Raven, New York.
8. Taube, H. (1965). Mechanisms of oxidation with oxygen. *J. Gen. Physiol.* **49**:29.
9. Antonini, E., Brunori, M., Greenwood, C., and Malmstrom, B. G. (1970). Catalytic mechanism of cytochrome oxidase. *Nature (London)* **228**:936.
10. Britton, L., Malinowski, D. P., and Fridovich, I. (1978). Superoxide dismutase and oxygen metabolism in streptococcus faecalis and comparisons with other organisms. *J. Bacteriol.* **134**:229.
11. Misra, H. P., and Fridovich, I. (1972). The univalent reduction of oxygen by reduced flavins and quinones. *J. Biol. Chem.* **247**:188.
12. Ballou, D., Palmer, G., and Massey, V. (1969). Direct demonstration of superoxide anion production during the oxidation of reduced flavin and of its catalytic decomposition by erythrocuprein. *Biochem. Biophys. Res. Commun.* **36**:898.

13. Misra, H. P., and Fridovich, I. (1972). The role of superoxide anion in the autoxidation of epinephrine and a simple assay for superoxide dismutase. *J. Biol. Chem.* **247:**3170.
14. Cohen, G., and Heikkila, R. (1974): The generation of hydrogen peroxide, superoxide radical, and hydroxyl radical by 6-hydroxydopamine, dialuric acid, and related cytotoxic agents. *J. Biol. Chem.* **249:**2447.
15. Misra, H. P. (1974). Generation of superoxide free radical during the autoxidation of thiols. *J. Biol. Chem.* **249:**2151.
16. Fisher, D. B., and Kaufman, S. (1973). Tetrahydropterin oxidation without hydroxylation catalyzed by rat liver phenylalanine hydroxylase. *J. Biol. Chem.* **248:**4300.
17. Misra, H. P., and Fridovich, I. (1971). The generation of superoxide radical during the autoxidation of ferredoxins. *J. Biol. Chem.* **246:**6886.
18. Misra, H. P., and Fridovich, I. (1972). The generation of superoxide radical during the autoxidation of hemoglobin. *J. Biol. Chem.* **247:**6960.
19. Gotoh, T., and Shikama, K. (1976). Generation of the superoxide radical during autoxidation of oxymyoglobin. *J. Biochem.* *(Tokyo)* **80:**397.
20. Hamilton, G. A., and Libby, R. D. (1973). The valence of copper and the role of superoxide in the D-galactose oxidase catalyzed reaction. *Biochem. Biophys. Res. Commun.* **55:**333.
21. Hirata, F., and Hayaishi, O. (1975). Studies on indoleamine 2,3-dioxygenase. I. Superoxide anion as substrate. *J. Biol. Chem.* **250:**5960.
22. Kido, T., Soda, K., Suzuki, T., and Asada, K. (1976). A new oxygenase, 2-nitropropane dioxygenase of Hansenula mrakii. Enzymologic and spectrophotometric properties. *J. Biol. Chem.* **251:**6994.
23. Loschen, G., Azzi, A., Richler, C., and Flohé, L. (1974). Superoxide radicals as precursors of mitochondrial hydrogen peroxide. *FEBS Lett.* **42:**68.
24. Boveris, A. (1977). Mitochondrial production of superoxide radical and hydrogen peroxide. *Adv. Exp. Med. Biol.* **78:**67.
25. Asada, K., and Kiso, K. (1973). Initiation of aerobic oxidation of sulfite by illuminated spinach chloroplasts. *J. Biochem.* *(Tokyo)* **33:**253.
26. Epel, B. L., and Neumann, J. (1973). The mechanism of the oxidation of ascorbate and MN2 + by chloroplasts. The role of the radical superoxide. *Biochim. Biophys. Acta* **325:**520.
27. Halliwell, B. (1975). Hydroxylation of P-coumaric acid by illuminated chloroplasts. The role of superoxide. *Eur. J. Biochem.* **55:**355.
28. Cheson, B. D., Curnutte, J. T., and Babior, B. M. (1977). The oxidative killing mechanisms of the neutrophil. *Prog. Clin. Immunol.* **3:**1.
29. Lavelle, F., Michelson, A. M., and Dimitrejevic, L. (1973). Biological protection by superoxide dismutase. *Biochem. Biophys. Res. Commun.* **55:**350.
30. Kellogg, E. W., III, and Fridovich, I. (1975). Superoxide, hydrogen peroxide, and singlet oxygen in lipid peroxidation by a xanthine oxidase system. *J. Biol. Chem.* **250:**8812.
31. Goldberg, B., and Stern, A. (1976). Superoxide anion as a mediator of drug-induced oxidative hemolysis. *J. Biol. Chem.* **251:**6468.
32. Kellogg, E. W., III, and Fridovich, I. (1977). Liposome oxidation and erythrocyte lysis by enzymically generated superoxide and hydrogen peroxide. *J. Biol. Chem.* **252:**6721.
33. Michelson, A. M., and Buckingham, M. E. (1974). Effects of superoxide radicals on myoblast growth and differentiation. *Biochem. Biophys. Res. Commun.* **58:**1079.
34. Beauchamp, C., and Fridovich, I. (1970). A mechanism for the production of ethylene from methional. The generation of the hydroxyl radical by xanthine oxidase. *J. Biol. Chem.* **245:**4641.
35. Haber, F., and Weiss, J. (1934). The catalytic decomposition of hydrogen peroxide by iron salts. *Proc. R. Soc. London, Ser. A* **47:**332.

36. Halliwell, B. (1976). An attempt to demonstrate a reaction between superoxide and hydrogen peroxide. *FEBS Lett.* **72**:8.
37. McCord, J. M., and Day, E. D. (1978). Superoxide-dependent production of hydroxyl radical catalyzed by iron-EDTA complex. *FEBS Lett.* **86**:139.
38. Peters, J. W., and Foote, C. S. (1976). Chemistry of superoxide anion. II. Reaction with hydroperoxides. *J. Am. Chem. Soc.* **98**:873.
38a. Ambruso, D. R., and Johnston, R. B. (1981). Lactoferrin enhances hydroxyl radical production by human neutrophil, neutrophil particulate fractions, and an enzymatic generating system. *J. Clin. Invest.* **67**:352.
39. Steinman, H. M., and Hill, R. L. (1973). Sequence homologies among bacterial and mitochondrial superoxide dismutases. *Proc. Natl. Acad. Sci. U.S.A.* **70**:3725.
40. Puget, K., and Michelson, A. M. (1974). Isolation of a new copper-containing superoxide dismutase bacteriocuprein. *Biochem. Biophys. Res. Commun.* **58**:830.
41. Reichelt, J. L., Nealson, K., and Hastings, J. W. (1977). The specificity of symbiosis: Ponyfish and luminescent bacteria. *Arch. Microbiol.* **112**:157.
41a. Martin, J. P., Jr., and Fridovich, I. (1981). Evidence for a natural gene transfer from the ponyfish to its bioluminescent bacterial symbiont *Photobacter leiognathi. J. Biol. Chem.* **256**:6080.
42. Ravindranath, S. D., and Fridovich, I. (1975). Isolation and characterization of a manganese-containing superoxide dismutase from yeast. *J. Biol. Chem.* **250**:6107.
43. Giannopolitis, C. N., and Ries, S. K. (1977). Superoxide dismtuases. I. Occurrence in higher plants. *Plant Physiol.* **59**:309.
44. Fridovich, S. E., Misra, H. P., and Fridovich, I. Unpublished observations.
45. Weisiger, R. A., and Fridovich, I. (1973). Superoxide dismutase. Organelle specificity. *J. Biol. Chem.* **248**:3582.
46. Peeters-Joris, C., Vandervoorde, A. M., and Baudhuin, P. (1973). Intracellular localization of superoxide dismutase in rat liver. *Arch. Int. Physiol. Biochim.* **81**:981.
47. McCord, J. M., Boyle, J. A., Day, E. D., Jr., Rizzolo, L. J., and Salin, M. L. (1977). A manganese-containing superoxide dismutase from human liver. *In* "Superoxides and Superoxide Dismutases" (A. M. Michelson, J. M. McCord, and I. Fridovich, eds.), p. 129. Academic Press, New York.
48. Rabani, J., and Nielson, S. O. (1969). Absorption spectrum and decay kinetics of O_2^- and HO_2 in aqueous solutions by pulse radiolysis. *J. Phys. Chem.* **73**:3736.
49. Behar, D., Czapski, G., Dorfman, L. M., Rabani, J., and Schwarz, H. A. (1970). The acid dissociation constant and decay kinetics of the perhydroxyl radical. *J. Phys. Chem.* **74**:3209.
49a. Marklund, S. (1976). Spectrophotometric study of spontaneous disproportionation of superoxide anion radical and sensitive direct assay for superoxide dismutase. *J. Biol. Chem.* **251**:7504.
49b. Bielski, B. H. J., and Allen, A. O. (1977). Mechanism of the disproportionation of superoxide radical. *J. Phys. Chem.* **81**:1048.
50. Klug, D., Rabani, J., and Fridovich, I. (1972). A direct demonstration of the catalytic action of superoxide dismutase through the use of pulse radiolysis. *J. Biol. Chem.* **247**:4839.
51. Rotilio, G., Bray, R. C., and Fielden, E. M. (1972). A pulse radiolysis study of superoxide dismutase. *Biochim. Biophys. Acta* **268**:605.
52. Klug, D., Fridovich, I., and Rabani, J. (1973). Pulse radiolytic investigations of superoxide catalyzed disproportionation. *J. Am. Chem. Soc.* **95**:2786.
53. Pick, M., Rabani, J., Yost, F., and Fridovich, I. (1974). The catalytic mechanism of the manganese-containing superoxide dismutase of *Escherichia coli* studied by pulse radiolysis. *J. Am. Chem. Soc.* **96**:7329.

54. McAdam, M. E., Fox, R. A., Lavelle, F., and Fielden, E. M. (1977). A pulse-radiolysis study of the manganese-containing superoxide dismutase from *Bacillus stearothermophilus*. A kinetic model for the enzyme action. *Biochem. J.* **165**:71.

54a. McAdam, M. E., Fox, R. A., Lavelle, F., and Fielden, E. M. (1977). A pulse-radiolysis study of the manganese-containing superoxide dismutase from *Bacillus stearothermophilus*. Further studies on the properties of the enzyme. *Biochem. J.* **165**:81.

55. Lavelle, F., McAdam, M. E., Fielden, E. M., Roberts, P. B., Puget, K., and Michelson, A. M. (1977). A pulse-radiolysis study of the catalytic mechanism of the iron-containing superoxide dismutase from *Photobacterium leiognathi*. *Biochem. J.* **161**:3.

56. McCord, J. M., Keele, B. B., Jr., and Fridovich, I. (1971). An enzyme-based theory of obligate anaerobiosis: The physiological function of superoxide dismutase. *Proc. Natl. Acad. Sci. U.S.A.* **68**:1024.

57. Gregory, E. M., and Fridovich, I. (1974). Oxygen metabolism in *Lactobacillus plantarum*. *J. Bacteriol.* **117**:166.

57a. Archibald, F. S., and Fridovich, I. (1981). Manganese and defenses against oxygen toxicity in *Lactobacillus plantarum*. *J. Bacteriol.* **145**:442.

57b. Archibald, F. S., and Fridovich, I. (1981). Manganese, superoxide dismutase, and oxygen tolerance in some lactic acid bacteria. *J. Bacteriol.* **146**:928.

58. Hassan, H. M., and Fridovich, I. (1977). Enzymatic defenses against the toxicity of oxygen and of streptonigrin in *Escherichia coli*. *J. Bacteriol.* **129**:1574.

59. Hassan, H. M., and Fridovich, I. (1977). Physiological function of superoxide dismutase in glucose-limited chemostat cultures of *Escherichia coli*. *J. Bacteriol.* **130**:805.

60. Hassan, H. M., and Fridovich, I. (1977). Regulation of superoxide dismutase synthesis in *Escherichia coli*: Glucose effect. *J. Bacteriol.* **132**:505.

61. Hassan, H. M., and Fridovich, I. (1977). Regulation of the synthesis of superoxide dismutase in *Escherichia coli*. Induction by methyl viologen. *J. Biol. Chem.* **252**:7667.

61a. Hassan, H. M., and Fridovich, I. (1979). Intracellular production of superoxide radical and of hydrogen peroxide by redox active compounds. *Arch. Biochem. Biophys.* **196**:385.

61b. Hassan, H. M., and Fridovich, I. (1980). Mechanism of the antibiotic action of pyocyanine. *J. Bacteriol.* **141**:156.

62. McCord, J. M., Beauchamp, C. O., Goscin, S., Misra, H. P., and Fridovich, I. (1973). Superoxide and superoxide dismutase. *In* "Oxidases and Related Redox Systems" (T. E. King, H. S. Mason, and M. Morrison, eds.), p. 51. University Park Press, Baltimore, Maryland.

63. Yost, F. J., Jr., and Fridovich, I. Unpublished observations.

64. Hassan, H. M. (1976). Obligately anaerobic mutants of *Escherichia coli*, K12. *Fed. Proc., Fed. Am. Soc. Exp. Biol.* **35**:1630.

64a. Hassan, H. M., and Fridovich, I. (1979). Superoxide, hydrogen peroxide, and oxygen tolerance of oxygen-sensitive mutants of *Escherichia coli*. *Rev. Infect. Dis.* **1**:357.

65. Goscin, S. A., and Fridovich, I. (1972). The role of superoxide radical in a nonenzymatic hydroxylation. *Arch. Biochem. Biophys.* **153**:778.

66. Van Hemmen, J. J., and Meuling, W. J. A. (1975). Inactivation of biologically active DNA by gamma-ray-induced superoxide radicals and their dismutation products singlet molecular oxygen and hydrogen peroxide. *Biochim. Biophys. Acta* **402**:133.

67. Oberley, L. W., Lindgren, A. L., Baker, S. A., and Stevens, R. H. (1976). Superoxide ion as the cause of the oxygen effect. *Radiat. Res.* **68**:320.

68. Petkau, A., Chelack, W. S., and Pleskach, S. D. (1976). Letter: Protection of post-irradiated mice by superoxide dismutase. *Int. J. Radiat. Biol.* **29**, 297.

69. Watson, J. D. (1952). Properties of X-ray inactivated bacteriophage; inactivation by indirect effects. *J. Bacteriol.* **63**:473.
70. Misra, H. P., and Fridovich, I. (1976). Superoxide dismutase and the oxygen enhancement of radiation lethality. *Arch. Biochem. Biophys.* **176**:577.
70a. Samuni, A., and Czapski, G. (1978). Radiation-induced damage in *Escherichia coli* B: The effect of superoxide radicals and molecular oxygen. *Radiat. Res.* **76**:624.
70b. Mitchell, R. E. (1979). On the mechanism of oxygen protection against ionizing radiation damage in the cell wall of *Micrococcus radiodurans*. *Radiat. Res.* **79**:63.
71. McCord, J. M. (1974). Free radicals and inflammation: Protection of synovial fluid by superoxide dismutase. *Science* **185**:529.
72. Salin, M. L., and McCord, J. M. (1975). Free radicals and inflammation. Protection of phagocytosing leukocyte by superoxide dismutase. *J. Clin. Invest.* **56**:1319.
73. Carson, S., Vogin, E. E., Huber, W., and Schulte, T. (1973). Safety tests of orgotein, as antiinflammatory protein. *Toxicol. Appl. Pharmacol.* **26**:184.
74. Edsmyr, F., Huber, W., and Menander, K. B. (1976). Orgotein efficacy in ameliorating side effects due to radiation therapy. I. Double-blind, placebo-controlled trial in patients with bladder tumors. *Curr. Ther. Res.* **19**:198.
75. Ôyanagui, Y. (1976). Participation of superoxide anions at the prostaglandin phase of carrageenan foot-edema. *Biochem. Pharmacol.* **25**:1465.
76. Boxer, L. A., Yoder, M., Bonsib, S., Schmidt, M., Ho, P., Jersild, R., and Baehner, R. L. (1979). Effects of a chemotactic factor, N-formyl methionyl peptide, on adherence, O_2^--generation, phagocytosis and microtubule assembly of human polymorphonuclear leukocytes. *J. Lab. Clin. Med.* **93**:506.
77. Turner, S. R., Campbell, J. A., and Lynn, W. S. (1975). Biogenesis of chemotactic molecules by the arachidonate lipoxygenase system of platelets. *Nature (London)* **257**:680.
78. Perez, H. D., and Goldstein, I. M. (1979). Generation of a chemotactic lipid from arachidonic acid by exposure to a superoxide-generating system. *Fed. Proc., Fed. Am. Soc. Exp. Biol.* **38**:1170 (abstr.).
79. Petrone, W. F., English, D. K., Wong, K., and McCord, J. M. (1980). Free radicals and inflammation: Superoxide-dependent activation of a neutrophil chemotactic factor in plasma. *Proc. Natl. Acad. Sci. U.S.A.*, **77**:1159.

DISCUSSION

BUETTNER: What fraction of the electron flow will produce O_2^-?

FRIDOVICH: Boveris and Chance [*Biochem. J.* (1973) 134:707–716] have estimated that, in isolated mitochondria, between 2 and 5% of the electron flow goes to produce O_2^- and then H_2O_2. In *E. coli* we arrive at a similar estimate by measuring cyanide-resistant respiration. Paraquat greatly increases this cyanide-resistant respiration and thus the intracellular production of O_2^-.

MEHDI: You indicated that the *E. coli* superoxide dismutase was inducible. Have you come across constitutive mutants? With reference to the catabolite repression of this system, have you examined the effect of cyclic AMP in the presence and absence of paraquat?

FRIDOVICH: The *E. coli* MnSOD is inducible; the FeSOD appears to be constitutive. We have not yet found constitutive mutants that always have derepressed levels of the MnSOD. Such mutants would be very useful for clarifying the physiological function of this enzyme. We have reported mutants with defects in MnSOD, and they behave like obligate anaerobes. We have also reported a mutant with a very high level of FeSOD, and it was unusually tolerant of hyperbaric oxygen. Cyclic AMP has no role in the induction of MnSOD by paraquat.

PIETTE: As you reported, the mechanism of toxicity of paraquat is thought to be dependent on its reduction and reoxidation by O_2 to form O_2^-. How is paraquat actually reduced? Is the mechanism the same as that for some of the diazo dyes and the azoreductases?

FRIDOVICH: We presume that paraquat is reduced inside the cells by the action of an NAD(P)H diaphorase. We are in the process of isolating such an enzyme from *E. coli*.

DEL MAESTRO: Since paraquat increases the flux of electrons through the univalent pathway, have experiments been carried out in which sublethal doses of paraquat have been used to induce the production of superoxide dismutase and then the protective effects of this treatment on hyperoxia and hypoxia have been assessed?

FRIDOVICH: Yes; *E. coli* induced by paraquat and then freed of paraquat by washing are very resistant to hyperoxia and the aerobic lethality of streptonigrin. Conversely, *E. coli* induced with respect to MnSOD by hyperoxia or by pyocyanine are thereby rendered resistant to the lethal effects of paraquat.

DEMOPOULOS: The toxicity of paraquat in mice can be ameliorated by barbiturates. Might this involve free radicals?

FRIDOVICH: Perhaps barbiturates afford protection through their effects on the endoplasmic reticulum hydroxylase system. They may also protect by depressing respiration.

DEL MAESTRO: During experiments in which we depolymerized hyaluronic acid using the hypoxanthine–xanthine oxidase system, we observed a decrease in the rate and total amount of depolymerization when barbituric acids such as phenobarbital were added to the system. This may suggest a possible radical-scavenging role for phenobarbital.

PIETRONIGRO: Do you have any evidence concerning the capacity of paraquat to redox-cycle in eukaryotes? That is, do you think enzymes in the cytosol would be responsible for this, or would the activity be associated with either the endoplasmic reticulum or the mitochondria?

FRIDOVICH: Paraquat has been shown by other workers to cause increased O_2^- production in a liver microsome preparation supplied with reduced pyridine coenzymes. I do not, however, know of a thorough study of subcellular fractions undertaken to ascertain the most significant site of paraquat reduction in eukaryotic cells. In *E. coli* a cytoplasmic diaphorase catalyzes this reaction.

Chapter 2

Light, Oxygen, and Toxicity

CHRISTOPHER S. FOOTE

INTRODUCTION

Light and oxygen are toxic to many organisms. Environmental chemicals or natural cell constituents (such as porphyrins or flavins) can sensitize an organism to this damage. Examples of such sensitization in man include photosensitive porphyrias, drug photosensitivity, and photoallergy. Several diseases, such as aging of sun-exposed skin and sensitized carcinogenesis, may be related to these processes (1–5).

BASIC PHOTOCHEMISTRY (6)

Organic molecules are converted to chemically reactive, electronically excited states on absorption of light. Only light that is absorbed can cause photochemical reactions. Electrons are confined to distinct energy levels referred to as orbitals. These levels are filled from the bottom up in the ground state, the most stable electronic state of a molecule. In almost all molecules, the electrons are paired with electrons of opposite spin. A molecule with no net unpaired spins is in a singlet state. Absorption of

21

PATHOLOGY OF OXYGEN
ISBN 0-12-068620-1

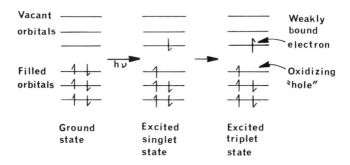

light promotes an electron to a higher orbital without change of spin; thus, the first state formed is also a singlet, in which there are no unpaired spins. In many cases the singlet undergoes a spin inversion very rapidly to give the triplet state, which has two unpaired electrons. Usually, the triplet state has a much longer lifetime than the singlet. Both states involve electrons that have been promoted to higher orbitals. Because these orbitals bind the electrons less strongly than do those of the ground state, electrons in higher orbitals are more readily removed by oxidizing agents than are those in the ground state. Similarly, the "holes" left by the promoted electron are located in orbitals that bind electrons strongly; for this reason, electronically excited molecules are more readily reduced than are molecules in the ground state.

Photosensitized oxidations of organic compounds have been studied for many years (7–9). Chemists were originally attracted to these reactions by the observations of biologists that the combination of sensitizing dyes, light, and oxygen is capable of damaging organisms of virtually all classes (1–3). The effects, collectively referred to as photodynamic action, include membrane damage, mutagenesis, interference with metabolism, and death. The chemical basis of these effects has been traced to damage of many different cell constituents, including lipids (which are peroxidized) and certain enzymes and peptides (of which methionine, histidine, tryptophan, and tyrosine are the most susceptible to photosensitized oxidation), and to nucleic acids (of which the guanine residues are the most sensitive) (1–3). Recent studies have led to greatly improved understanding in this area. It is now possible to recognize several distinct mechanistic pathways and to begin predicting which mechanism will occur in a given case (4,5).

PRIMARY PROCESSES

The classification of photooxidation mechanisms is important because it is now known that several types of biological molecules prevent damage by various intermediates, and it should be possible to design systems that protect against damage if the mechanism is known. At least one successful therapeutic method has already been designed on the basis of these considerations and is discussed below (10,11).

Photooxidations are of two classes: direct oxidations, in which the excited molecule is oxidized directly, and sensitized oxidations, in which the initially excited molecule ("sensitizer") indirectly promotes the oxidation of another molecule. An example of a direct photooxidation is the direct expulsion of an electron from a photoexcited molecule (M); the electron (e^-) can subsequently be trapped by oxygen to give superoxide

$$M \xrightarrow{h\nu} M^{+} + e^- \xrightarrow{O_2} M^{+} + O_2^-$$

ion (O_2^-) (12). Many processes induced by X rays and γ rays involve reactions of this type. It is reasonable to speculate that this process may be involved in some aspects of sunburning and light-induced elastin cross-linking, although this has not been demonstrated.

Sensitized oxidations can proceed by several different mechanisms. In one of these, the excited sensitizer interacts with another molecule directly, usually with transfer of a hydrogen atom or an electron. The radicals thus formed undergo further reaction with oxygen or other organic molecules. This is called a type I reaction. In a second class of reaction,

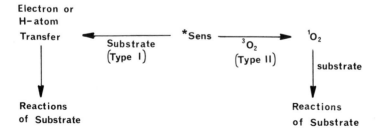

type II, the sensitizer triplet interacts with oxygen, most commonly by energy transfer, to give an excited electronic state of oxygen,* singlet molecular oxygen, which reacts further with various acceptors in solution. The sensitizer itself is often recovered unchanged (4,5).

TYPE I REACTIONS

An example of a type I reaction that is readily initiated by photoexcited molecules, particularly ketones and quinones and probably many flavins as well, is a hydrogen abstraction from suitable donors, for example, polyunsaturated fatty acids (see the section on radical chain processes, below). Free radicals are organic molecules with an odd number of elec-

$$R_2C{=}O^* \; + \; R{-}\underset{\underset{R}{|}}{\overset{\overset{R}{|}}{C}}{-}H \; \longrightarrow \; R_2\dot{C}{-}OH \; + \; R{-}\underset{\underset{R}{|}}{\overset{\overset{R}{|}}{C}}\cdot$$

excited ketone	abstractable hydrogen	free radicals

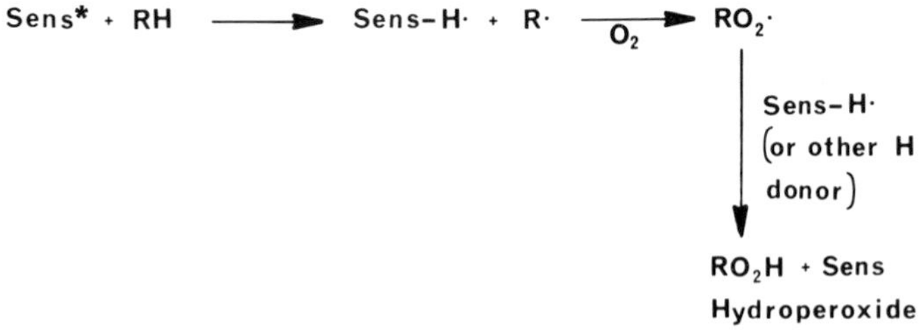

trons. Since the valence is not saturated, they are very reactive. They react rapidly with oxygen and ultimately produce hydroperoxides. The free radicals that result from the hydrogen abstraction reaction shown above can also enter chain reactions (see the section on radical chain processes, below).

$$\text{Sens}^* \; + \; \text{RH} \; \longrightarrow \; \text{Sens-H}\cdot \; + \; \text{R}\cdot \; \xrightarrow{O_2} \; RO_2\cdot$$

$$\Big\downarrow \begin{array}{l} \text{Sens-H}\cdot \\ \big(\text{or other H} \\ \text{donor}\big) \end{array}$$

$$RO_2H \; + \; \text{Sens}$$
Hydroperoxide

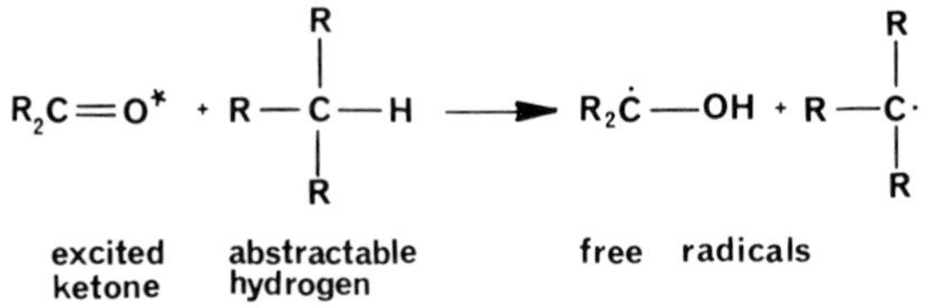

* The ground state of oxygen is one of the very few stable triplet molecules.

A recently discovered sensitized type I reaction is the oxidation of substrates photosensitized by 9,10-dicyanoanthracene (DCA) (13–15). The reaction appears to proceed by the mechanism shown below with a wide variety of electron-donating substrates (D). The only requirement is that the oxidation potential of the substrate be sufficiently low that electron transfer to singlet excited dicyanoanthracene (^{1}DCA) is exothermic. The products, DO_2, incorporate oxygen and are much like those with singlet oxygen (see the section on type II reactions, below).

^{1}DCA + D $\longrightarrow$ D$^+$ + DCA$^-$

O_2

DO_2

O_2^- + DCA

TYPE II REACTIONS

The type II reactions that occur with singlet O_2 are of several different classes (4,5,7–9). Typically, peroxides are the initial products. Two classes of singlet oxygen reactions are best known: additions to olefins, giving allylic hydroperoxides, analogous to the Alder "ene" reaction [reaction (1)], and additions to diene systems to produce endoperoxides, analogous to the Diels–Alder reaction [reaction (2)] (4,5,7–9,16,17). Reaction of unsaturated fatty acids to give the corresponding hydroperoxides is an example of the first class of reaction. An example of the second class is the reaction of certain heterocyclic compounds, such as the amino

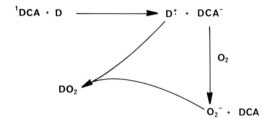

(1)

(2)

acid histidine, to give unstable endoperoxides as the primary product (4,5).

Three other classes of reaction with singlet oxygen have been discovered more recently. The first is a [2 + 2] cycloaddition to electron-rich olefins to produce dioxetanes, which are sometimes of moderate stability but readily cleave into two carbonyl-containing fragments (4,5) [reaction (3)]. Many heterocyclic compounds undergo this type of reaction. The second reaction involves oxidation of certain heteroatoms, notably sulfur (18,19), and is exemplified by the oxidation of methionine to its sulfoxide (20), where by 2 mol of sulfoxide are formed for each mole of oxygen consumed [reaction (4)]. The third reaction, involving phenols, is discussed in the section on phenols, below.

$$\text{(3)}$$

$$2CH_3-S-CH_2-CH_2-\underset{\underset{R}{\overset{|}{NH}}}{\overset{|}{CH}}-\overset{\overset{O}{\|}}{C}-R' \xrightarrow{{}^1O_2} 2CH_3-\overset{\overset{O^-}{|}}{\overset{+}{S}}-CH_2-CH_2-\underset{\underset{R}{\overset{|}{NH}}}{\overset{|}{CH}}-\overset{\overset{O}{\|}}{C}-R' \qquad \text{(4)}$$

QUENCHING (21)*

One other significant interaction of organic molecules with singlet oxygen has been established. One of the functions of carotenes in photosynthetic organisms appears to be protection of the organisms against photodynamic damage by natural sensitizers (22). For example, carotenoidless mutants or plants, in which carotene synthesis is blocked, are killed by light and oxygen under conditions that are normally harmless. Carotenoids also protect organisms against exogenous sensitizers. Carotenes (car) quench triplet molecules (e.g., chlorophyll) at a very high rate, but we have shown that they are also extremely efficient quenchers of

---

* Quenching is a process in which an excited molecule is converted to the ground state with no net chemical reaction.

singlet oxygen (23,24). Quenching of singlet oxygen may be an important mechanism of protection against the photodynamic effect. We originally proposed an energy transfer mechanism for this quenching, although other mechanisms were not ruled out (24). This mechanism has since been confirmed (25–27).

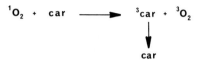

Nickel complexes (28–30) and polymethine dyes (31,32) are also excellent quenchers of singlet oxygen. These compounds may quench by an energy transfer mechanism, although definite evidence for this is still lacking. Other compounds can also quench singlet oxygen, although not as efficiently as those noted above. For example, 1,4-diazabicyclooctane (DABCO) has been shown by several groups to quench singlet oxygen (33–35). Other amines both quench singlet oxygen and react with it, de-

$$^1O_2 + Q \longrightarrow (O_2^- + Q^{\cdot+}) \longrightarrow {}^3O_2 + Q$$

pending on the conditions (36,37). These and other electron-rich compounds probably quench by a different mechanism, one involving charge transfer in which the quencher (Q) donates an electron.

PHENOLS

Phenols quench singlet oxygen (38), and some phenols also react chemically with it. Vitamin E (α-tocopherol) is a particularly interesting compound since it quenches singlet oxygen at a high rate in all solvents but is appreciably converted to products only in polar solvents (39–42). The initial product of the chemical reaction is the very unstable hydroperoxydienone (43). It is tempting to suggest that some of the biological activity of vitamin E is due to this quenching reaction; probably much more important chemically, however, is its capacity to terminate radical chain reactions (see below) (43,44).

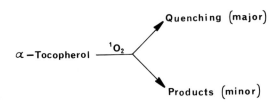

RADICAL CHAIN PROCESSES

In all of the above reactions, peroxides (ROOH or ROOR) are produced. Peroxides contain a weak O—O bond that is easily broken thermally, particularly in the presence of transition metals. The products of this breakdown are alkoxy radicals (RO·). Alkoxy radicals, like many electronically excited molecules, react rapidly with compounds with abstractable hydrogen atoms (R″H) to give alkyl radicals (R″). These react rapidly with oxygen to give alkylperoxy radicals (R″OO·), which can in turn attack a new R″H to give a radical chain autoxidation reaction. Fatty acids and cholesterol are examples of compounds attacked in this process. The hydroperoxides (R″OOH) formed eventually cause damage to membranes, among other effects.

$$
\begin{array}{lll}
\text{ROOR}' & \longrightarrow & \text{RO·} \;+\; \text{RO}'_! \\[4pt]
\text{RO·} \;+\; \text{R}''\text{H} & \longrightarrow & \text{R·}'' \;+\; \text{ROH}
\end{array}
\left.\begin{array}{l} \\ \\ \end{array}\right\} \begin{array}{l}\text{initiation of}\\ \text{chain}\end{array}
$$

$$
\text{R·}'' \;+\; \text{O}_2 \longrightarrow \text{R}''\text{OO·}
$$

$$
\text{R}''\text{OO·} \;+\; \text{R}''\text{H} \longrightarrow \text{R}''\text{OOH} \;+\; \text{R·}'' \qquad (\text{chain})
$$

Thus, a compound (e.g., R″H) not initially attacked in any of the photochemical processes can subsequently be attacked in this quite nonselective autoxidation. Many molecules of R″H can be attacked for each RO·

formed. Membranes are easily damaged by this mechanism. Many compounds, such as tocopherols and other phenols, protect against oxidative damage by terminating the radical chain, as shown below:

$$RO\cdot + XH \longrightarrow ROH + X\cdot$$

In this reaction, XH is a compound with a weak bond, such as the phenolic OH; the X radical is too unreactive to attack a stronger CH bond (e.g., in R″H in the chain reaction above) and the chain is broken. One phenol molecule can thus protect many molecules of R″H.

A second type of biological protection is afforded by such systems as glutathione peroxidase, which acts by reducing the initial peroxide to an unreactive alcohol, thus preventing the initiation step (45).

$$ROOR' \xrightarrow[\text{[H]}]{} ROH + R'OH$$

SINGLET OXYGEN FORMATION

In photochemical reactions, singlet oxygen is produced by energy transfer from triplet molecules that are formed after the absorption of light by a sensitizer (4,5,7–9). In 1964, it was found that the reactions produced by singlet oxygen in solution were the same as those produced by the reactive intermediate in dye-sensitized photooxygenations. The intermediacy of singlet oxygen in these reactions has since been unequivocally demonstrated. Singlet oxygen is also formed in numerous nonphotochemical reactions (4,5,46). Its importance in many pathological biological side reactions has been suggested but not yet clearly established. This question is discussed in subsequent sections.

It can be difficult to distinguish among the many mechanisms introduced above and among combinations of them, which often occur in competition. Devising quantitative and careful studies with traps, quenchers, and inhibitors for various processes is a first step, but it is important to recognize that most such reagents are not completely specific for a given process (46).

COMPARISON OF REACTIONS WITH OTHER
SOURCES OF SINGLET OXYGEN

If singlet oxygen is believed to be the intermediate in a given reaction, it may be useful to compare the products and/or kinetics with those of chemically produced singlet oxygen (4,5,46). Indeed, such studies were first used to demonstrate the intermediacy of singlet oxygen in photooxidations. Both products and kinetics must also be independent of the sensitizing dye if singlet oxygen is the intermediate. Unfortunately, many biological substrates are so easily oxidized that their direct reaction with the reagents used to generate singlet oxygen may be a problem; for example, NaOCl, H_2O_2, and triphenyl phosphite ozonide are powerful oxidants in their own right. Similar drawbacks attend the use of virtually all of the nonphotochemical sources of singlet oxygen. Nevertheless, these techniques have been used, for example, with phenols (47–49), tocopherols (50), and nucleic bases (51–53) to indicate that reaction occurs with singlet oxygen. Of course, the observation of reaction with singlet oxygen is not, by itself, proof that singlet oxygen is the intermediate in photooxygenation. Another problem is that products of singlet oxygen reactions and autoxidation may be identical, for example, in the case of phenols.

KINETICS

One of the most powerful techniques for demonstrating the intermediacy of singlet oxygen involves competitive inhibition with a known singlet oxygen acceptor that is not a good type I substrate (4,5,21). However, to be most useful, the results should be obtained under conditions which demonstrate that quenching is competitive and should yield numerical values that can be compared with values determined from other studies. "One-point" experiments with quenchers are of very limited value, since most singlet oxygen quenchers are also capable of quenching sensitizer excited states or reacting with free radicals.

Kearns and associates have developed a technique for demonstrating singlet oxygen intermediacy based on the fact that the lifetime of singlet oxygen is much longer in D_2O than in H_2O; this can result in a higher rate of conversion of substrate in D_2O than in H_2O (54–56). However, several assumptions must be made before this technique can be used (4,5,46). Although there are several other kinetic techniques that can be used to test for the presence of singlet oxygen, they are too specialized to discuss in this chapter (4,5,46).

Chemiluminescence has been used frequently as an indicator of the presence of singlet oxygen (2). Singlet oxygen in the gas phase emits light at several specific wavelengths. However, this luminescence is exceedingly weak in solution, and there are many processes that give rise to luminescence without involving singlet oxygen (4,5). Unless the detailed spectrum is obtained and compared with that of singlet oxygen, chemiluminescence cannot be regarded as a positive indicator of the presence of this species (46).

TRAPS FOR SINGLET OXYGEN

An extensively employed technique for determining the intermediacy of singlet oxygen involves the use of chemical traps that react with singlet oxygen to give distinctive products. However, considerable caution is required. Furans are among the most commonly used traps for singlet oxygen in reactions of this type. The products of initial attack of singlet oxy-

gen on furans are endoperoxides, which are unstable and break down very rapidly to give diketones (57). Unfortunately, almost any oxidant will convert furans to diketones (for example, halogens, peracids, or air) (46); thus, this class of acceptors should not be used as a characteristic trap for singlet oxygen.

A better chemical trapping method for distinguishing between singlet oxygen reactions and radical chain autoxidations is the use of a chemical "fingerprint" such as cholesterol (46). Cholesterol reacts with singlet oxygen to give 5-α-hydroperoxycholesterol (5-αHPC) (1) (the double bond always shifts in this reaction). Reaction with radicals gives a complex product mixture, but no 5-αHPC is formed (58–64).

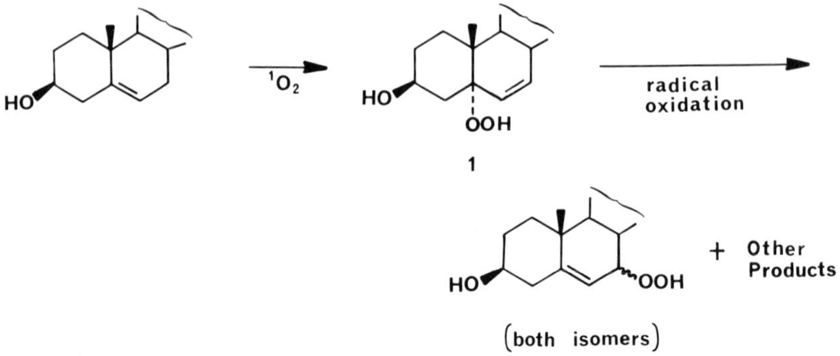

1

(both isomers)

SUPEROXIDE AND SINGLET OXYGEN

The chemistry of superoxide (O_2^-) has become a subject of active investigation in recent years (65,66). We have been interested in it for some time because of the damaging effects of superoxide and because of the possibility that singlet oxygen can be generated from superoxide (67–70) (see the chapter by Fridovich, this volume). Superoxide salts can be formed from oxygen by various electron transfer processes or prepared from potassium superoxide. Superoxide anion is stable in aprotic solvents but is rapidly decomposed by proton donors (e.g., water) to hydrogen peroxide and oxygen (67–74). There has been disagreement in the literature

$$2O_2^- \longrightarrow O_2 + H_2O_2$$

(67–74) concerning the amount of singlet oxygen formed in the spontaneous dismutation of O_2^- in water. Our recent conclusion is that, at most, about 1 part in 10^4 of the oxygen produced in the dismutation is singlet. We arrived at this figure using the cholesterol trapping system as a quantitative technique (75).

There are numerous medically important systems in which photooxidations are believed to be important. These are discussed in the next sections.

PORPHYRIA

Human porphyrias comprise several different syndromes that are caused by defects in the metabolism of blood porphyrins (76–78). Some porphyrias, especially erythropoietic protoporphyria (EPP), are associated with photosensitivity; patients with this disease tend to develop edema and erythema on exposure to light. The photosensitivity is caused by the deposition of photosensitizing porphyrins in the skin. There have been dramatic reports that the photosensitivity of patients with EPP can be largely relieved by orally administered β-carotene (10,11). The mechanism of this process is not known, but it is attractive to speculate that singlet oxygen is the active damaging species, formed by energy transfer from photoexcited protoporphyrin. The protective action of carotene could thus be understood as singlet oxygen quenching.

TREATMENT OF NEONATAL JAUNDICE

A common problem among newborn (especially premature) infants is jaundice, which, if untreated, may lead to brain damage (79,80). This disease involves an excess concentration of bilirubin, which is deposited in the skin and brain. The common treatment for neonatal jaundice is irradiation of the infant with light of wavelengths absorbed by bilirubin (centered at 450 nm). Irradiation bleaches the bilirubin in the skin and apparently prevents brain damage (81). A photooxidation is involved in at least part of the bilirubin loss, and the products (in vitro) are those that might be expected from singlet oxygen attack (82,83). Singlet oxygen, formed by bilirubin as sensitizer, has been shown to be the reactive intermediate in the destruction (84–87).

A recent study suggests that the major mechanism of action of jaundice phototherapy may not be photooxidation at all (88). Apparently, irradiation converts bilirubin to a short-lived photoisomer, which is much more water soluble than the natural form and can be rapidly excreted. Excretion of bilirubin in jaundiced rats increased dramatically immediately after irradiation.

TREATMENT OF HERPES SIMPLEX

Lesions caused by the herpes simplex virus have been effectively treated in man with neutral red followed by brief irradiation. The symptomatic improvement was superior to that obtained with any other therapy, and a decrease in the frequency of recurrences was noticed. Type 2 herpes genitalis appeared to be treated even more effectively in this way than type 1 virus (89,90). However, concern about the possible carcinogenicity of the technique has prevented its wide acceptance (90). The mechanism of action is unknown.

PHOTOCARCINOGENESIS

An association has been made repeatedly between photosensitizing capacity and carcinogenicity of polynuclear aromatic hydrocarbons, and many photodynamic photosensitizers are capable of producing tumors on prolonged irradiation (1–5,91). 3,4-Benzpyrene shows enhanced carcinogenicity in the presence of light (91,92). Several theories of carcinogenicity involving singlet oxygen have been proposed (92–94).

OTHER BIOLOGICAL IMPLICATIONS

Photooxidation reactions have numerous other medical implications, but only a few will be mentioned here. Psoriasis is commonly treated by the use of coal tar (which contains sensitizing hydrocarbons) and light (95). Recent studies have shown that certain photosensitizers are quite effective (96,97); however, the intermediacy of singlet oxygen is very uncertain in these systems.

Tumor cells can be killed photodynamically. It has been reported that malignant cells take up and bind hematoporphyrin to a greater extent than does normal tissue; irradiation then selectively kills the tumor cells (98–100). This approach, which has been used with several different tumor types, may be useful in the treatment of resistant tumors.

NONPHOTOCHEMICAL PRODUCTION OF
SINGLET OXYGEN

Several lines of evidence suggest that, in addition to the photochemical and nonphotochemical reactions mentioned above, singlet oxygen may be involved in numerous biological processes. Because the literature is so extensive, a complete review has not been attempted here [a reasonably recent review (4,5) and a critique (46) can be found elsewhere].

The question of whether singlet oxygen is produced in the lipoxygenase system has been debated a number of times (101–103). However, the finding that cholesterol oxidation gives rise to the radical product (104) seems to force one to the conclusion that singlet oxygen is not the major oxidizing species in this system.

It was also reported that both the peroxidase and synthase activity of sheep vesicular gland microscomes catalyzed the oxygenation of singlet oxygen traps. The traps were diphenylisobenzofuran, diphenylfuran, and bilirubin, which are readily oxidized by other oxidizing species. However, D_2O actually inhibited the reaction, an effect that was not adequately explained by the authors (105) and is not consistent with the intermediacy of singlet oxygen. Paine showed that riboflavin-sensitized oxygenation of liver cell cultures resulted in the stimulation of benzopyrene 3-monooxygenase, a cytochrome P-450-linked monooxygenase, and suggested on the basis of scavenging experiments that singlet oxygen was responsible (106). Similarly, King $et\ al.$ (107) showed that liver microsome oxidation of NADPH simultaneously caused the oxidation of diphenylfuran to dibenzoylethylene and concluded that singlet oxygen was the cause of this oxidation. However, this conclusion is subject to the caveats mentioned earlier.

An interesting recent finding is that chemiluminescence (suggested to be associated with singlet oxygen production) is associated with the killing of bacteria by leukocytes and macrophages (108–110). Several other authors have suggested that singlet oxygen is involved. Krinsky (111) found that carotenoids protected a microorganism against killing by leukocytes (58). Klebanoff (112,113) showed that furans are oxidized to diketones by the myeloperoxidase from these organisms and that this oxidation is inhibited by the singlet oxygen quenchers DABCO and tocopherol. Piatt $et\ al.$ (114) showed that the lactoperoxidase/H_2O_2 system also chemiluminesces and that diphenylisobenzofuran and diphenylfuran are oxidized by this system; DABCO and other singlet oxygen acceptors are powerful inhibitors of the reaction. Circumstantial evidence for the presence of singlet oxygen was obtained. However, hypochlorite is also believed to be present in the reaction and, since it is a strong oxidizing agent, it was not ruled out as the responsible agent. Superoxide ion has also been strongly implicated in the leukocyte system (115–117). There is clear evidence that powerful oxidants are produced (108–117), but their nature is far less clear; strong arguments have been advanced that they are not necessarily singlet oxygen (118,119).

In collaboration with Dr. Robert I. Lehrer of the UCLA Medical School, we have used the cholesterol trapping technique to search for singlet oxygen production by leukocytes (120). Human polymorphonuclear leukocytes ingested a mineral oil dispersion of radiolabeled cholesterol. After incubation, the cholesterol was extracted and reduced; unlabeled known products were added. The known spots were extracted from the thin-layer chromatogram and counted. No evidence for the formation of a singlet oxygen product was found; an upper limit of about 2% of the oxygen uptake could have appeared as singlet oxygen. Recent experiments using radiolabeled cholesterol adsorbed on polystyrene microbeads have produced similar negative results. Moreover, similar experiments using rat lung macrophages (in collaboration with Dr. Anne P. Autor, University of Iowa) have also yielded evidence that singlet oxygen is not produced (121).

It is obvious this field is in its infancy. More subtle and powerful techniques are urgently needed to sort out the complex chemistry involved in these biological systems.

ACKNOWLEDGMENTS

Original work reported in this chapter was supported by NSF Grant CHE77-21560 and NIH Grant GM20080. The experimental collaboration of numerous co-workers, mentioned in the references, is gratefully acknowledged.

REFERENCES

1. Spikes, J. D. (1968). Photodynamic action. *Photophysiology* **3**:33.
2. Spikes, J. D., and Livingston, R. (1969). The molecular biology of photodynamic action: Sensitized photoautoxidations in biological systems. *Adv. Radiat. Biol.* **3**:29.
3. Spikes, J. D., and MacKnight, M. L. (1970). Dye-sensitized photooxidation of proteins. *Ann. N.Y. Acad. Sci.* **171**:149.
4. Foote, C. S. (1968). Mechanisms of photosensitized oxidation. *Science* **162**:963.
5. Foote, C. S. (1976). Photosensitized oxidation and singlet oxygen: Consequences in biological systems. *In* "Free Radicals in Biology" (W. A. Pryor, ed.), Vol. 2, p. 85. Academic Press, New York.
6. Turro, N. J. (1978). "Modern Molecular Photochemistry." Benjamin/Cumming, Menlo Park, California.
7. Gollnick, K. (1968). Type II photooxygenation reactions in solution. *Adv. Photochem.* **6**:1.
8. Gollnick, K., and Schenck, G. O. (1967). Oxygenase dienophile. *In* "1,4-Cycloaddition Reactions" (J. Hamer, ed.), p. 255. Academic Press, New York.
9. Livingston, R. (1961). Photochemical autoxidation. *In* "Autoxidation and Antioxidants" (W. O. Lundberg, ed.), Vol. 1, p. 249. Wiley (Interscience), New York.
10. Deleo, V. A., Poh-Fitzpatrick, M., Mathews-Roth, M. M., and Harber, L. C. (1976). Erythropoietic protoporphyria. *Am. J. Med.* **60**:8.
11. Mathews-Roth, L. C., and Kass, E. H. (1970). β-carotene as a photoprotective agent in erythropoietic protoporphyria. *N. Engl. J. Med.* **282**:1231.

12. Grossweiner, L. I. (1976). Photochemical inactivation of enzymes. *Curr. Top. Radiat. Res. Q.* **11**:141.
13. Eriksen, J., and Foote, C. S. (1978). Electron-transfer fluorescence quenching and exciplexes of cyano-substituted anthracenes. *J. Phys. Chem.* **82**:2659.
14. Manring, L. E., Eriksen, J., and Foote, C. S. (1980). Electron-transfer photooxygenation. 4. Photooxygenation of *trans*-stilbene sensitized by methylene blue. *J. Am. Chem. Soc.* **102**:4275.
15. Eriksen, J., Foote, C. S., and Parker, T. L. (1977). Photosensitized oxygenation of alkenes and sulfides via a non-singlet oxygen mechanism. *J. Am. Chem. Soc.* **99**:6455.
16. Foote, C. S. (1968). Photosensitized oxygenations and the role of singlet oxygen. *Acc. Chem. Res.* **1**:104.
17. Kearns, D. R. (1971). Physical and chemical properties of singlet molecular oxygen. *Chem. Rev.* **71**:395.
18. Foote, C. S., and Peters, J. W. (1971). Photooxidation of sulfides. *Int. Cong. Pure Appl. Chem., Spec. Lect., 23rd, 1971.* Vol. 4, p. 129.
19. Foote, C. S., and Peters, J. W. (1971). Chemistry of singlet oxygen. XIV. A reactive intermediate in sulfide photoxidation. *J. Am. Chem. Soc.* **93**:3795.
20. Sysak, P. K., Foote, C. S., and Ching, T.-Y. (1977). Chemistry of singlet oxygen. XXV. Photooxygenations of methionine. *Photochem. Photobiol.* **26**:19.
21. Foote, C. S. (1978). Quenching of singlet oxygen. *In* "Singlet Oxygen" (H. H. Wasserman and R. W. Murray, eds.), p. 139. Academic Press, New York.
22. Krinsky, N. (1971). Function. *In* "Carotenoids" (O. Isler, ed.), p. 669. Birkhaeuser, Basel.
23. Foote, C. S., and Denny, R. W. (1968). Chemistry of singlet oxygen. VII. Quenching by β-carotene. *J. Am. Chem. Soc.* **90**:6233.
24. Foote, C. S., Chang, Y. C., and Denny, R. W. (1970). Chemistry of singlet oxygen. XI. Cis-trans isomerization of carotenoids by singlet oxygen and a probable quenching mechanism. *J. Am. Chem. Soc.* **92**:5218.
25. Farmilo, A., and Wilkinson, F. (1973). On the mechanism of quenching of singlet oxygen in solution. *Photochem. Photobiol.* **18**:447.
26. Breton, J., and Mathis, P. (1970). Mise en évidence de l'état triplet de la chlorophylle dans des lamelles chloroplastiques. *Hebd. Seances Acad. Sci., C. R. Ser. D* **271**:1094.
27. Mathis, P., and Kleo, J. (1973). The triplet state of beta-carotene of analog polyenes of different length. *Photochem. Photobiol.* **18**:343.
28. Carlsson, D. J., Mendenhall, G. D., Suprunchuk, T., and Wiles, D. M. (1972). Singlet oxygen ($^1\Delta$g) quenching in the liquid phase by metal (II) chelates. *J. Am. Chem. Soc.* **94**:8960.
29. Flood, J., Russell, K. E., and Wan, J. K. S. (1973). Quenching of singlet molecular oxygen by polyolefin additives in carbon disulfide solution. *Macromolecules* **6**:669.
30. Guillory, J. P., and Cook, C. F. (1973). Energy transfer processes involving ultraviolet stabilizers. Quenching of singlet oxygen. *J. Polym. Sci., Polym. Chem. Ed.* **11**:1927.
31. Merkel, P. B., and Kearns, D. R. (1972). Radiationless decay of singlet molecular oxygen in solution. An experimental and theoretical study of electronic-to-vibrational energy transfer. *J. Am. Chem. Soc.* **97**:7244.
32. Smith, W. F., Herkstroeter, W. G., and Eddy, K. L. (1975). Quenching of singlet molecular oxygen in solution by azomethine dyes. *J. Am. Chem. Soc.* **97**:2764.
33. Foote, C. S., Denny, R. W., Weaver, L., Chang, Y., and Peters, J. (1970). Quenching of singlet oxygen. *Ann. N.Y. Acad. Sci.* **171**:139.
34. Oannès, C., and Wilson, T. (1968). Quenching of singlet oxygen by tertiary aliphatic-amines. Effects of DABCO. *J. Am. Chem. Soc.* **90**:6527.

35. Ogryzlo, E. A., and Tang, C. W. (1970). Quenching of oxygen ($^1\Delta g$) by amines. *J. Am. Chem. Soc.* **92**:5034.
36. Dalle, J. O., Magous, R., and Mousseron-Canet, M. (1972). Inhibition de l'oxygen singulet. *Photochem. Photobiol.* **15**:411.
37. Smith, W. F., Jr. (1972). Kinetic evidence for both quenching and reaction of singlet oxygen with triethylamine in pyridine solution. *J. Am. Chem. Soc.* **94**:186.
38. Thomas, M. J., and Foote, C. S. (1978). Chemistry of singlet oxygen. XXVI. Photooxygenation of phenols. *Photochem. Photobiol.* **27**:683.
39. Fahrenholtz, S. R., Doleiden, F. H., Trozzolo, A. M., and Lamola, A. A. (1974). On the quenching of singlet oxygen by alpha-tocopherol. *Photochem. Photobiol.* **20**:505.
40. Foote, C. S., Ching, T.-Y., and Geller, G. G. (1974). Chemistry of singlet oxygen. XVIII. Rates of reaction and quenching of α-tocopherol and singlet oxygen. *Photochem. Photobiol.* **20**:511.
41. Grams, G. W., and Eskins, K. (1972). Dye-sensitized photooxidation of tocopherols. Correlation between singlet oxygen reactivity and vitamin E activity. *Biochemistry* **11**:606.
42. Stevens, B., Small, R. D., Jr., and Perez, S. R. (1974). The photopheroxidation of unsaturated organic molecules. XIII. O_2-$^1\Delta g$ quenching by α-tocopherol. *Photochem. Photobiol.* **20**:515.
43. Clough, R. L., Yee, B. G., and Foote, C. S. (1979). Chemistry of singlet oxygen. XXX. The unstable primary product of tocopherol photooxidation. *J. Am. Chem. Soc.* **101**:683.
44. Pryor, W. A. (1976). The role of free radical reactions in biological systems. *In* "Free Radicals in Biology" (W. A. Pryor, ed.), Vol. 1, p. 1. Academic Press, New York.
45. Kosower, N. S., and Kosower, E. M. (1976). The glutathione-glutathione disulfide system. *In* "Free Radicals in Biology" (W. A. Pryor, ed.), Vol. 2, p. 55. Academic Press, New York.
46. Foote, C. S. (1979): Detection of singlet oxygen in complex systems: A critique. *In* "Oxygen: Biochemical and Clinical Aspects" (W. S. Caughey, ed.), p. 603. Academic Press, New York.
47. Matsuura, T., Yoshimura, N., Nishinaga, A., and Saito, I. (1972). Participation of singlet oxygen in the hydrogen abstraction from a phenol in the photosensitized oxygenation. *Tetrahedron* **28**:4933.
48. Pfoertner, K., and Bose, D. (1970). Die photosensibiliserte oxydation einwertiger phenole zu chinonen. *Helv. Chim. Acta* **53**:1553.
49. Saito, I., Kato, S., and Matsuura, T. (1970). Photoinduced reactions. XL. Addition of singlet oxygen to monocyclic aromatic ring. *Tetrahedron Lett.* p. 239.
50. Grams, G. W. (1971). Oxidation of α-tocopherol by singlet oxygen. *Tetrahedron Lett.* p. 4823.
51. Clagett, D. C., and Galen, T. J. (1971). Ribonucleoside reactivities with singlet (one-delta g) molecular oxygen. *Arch. Biochem. Biophys.* **146**:196.
52. Hallett, F. R., Hallett, B. P., and Snipes, W. (1970). Reactions between singlet oxygen and the constituents of nucleic acids. Importance of reactions in photodynamic processes. *Biophys. J.* **10**:305.
53. Rosenthal, I., and Pitts, J. N., Jr. (1971). Reactivity of purine and pyrimidine bases toward singlet oxygen. *Biophys. J.* **11**:963.
54. Merkel, P. B., and Kearns, D. R. (1972). Remarkable solvent effects on the lifetime of $^1\Delta g$ oxygen. *J. Am. Chem. Soc.* **94**:1029.
55. Merkel, P. B., Nilsson, R., and Kearns, D. R. (1972). Deuterium effects on singlet oxygen lifetime in solutions. A new test of singlet oxygen reactions. *J. Am. Chem. Soc.* **94**:1030.

56. Nilsson, R., Merkel, P. B., and Kearns, D. R. (1972). Unambiguous evidence for the participation of singlet oxygen in photodynamic oxidation of amino acids. *Photochem. Photobiol.* **16:**117.
57. Foote, C. S., Wuesthoff, M. T., Wexler, S., Burstain, I. G., Denny, R., Schenck, G. O., and Schulte-Elte, K.-H. (1967). Photosensitized oxygenation of alkyl-substituted furans. *Tetrahedron* **23:**2583.
58. Kulig, M. J., and Smith, L. L. (1973). Sterol metabolism. XXV. Cholesterol oxidation by singlet molecular oxygen. *J. Org. Chem.* **38:**3639.
59. Nickon, A., and Bagli, J. F. (1959). Photosensitized oxygenation of mono-olefins. *J. Am. Chem. Soc.* **81:**6330.
60. Nickon, A., and Bagli, J. F. (1961). Reactivity and geometry in allylic systems. I. Stereochemistry of photosensitized oxygenation of mono-olefins. *J. Am. Chem. Soc.* **83:**1498.
61. Schenck, G. O., Gollnick, K., and Neumüller, O.-A. (1957). Darstelling von steroid-hydroperoxyden mittels phototoxischer photosensibilisatoren. *Justus Liebigs Ann. Chem.* **603:**46.
62. Schenck, G. O., and Neumüller, O.-A. (1958). Synthese tertiärer steroid-hydroperoxide, insbesondere des Δ-allopregnen-3-β-ol-20-5-α-hydroperoxyds. *Justus Liebigs Ann. Chem.* **618:**194.
63. Smith, L. L., and Hill, F. L. (1972). Detection of sterol hydroperoxides on thin-layer chromatoplates by means of the Wurster dyes. *J. Chromatogr.* **66:**101.
64. Smith, L. L., Teng, J. I., Kulig, M. J., and Hill, F. L. (1973). Sterol metabolism. XXIII. Cholesterol oxidation by radiation-induced processes. *J. Org. Chem.* **38:**1763.
65. Fridovich, I. (1972). Superoxide radical and superoxide dismutase. *Acc. Chem. Res.* **5:**321.
66. Fridovich, I. (1976). Oxygen radicals, hydrogen peroxide, and oxygen toxicity. In "Free Radicals in Biology" (W. A. Pryor, ed.), Vol. 1, p. 239. Academic Press, New York.
67. Khan, A. U. (1970). Singlet molecular oxygen from superoxide anion and sensitized fluorescence of organic molecules. *Science* **168:**476.
68. Khan, A. U., (1976). Singlet molecular oxygen. A new kind of oxygen. *J. Phys. Chem.* **80:**2219.
69. Mayeda, E. A., and Bard, A. J. (1974). Singlet oxygen. The suppression of its production in dismutation of superoxide ion by superoxide dismutase. *J. Am. Chem. Soc.* **96:**4023.
70. Zimmerman, R., Flohé, L., Weser, U., and Hartmann, H.-J. (1973). Inhibition of lipid peroxidation in isolated inner membrane of rat liver mitochondria by superoxide dismutase. *FEBS Lett.* **29:**117.
71. Guiraud, H. J., and Foote, C. S. (1976). Chemistry of superoxide ion. III. Quenching of singlet oxygen. *J. Am. Chem. Soc.* **98:**1984.
72. Nakano, M., Takayama, K., Shimizu, Y., Tsuji, Y., Inaba, H., and Migita, T. (1976). Spectroscopic evidence for the generation of singlet oxygen in self-reaction of *sec*-peroxy radicals. *J. Am. Chem. Soc.* **98:**1974.
73. Nilsson, R., and Kearns, D. R. (1974). Role of singlet oxygen in some chemiluminescence and enzyme oxidation reactions. *J. Phys. Chem.* **78:**1681.
74. Poupko, R., and Rosenthal, I. (1973). Electron-transfer interactions between superoxide ion and organic compounds. *J. Phys. Chem.* **77:**1722.
75. Foote, C. S., Shook, F. C., Abakerli, R. B. (1980). Chemistry of superoxide ion. 4. Singlet oxygen is not a major product of dismutation. *J. Am. Chem. Soc.* **102:**2503.
76. Fitzpatrick, T. B., Arndt, K. A., Clark, W. H., Jr., Eisen, A. Z., Van Scott, E. J., and

Vaughn, J. H., ed. (1971). "Dermatology in General Medicine." McGraw-Hill, New York.

77. Magnus, I. A. (1972). Photodynamic action in the skin. *Res. Prog. Org.-Biol. Med. Chem.* **3,** 571.

78. Marver, H. S., and Schmid, R. (1972). Postreplication repair in the xeroderma pigmentasum variant and the role of caffeine in DNA repair. *In* "The Metabolic Basis of Inherited Disease" (J. B. Stanbury, J. B. Wyngaarden, and D. S. Fredrickson, eds.), 3rd ed., p. 1087. McGraw-Hill, New York.

79. Bergsma, D., Hsia, D. Y.-Y., and Jackson, C., eds. (1970). "Bilirubin Metabolism in the Newborn." Williams & Wilkins, Baltimore, Maryland.

80. Odell, G. B., Schaffer, R. P., and Simopoulos, A. P., ed. (1972). "Phototherapy in the Newborn: An Overview." National Academy of Sciences, Washington, D.C.

81. Cremer, R. J., Perryman, P. W., and Richards, D. H. (1957). Influence of light on the hyperbilirubinaemia of infants. *Lancet* **1:**1094.

82. Bonnett, R., and Stewart, J. C. M. (1972). Photo-oxidation of bilirubin in hydroxylic solvents: Propentdyopent adducts as major products. *J. Chem. Soc., Chem. Commun.* p. 596.

83. Lightner, D. A., and Quistad, G. B. (1972). Hematinic acid and propentdyopents from bilirubin photo-oxidized *in vitro. FEBS Lett.* **25:**94.

84. Bonnett, R., and Stewart, J. C. M. (1972). Singlet oxygen in the photooxidation of bilirubin in hydroxylic solvents. *Biochem. J.* **130:**895.

85. McDonagh, A. F. (1971). The role of singlet oxygen in bilirubin photooxidation. *Biochem. Biophys. Res. Commun.* **44:**1306.

86. McDonagh, A. F. (1972). The photochemistry and photometabolism of bilirubin. *In* "Phototherapy in the Newborn: An Overview" (G. B. Odell, R. P. Schaffer, and A. P. Simonpoulos, eds.), p. 56. National Academy of Sciences, Washington, D.C.

87. Foote, C. S., and Ching, T.-Y. (1975). Chemistry of singlet oxygen. XXI. Kinetics of bilirubin photoxygenation. *J. Am. Chem. Soc.* **97:**6209.

88. McDonagh, A. F., and Ramonas, L. M. (1978). Jaundice phototherapy: Micro flow-cell photometry reveals rapid biliary response of Gunn rats to light. *Science* **201:**829.

89. Felber, T. D., Smith, E. B., Knox, M., Wallis, C., and Melnick, J. L. (1973). Photodynamic inactivation of *Herpes simplex:* Report of a clinical trial. *JAMA, J. Am. Med. Assoc.* **223:**289.

90. Symposium on Dye-Light Therapy for *Herpes simplex* Lesions (1977). 4th Annual Meeting of the American Society for Photobiology, February 1976. *Photochem. Photobiol.* **25:**333.

91. Santamaria, L. (1972). Further considerations on photodynamic action and carcinogenicity. *Res. Prog. Org.-Biol. Med. Chem.* **3:**671.

92. Khan, A. U., and Kasha, M. (1970). An optical-residue singlet-oxygen theory of carcinogenicity. *Ann. N.Y. Acad. Sci.* **171:**24.

93. Cavalieri, E., and Calvin, M. (1971). Photochemical coupling of benzo[a]pyrene with 1-methylcytosine: Photoenhancement of carcinogenicity. *Photochem. Photobiol.* **14:**641.

94. Foote, C. S. (1972). Chemical reactivity of polycyclic aromatic hydrocarbons and azaarenes. *In* "Particulate Polycyclic Organic Matter," p. 63. Committee on Biological Effects of Atmospheric Pollutants, National Academy of Sciences, Washington, D.C.

95. Farber, E. M., and Cox, A. H., ed. (1971). "Psoriasis." Stanford Univ. Press, Stanford, California.

96. Parrish, J. A., Fitzpatrick, T. B., Tanenbaum, L., and Pathak, M. A. (1974). Photochemotherapy of psoriasis with oral methoxsalen and longwave ultraviolet light. *N. Engl. J. Med.* **291:**1207.

97. Weber, G. (1974). Combined g-methoxypsoralen and black light therapy of psoriasis. *Br. J. Dermatol.* **90:**317.
98. Diamond, I., McDonagh, A. F., Wilson, C. B., Granelli, S. G., Nielsen, S., and Jaenicke, R. (1972). Photodynamic therapy of malignant tumors. *Lancet* **2:**1175.
99. Doherty, T. J., Grindley, G. B., Fiel, R., Weishaupt, K. R., and Boyle, D. G. (1975). Photoradiation therapy. II. Cure of animal tumors with hematoporphyrin and light. *JNCI, J. Natl. Cancer Inst.* **55:**115.
100. Granelli, S. G., Diamond, I., McDonagh, A. F., Wilson, C. B., and Nielsen, S. L. (1975). Photochemotherapy of glioma cells by visible light and hematoporphyrin. *Cancer Res.* **35:**2567.
101. Baldwin, J. E., Swallow, J. C., and Chan, H. W.-S. (1971). Oxygen insertion reactions. A re-investigation of the reaction of chromium pentoxide etherate with tetracyclone. *J. Chem. Soc., Chem. Commun.* p. 1407.
102. Chan, H. W.-S. (1971). Singlet oxygen analogs in biological systems. Coupled oxygenation of 1,3-dienes by soybean lipoxidase. *J. Am. Chem. Soc.* **93:**2357.
103. Faria Oliveira, O. M. M., Sanioto, D. L., and Cilento, G. (1974). Singlet oxygen generation by the lipoxidase system. *Biochem. Biophys. Res. Commun.* **58:**391.
104. Teng, J. I., and Smith, L. L. (1973). Sterol metabolism. XXIV. On the unlikely participation of singlet molecular oxygen in several enzyme oxygenations. *J. Am. Chem. Soc.* **95:**4060.
105. Rahimtula, A., and O'Brien, P. J. (1976). The possible involvement of singlet oxygen in prostaglandin biosynthesis. *Biochem. Biophys. Res. Commun.* **70:**893.
106. Paine, A. J. (1976). Induction of benzo[a]pyrene monooxygenase in liver cell culture by the photochemical generation of active oxygen species. *Biochem. J.* **158:**109.
107. King, M. M., Lai, E. K., and McCay, P. B. (1975). Singlet oxygen production associated with enzyme-catalyzed lipid peroxidation in liver microsomes. *J. Biol. Chem.* **250:**6496.
108. Allen, R. C., Sternholm, R. L., and Steele, R. H. (1972). Evidence for the generation of an electronic excitation state(s) in human polymorphonuclear leukocytes and its participation in bactericidal activity. *Biochem. Biophys. Res. Commun.* **47:**679.
109. Allen, R. C., Yevich, S. Y., Orth, R. W., and Steele, R. H. (1974). The superoxide anion and singlet molecular oxygen: Their role in the microbicidal activity of the polymorphonuclear leukocyte. *Biochem. Biophys. Res. Commun.* **60:**909.
110. Maugh, T. H. (1973). Singlet oxygen: A unique microbicidal agent in cells. *Science* **182:**44.
111. Krinsky, N. (1974). Singlet excited oxygen as a mediator of the antibacterial action of leukocytes. *Science* **186:**363.
112. Klebanoff, S. J. (1975). Antimicrobial systems of the polymorphonuclear leukocyte. *In* "The Phagocytic Cell in Host Resistance" (J. A. Bellanti and D. H. Dayton, eds.), p. 45. Raven, New York.
113. Rosen, H., and Klebanoff, S. J. (1976). Chemiluminescence and superoxide production by myeloperoxidase-deficient leukocytes. *J. Clin. Invest.* **58:**50.
114. Piatt, J. F., Cheema, A. S., and O'Brien, P. J. (1977). Peroxidase catalyzed singlet oxygen formation from hydrogen peroxide. *FEBS Lett.* **74:**251.
115. Klebanoff, S. J. (1975). Antimicrobial mechanisms in neutrophilic polymorphonuclear leukocytes. *Semin. Hematol.* **12:**117.
116. Sagone, A. L., Jr., King, G. W., and Metz, E. N. (1976). A comparison of the metabolic response to phatocytosis in human granulocytes and monocytes. *J. Clin. Invest.* **57:**1352.
117. Yost, F. J., Jr., and Fridovich, I. (1974). Superoxide radicals and phagocytosis. *Arch. Biochem. Biophys.* **161:**395.

118. Harrison, J. E., Watson, B. D., and Schultz, J. (1978). Myeloperoxidase and singlet oxygen: A reappraisal. *FEBS Lett.* **92**:327.
119. Held, A. M., and Hurst, J. K. (1978). Ambiguity associated with use of singlet oxygen trapping agents in myeloperoxidase-catalyzed oxidations. *Biochem. Biophys. Res. Commun.* **81**:878.
120. Foote, C. S., Abakerli, R. B., Clough, R. L., and Lehrer, R. I. (1980). On the question of singlet oxygen production in polymorphonuclear leucocytes. *In* "Bioluminescence and Chemiluminescence" (M. A. DeLuca and W. D. McElroy, eds.) p. 81. Academic Press, New York.
121. Abakerli, R. B., Foote, C. S., Stevens, and Autor, A. P. (1982). In preparation.

DISCUSSION

DEL MAESTRO: Is singlet oxygen a radical since it has a single electron in its outermost orbital?

FOOTE: The question is largely semantic. Its reactivity is different from that of most radicals, and we do not usually refer to it as a radical. A radical is normally defined as having a single unpaired electron ("doublet"). Oxygen is a complex case: The spins of the two electrons are either parallel (triplet state, ↑↑) or antiparallel (singlet state, ↑↓); in each case, the spins interact. The singlet does not have radical-like reactivity.

McGINNESS: The definition of a radical used in organic chemistry does not make sense to physicists. Would you explain why the angular momentum (spin–orbit coupling) is ignored? Would you also outline the role of hyperfine interactions and the apparent restriction of the G value to nearly 2 in the spectra obtained from electron spin resonance analysis?

FOOTE: The definition of "radical" is perhaps most simple if it is limited to "doublets," i.e., those species with a single unpaired electron. In organic systems, such species have a G value of nearly 2. Hyperfine interactions and angular momentum usually have only small effects on reactions of such species (except *between* radicals or in a magnetic field). Compounds with more than a single unpaired spin may or may not behave like simple free radicals since the spins may interact strongly (e.g., carbenes, triplet molecules).

ŌYANAGUI: Is there a possibility that β-carotene acts as a singlet-oxygen-producing agent at some specific concentration?

FOOTE: There is evidence that it can in polar systems. This does not happen in nonpolar solvents, where carotene is soluble.

FRIDOVICH: When methionine is oxidized by singlet oxygen, what happens to the other oxygen atom?

FOOTE: Two molecules of R_2S are oxidized. Apparently, there is a reactive intermediate formed which can be trapped:

$$R_2S + {}^1O_2 \longrightarrow R_2\overset{+}{S}OO^- \xrightarrow{R_2'S} R_2\overset{+}{S}-O^- + R_2'\overset{+}{S}-O^-$$

$$\downarrow R_2S \quad \text{(trap)}$$

$$2\,R_2\overset{+}{S}-O^-$$

PIETTE: Do you think that singlet oxygen is important as a toxic agent in biological systems? Most data to date seem to indicate that singlet oxygen is not present in biological systems.

FOOTE: I would like to know the answer to this question. I believe that in some instances of photodynamic damage the answer is yes. I am uncertain about most of the thermal and enzymatic systems.

BUETTNER: We have recently seen that protoporphyrin produces O_2^- and $HO\cdot$ as well as ${}^1O_2$ upon illumination. Could β-carotene also be an effective quencher of the excited state of protoporphyrin?

FOOTE: Yes, it does quench triplets, but a higher concentration is required. By the way, the nitroxide spin trap used to detect O_2^- and $HO\cdot$ also quenches ${}^1O_2$. It is possible that an oxidized intermediate could give both spin adducts:

MICHELSON: Are any enzymatic reactions known that unequivocally produce singlet oxygen?

FOOTE: Many have been suggested, but the evidence does not impress me as being unequivocal.

SCHMIDT: What is the mechanism of action for the photosensitivity caused by semisynthetic tetracycline and other antibiotics?

FOOTE: As I recall, this is probably a type I photooxidation, although some drugs are capable of type II chemistry.

SCHMIDT: What is the protective effect of the retinols (retinions, retinoic acid) on cell membranes? Is it related to oxygen toxicity?

FOOTE: It is probably not singlet oxygen quenching. It could involve a radical inhibitor, but I'm not sure.

PROCTOR: Retinoids appear to be weak photosensitizers. Do you have any comments on this?

FOOTE: This is suggested to be important in some eye diseases (e.g., retinitis pigmentosa).

PROCTOR: Do you think that melanins may act as quenchers of singlet oxygen?

FOOTE: This is a very complex system since melanins also react with excited molecules and radicals. They should be excellent electron transfer catalysts and "sinks" for electronic excitation. Eumelanins (from redheaded individuals) have been suggested to act as photosensitizers; this action may account for the sun sensitivity of redheads.

COHEN: Do you think that you may be underestimating singlet oxygen production by phagocytes because your detector is already present in a vacuole, whereas the entire outer membrane of the phagocyte is active? Under these conditions, you may be measuring only 1% or less of singlet oxygen, compared to 100% of the O_2 consumption.

FOOTE: Possibly. We are now looking at material formed both intra- and extracellularly, and this should answer the question.

Chapter 3

The Role of Active Oxygen in Microbial Killing by Phagocytes

BERNARD M. BABIOR

INTRODUCTION

Phagocytes (neutrophils, eosinophils, and mononuclear phagocytes) are important participants in the defense of the host against invading pathogens. Their role is to kill the invading organisms, a task they accomplish by establishing close contact with the organisms and then attacking them with a battery of highly noxious chemical agents. Among these agents is a group of reactive oxidants generated by the partial reduction of oxygen. What these oxidants are, how they are made, and how they are used to kill invading organisms are the subjects of this chapter. The neutrophil is used here as the representative phagocyte, although all classes of phagocytes have been shown to produce these oxidizing agents under appropriate circumstances (1–3).

INTERACTION BETWEEN NEUTROPHILS AND THEIR TARGETS

The interaction between neutrophils and invading microorganisms can be broken down into three sequential stages: approach, contact, and de-

PATHOLOGY OF OXYGEN

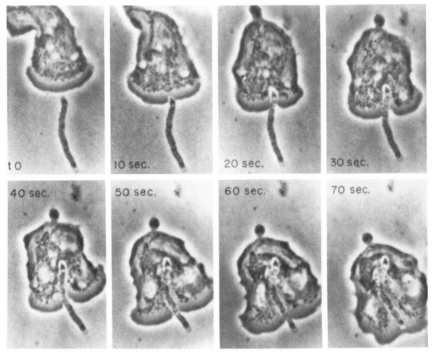

Fig. 1.   Phagocytosis. From Hirsch (4).

struction (1). *Approach* occurs by a process termed chemotaxis, in which the neutrophil "senses" the concentration gradient of diffusible substances released in the vicinity of the invading organism and migrates toward their source. On reaching the invader, which by this time has become coated with serum-derived proteins (opsonins) that identify it as a target, the neutrophil establishes intimate *contact*, either by engulfing the organism through phagocytosis (Fig. 1) (4) or, if it is large, by spreading onto its surface. Two mechanisms designed to *destroy* the microorganism then begin operation. One involves the fusion of lysosomes with the region of plasma membrane in contact with the target (Fig. 2), a process that results in the discharge of the lysosomal contents onto the surface of the invading organism (5). This process is termed degranulation. The other process is the manufacture of cytotoxic oxidants by the neutrophil.

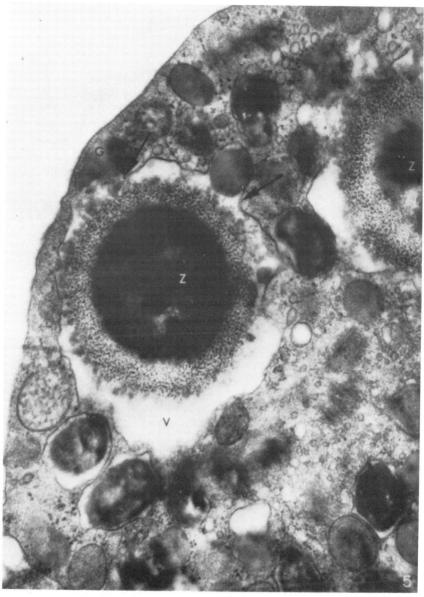

Fig. 2. Degranulation. G, granules; Z, zymosan; V, vesicle. The arrows indicate the vesicular membrane. From Zucker-Franklin and Hirsch (5).

PRODUCTION OF OXIDANTS BY THE
NEUTROPHIL: THE RESPIRATORY BURST

The resting neutrophil is a cell that consumes very little oxygen, relying mainly on glycolysis for energy production (6). On exposure to the appropriate stimuli, however, the cell undergoes a remarkable change in its oxygen metabolism. Oxygen uptake is greatly increased (7), exceeding the resting value by as much as 50-fold under favorable circumstances. Concomitantly, there is an abrupt surge of O_2^- (8) and H_2O_2 (9) production, and glucose consumption via the hexose monophosphate shunt rises sharply. These events and the underlying alterations in neutrophil metabolism are known collectively as the "respiratory burst" (7). It is during the respiratory burst that the oxidants used for the killing of pathogens are produced.

The respiratory burst in whole neutrophils is a transient event the time course of which is characterized by an initial lag of about 1 min between the exposure to the stimulus and the onset of the burst (10,11) and a late decline, during which burst activity falls to nearly resting levels (Fig. 3) (8,12). The initial lag suggests that activation must be a complex process requiring many steps, but beyond this very little is known. It has been

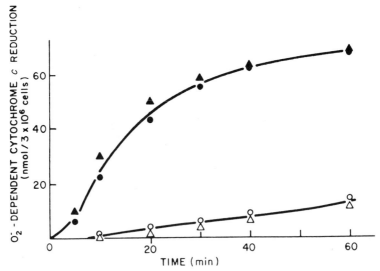

Fig. 3. Production of O_2^- by resting (open symbols) and stimulated (closed symbols) neutrophils as a function of time. The early lag and late decline are evident in the curve obtained with stimulated cells. From Curnutte and Babior (8).

shown that activation is independent of phagocytosis and degranulation (13,14), that it is reversible (14), and that it requires energy (11). A newly described membrane-bound cytochrome may or may not participate in this process (15). These sketchy conclusions represent the sum of current knowledge regarding the activation process. It is evident that the surface of this fascinating problem has barely been scratched.

More is known about the late decline in burst activity (14). A recent study has suggested that this decline results from the destruction of the plasma-membrane-bound enzyme responsible for the burst (see below). Destruction occurs by two mechanisms: oxidative inactivation by the products of the respiratory burst and inactivation by an oxygen-independent mechanism after internalization by phagocytosis.

The respiratory burst obviously does not occur under conditions of strict anerobiosis. It has been shown, however, that a vigorous burst takes place at surprisingly low oxygen tensions (16). Figure 4 shows that O_2^- production by stimulated neutrophils in 1% oxygen is nearly 70% that in room air. A reduction in the oxygen concentration to 0.35% is required before the rate of O_2^- production declines to half that occurring in room air. It is clear, then, that neutrophils can use oxidizing agents to destroy pathogens under very hypoxic conditions.

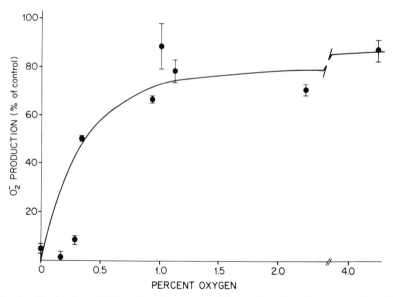

Fig. 4. Production of O_2^- by stimulated neutrophils as a function of oxygen tension. Control refers to the value obtained in room air.

BIOCHEMICAL BASIS FOR THE
RESPIRATORY BURST

The respiratory burst results from the activation of a flavoprotein oxidase, dormant in resting cells, which catalyzes the reduction of oxygen to O_2^- at the expense of a reduced pyridine nucleotide (17–19):

$$2O_2 + NAD(P)H \rightarrow 2O_2^- + NAD(P)^+ + H^+$$

NADPH is the favored substrate, showing a high affinity for the oxidase (K_m of 33 μM), but NADH (K_m of 0.4 mM) is also a substrate and could conceivably be of importance *in vivo* under certain circumstances.

As mentioned above, the oxidase is located in the plasma membrane of the neutrophil (20–23). Teleologically, this location is very reasonable since the lining of a phagocytic vesicle containing an ingested microorganism is composed largely of what was formerly the plasma membrane, and the presence of the oxidase in this membrane ensures that the lethal oxidizing agents are generated as close as possible to the target.

The action of the oxidase thus accounts for the uptake of oxygen and the liberation of O_2^- by activated neutrophils. The other manifestations of the respiratory burst are consequences of these events. Hydrogen peroxide is formed by the dismutation of the O_2^- generated during the burst (24):

$$2O_2^- + 2H^+ \rightarrow H_2O_2 + O_2$$

Part of this H_2O_2 appears in the phagocytic vesicle, where it is used in the killing of bacteria. Another portion is released from the cell and appears in the medium. The remainder diffuses back into the cytoplasm, where it is destroyed by a glutathione-dependent detoxifying system according to the following scheme (25):

$$2GSH + H_2O_2 \xrightarrow{\text{glutathione peroxidase}} GSSG + 2H_2O$$

$$GSSG + NADPH \xrightarrow{\text{glutathione reductase}} 2GSH + NADP$$

The NADP produced in this reaction is rereduced to NADPH by the first two reactions of the hexose monophosphate shunt:

Glucose 6-phosphate + NADP → 6-phosphogluconate + NADPH
6-Phosphogluconate + NADP → ribulose 5-phosphate + NADPH + CO_2

Part of the increase in hexose monophosphate shunt activity during the respiratory burst is therefore a result of the activity of the glutathione-dependent H_2O_2-detoxifying system. The rest of this increase, of course, is due to the activity of the oxidase itself, which produces NADP when it reduces oxygen to O_2^-.

OXYGEN-DEPENDENT
BACTERICIDAL MECHANISMS

There appear to be two microbicidal mechanisms that employ the agents produced in the respiratory burst: the halide–peroxide–myeloperoxidase mechanism and a mechanism based on the production of highly reactive oxidizing radicals from O_2^- and various peroxides. These two mechanisms may be interconnected.

Of these two mechanisms, the first to be discovered was the myeloperoxidase mechanism (26). Myeloperoxidase, a heme enzyme of MW 150,000 (27), is present in large quantities in the azurophil granules (28), one of two classes of lysosomes present in neutrophils, and is delivered into the phagocytic vesicle during degranulation. The phagocytic vesicle also contains H_2O_2, produced during the respiratory burst, and this oxidant plus myeloperoxidase, in the presence of a halide ion [probably Cl^-, which is present in neutrophils at a concentration of about 90 mM (29)], constitutes an exceedingly potent microbicidal system.

Current studies leave little doubt as to the importance of the myeloperoxidase-dependent system in neutrophil physiology. Less certain is the mechanism by which this system destroys bacteria. Halogenation of macromolecular constituents of the microorganism (29,30) and oxidation of its amino acids (31) have both been proposed as microbicidal mechanisms, but it has also been shown that bacteria are efficiently killed by myeloperoxidase when both of these processes are blocked (32). The production of singlet oxygen by the myeloperoxidase system has also been postulated as the basis for its bactericidal action, but the evidence for this proposal is ambiguous and difficult to interpret (1,33). It is probably fair to say that, at present, the mechanism of bacterial killing by the myeloperoxidase system is not understood.

The existence of the other oxygen-requiring bactericidal mechanism, which appears to use highly reactive oxidizing radicals, was proposed as soon as it became apparent that O_2^- was a product of the respiratory burst. In its initial version, this mechanism was postulated to involve the reaction of O_2^- with H_2O_2 to yield hydroxyl radical (the Haber–Weiss reaction) (34):

$$O_2^- + H_2O_2 \rightarrow HO^{\cdot} + O_2 + OH^-$$

The hydroxyl radical, an exceedingly reactive species that oxidizes virtually any organic compound it comes into contact with, was proposed to serve as the proximate killing agent. Evidence supporting this hypothesis appeared rapidly. Studies of O_2^--generating systems, including human neutrophils, revealed that these systems killed bacteria and that bacterial killing could be prevented by either superoxide dismutase or catalase (35–38) (it should be recalled that H_2O_2 accumulates rapidly in any O_2^--forming system because of the exceedingly facile spontaneous dismutation of O_2^- to H_2O_2 and oxygen). This finding shows that the bactericidal agent is produced in a reaction (or series of reactions) in which O_2^- and H_2O_2 both participate as substrates. At the same time, direct evidence that neutrophils manufacture HO˙ (or oxidants of similar reactivity) was obtained by the use of trapping agents (39,40). It is now well established that oxidizing radicals participate in bacterial killing by neutrophils.

As the evidence concerning oxidizing radicals emerged, two areas of confusion developed. One dealt with the identity of the oxidizing species and the other with the reaction responsible for its (their) production. With regard to the second point, many expressed concern as to whether the Haber–Weiss reaction could be the source of the HO˙ produced by neutrophils, since it had been convincingly demonstrated that, *in pure water,* this reaction is exceedingly slow (41). In reply, the defenders of the proposal made the reasonable point that biological systems are not composed of pure water, and recent experiments have shown that HO˙ is efficiently produced by an *iron-catalyzed* Haber–Weiss reaction (42,43). Since it is likely that the neutrophil contains some iron, it would seem that in this cell the Haber–Weiss reaction could serve in principle as a source of HO˙.

However, is HO˙ the only reactive oxidizing radical made by the neutrophil? Although no direct evidence on this point is available, it seems *a priori* to be quite unlikely. First, the trapping agents used to demonstrate oxidizing radical production are not specific for HO˙ but react with alkoxy, alkyl, and acyl radicals as well (44). Second, alkyl hydroperoxides, which react rapidly with O_2^- to generate alkyl radicals (45),

$$O_2^- + ROOH \rightarrow RO˙ + O_2 + OH^-$$

are produced by the oxidation of polyunsaturated fatty acids in neutrophils undergoing the respiratory burst, so that a potential source of alkoxyl radicals is present in activated neutrophils (46,47). Third, alkyl radicals may arise via secondary reactions involving HO˙ (or RO˙) and hydrocarbon residues. Oxidizing radical production in neutrophils is therefore likely to be a highly complex process the details of which will require many years to work out.

A TWO-EDGED SWORD

The inflammatory process, designed to dispose of invading pathogens, inflicts damage on host tissues as well. Tissue damage results largely from the action of destructive agents released by phagocytes into the surrounding environment (48). These agents include the products of the respiratory burst, and a number of studies have suggested that at least a portion of the damage occurring at inflammatory sites is likely to be caused by these oxidants. It has been shown, for example, that the killing of tumor cells by macrophages exposed to opsonized zymosan, a particulate stimulus that activates the respiratory burst, is mediated by the myeloperoxidase-dependent microbicidal system (49). Similarly, endothelial cells are injured by stimulated neutrophils, injury in this case resulting from the action of oxidizing radicals released from the phagocytes (50). Neutrophils themselves have been shown to be damaged by the products of their own respiratory burst (51). From these observations, it is reasonable to propose that oxygen radicals are most likely responsible for much of the injury that takes place in regions of inflammation.

There is a corollary to this proposal that may be of therapeutic significance: Agents that can destroy the oxidants liberated from neutrophils into surrounding tissues may be able to restrict tissue injury in the neighborhood of an inflammatory process without impairing the ability of the neutrophil to destroy ingested microorganisms. A number of these agents are under active investigation, and it is to be hoped that one or more of them will prove useful in this capacity.

ACKNOWLEDGMENT

Work by the author cited here was supported in part by Grant AM-11827 from the National Institutes of Health.

REFERENCES

1. Babior, B. M. (1978). Oxygen-dependent microbial killing by phagocytes. *N. Engl. J. Med.* **298**:659.
2. Sagone, A. L. Jr., King, G. W., and Metz, E. N. (1976). A comparison of the metabolic response to phagocytosis in human granulocytes and monocytes. *J. Clin. Invest.* **57**:1352.
3. DeChatelet, L. R., Shirley, P. S., McPhail, L. D., Huntley, C. C., Muss, H. B., and Bass, D. A. (1977). Oxidative metabolism of the human eosinophil. *Blood* **50**:525.
4. Hirsch, J. G. (1962). Cinemicrophotographic observations on granule lysis in polymorphonuclear leucocytes during phagocytosis. *J. Exp. Med.* **116**:827.
5. Zucker-Franklin, D., and Hirsch, J. G. (1964). Electron microscope studies on the degranulation of rabbit peritoneal leukocytes during phagocytosis. *J. Exp. Med.* **120**:569.
6. Karnovsky, M. L. (1968). The metabolism of leukocytes. *Semin. Hematol.* **5**:156.
7. Sbarra, A. J., and Karnovsky, M. L. (1959). The biochemical basis of phagocytosis. I.

Metabolic changes during the ingestion of particles by polymorphonuclear leukocytes. *J. Biol. Chem.* **234:**1355.

8. Curnutte, J. T., and Babior, B. M. (1974). Biological defense mechanisms. The effect of bacteria and serum on superoxide production by granulocytes. *J. Clin. Invest.* **53:**1662.

9. Iyer, G. Y., Islam, M. F., and Quastel, J. H. (1961). Biochemical aspects of phagocytosis. *Nature (London)* **192:**535.

10. Root, R. K., Metcalf, J., Oshino, N., and Chance, B. (1975). H_2O_2 release from human granulocytes during phagocytosis. *J. Clin. Invest.* **55:**945.

11. Cohen, H. J., and Chovaniec, M. E. (1978). Superoxide generation by digitonin-stimulated guinea pig granulocytes. *J. Clin. Invest.* **61:**1081.

12. Jandl, R. C., André-Schwartz, J., Borges-DuBois, L., Kipnes, R. S., McMurrich, B. J., and Babior, B. M. (1978). Termination of the respiratory burst in human neutrophils. *J. Clin. Invest.* **61:**1176.

13. Goldstein, I. M., Roos, D., Kaplan, H. B., and Weissmann, G. (1975). Complement and immunoglobulins stimulate superoxide production by human leukocytes independently of phagocytosis. *J. Clin. Invest.* **56:**1155.

14. Curnutte, J. T., Babior, B. M., and Karnovsky, M. L. (1979). Fluoride-mediated activation of the respiratory burst in human neutrophils. A reversible process. *J. Clin. Invest.* **63:**637.

15. Segal, A. W., Webster, D., Jones, O. T. G., and Allison, A. C. (1978). Absence of a newly described cytochrome b from neutrophils of patients with chronic granulomatous disease. *Lancet* **2:**446.

16. Tauber, A. I., Gabig, T. G., and Babior, B. M. (1979). Evidence for production of oxidizing radicals by the particulate O_2^- forming system from human neutrophils. *Blood* **53:**666.

17. Babior, B. M., Curnutte, J. T., and McMurrich, B. J. (1976). The particulate superoxide-forming system from human neutrophils. Properties of the system and further evidence supporting its participation in the respiratory burst. *J. Clin. Invest.* **58:**989.

18. Babior, B. M., and Kipnes, R. S. (1977). Superoxide-forming enzyme from human neutrophils: evidence for a flavin requirement. *Blood* **50:**517.

19. Gabig, T. G., Kipnes, R. S., and Babior, B. M. (1978). Solubilization of the O_2^--forming activity responsible for the respiratory burst in human neutrophils. *J. Biol. Chem.* **253:**6663.

20. Briggs, R. T., Karnovsky, M. L., and Karnovsky, M. J. (1977). Hydrogen peroxide production in chronic granulomatous disease. A cytochemical study of reduced pyridine nucleotide oxidases. *J. Clin. Invest.* **59:**1088.

21. Goldstein, I. M., Cerquiera, J., Lind, S., and Kaplan, H. B. (1977). Evidence that the superoxide-generating system of human leukocytes is associated with the cell surface. *J. Clin. Invest.* **59:**249.

22. Root, R. K., and Metcalf, J. A. (1977). H_2O_2 release from human granulocytes during phagocytosis. Relationship to superoxide anion formation and cellular catabolism of H_2O_2: Studies with normal and cytochalasin B-treated cells. *J. Clin. Invest.* **60:**1266.

23. Dewald, B., Baggiolini, M., Curnutte, J. T., and Babior, B. M. (1979). Subcellular localization of the superoxide-forming enzyme in human neutrophils. *J. Clin. Invest.* **63:**21.

24. Bielski, B. H. J. (1978). Reevaluation of the spectral and kinetic properties of HO_2 and O_2^- free radicals. *Photochem. Photobiol.* **28:**645.

25. Reed, P. W. (1969). Glutathione and the hexose monophosphate shunt in phagocytizing and hydrogen peroxide-treated rat leukocytes. *J. Biol. Chem.* **244:**2459.

26. Klebanoff, S. J. (1967). Iodination of bacteria: A bactericidal mechanism. *J. Exp. Med.* **126:**1063.

27. Ehrenberg, A., and Agner, K. (1958). The molecular weight of myeloperoxidase. *Acta Chem. Scand.* **12**:95.
28. Bainton, D. F., and Farquhar, M. G. (1968). Differences in enzyme content of azurophil and specific granules of polymorphonuclear leucocytes. II. Cytochemistry and electron microscopy of bone marrow cells. *J. Cell Biol.* **39**:299.
29. Klebanoff, S. J., and Hamon, C. B. (1972). Role of myeloperoxidase-mediated antimicrobial systems in intact leukocytes. *J. Reticuloendothel. Soc.* **12**:170.
30. Zgliczynski, J. M., and Stelmaszynska, T. (1975). Chlorinating ability of human phagocytosing leukocytes. *Eur. J. Biochem.* **56**:157.
31. Strauss, R. R., Paul, B. B., Jacobs, A. A., and Sbarra, A. J. (1971). Role of the phagocyte in host-parasite interactions. XXVII. Myeloperoxidase-H_2O_2-Cl^--mediated aldehyde formation and its relationship to antimicrobial activity. *Infect. Immun.* **3**:595.
32. McCall, C. E., DeChatelet, L. R., Cooper, M. R., and Ashburn, P. (1971). The effects of ascorbic acid on bactericidal mechanisms of neutrophils. *J. Infect. Dis.* **124**:194.
33. Held, A. M., and Hurst, J. K. (1978). Ambiguity associated with use of singlet oxygen trapping agents in myeloperoxidase-catalyzed oxidations. *Biochem. Biophys. Res. Commun.* **81**:878.
34. Fridovich, I. (1974). Superoxide radical and the bactericidal action of phagocytes. *N. Engl. J. Med.* **290**:624.
35. Babior, B. M., Curnutte, J. T., and Kipnes, R. S. (1975). Biological defense mechanisms. Evidence for the participation of superoxide in bacterial killing by xanthine oxidase. *J. Lab. Clin. Med.* **85**:235.
36. Gregory, E. M., Yost, R. J., Jr., and Fridovich, I. (1973). Superoxide dismutases of Escherichia coli: Intracellular localization and functions. *J. Bacteriol.* **115**:987.
37. Johnston, R. B., Jr., Keele, B. B., Jr., Misra, H. P., Lehmeyer, J. E., Webb, L. S., Baehner, R. L., and Rajagopalan, R. V. (1975). The role of superoxide anion generation in phagocytic bactericidal activity. Studies with normal and chronic granulomatous disease leukocytes. *J. Clin. Invest.* **55**:1357.
38. Rosen, H., and Klebanoff, S. J. (1979). Bactericidal activity of a superoxide anion-generating system. A model for the polymorphonuclear leukocyte. *J. Exp. Med.* **149**:27.
39. Weiss, S. J., King, G. W., and LoBuglio, A. F. (1977). Evidence for hydroxyl radical generation by human monocytes. *J. Clin. Invest.* **60**:370.
40. Weiss, S. J., Rustagi, P. K., and LoBuglio, A. F. (1978). Human granulocyte generation of hydroxyl radical. *J. Exp. Med.* **147**:316.
41. Czapski, G., and Ilan, Y. A. (1978). On the generation of the hydroxylation agent from superoxide radical. Can the Haber-Weiss reaction be the source of ·OH radicals? *Photochem. Photobiol.* **28**:651.
42. McCord, J. M., and Day, E. D. (1978). Superoxide-dependent production of hydroxyl radical catalyzed by iron-EDTA complex. *FEBS Lett.* **86**:139.
43. Halliwell, B. (1978). Superoxide-dependent formation of hydroxyl radicals in the presence of iron chelates: Is it a mechanism for hydroxyl radical production in biochemical systems? *FEBS Lett.* **92**:321.
44. Pryor, W. A., and Tang, R. H. (1978). Ethylene formation from methional. *Biochem. Biophys. Res. Commun.* **81**:498.
45. Peters, J. W., and Foote, C. S. (1976). Chemistry of superoxide anion. II. Reaction with hydroperoxidases. *J. Am. Chem. Soc.* **98**:873.
46. Stossel, T. P., Mason, R. J., and Smith, A. L. (1974). Lipid peroxidation by human blood phagocytes. *J. Clin. Invest.* **54**:638.
47. Shohet, S. B., Pitt, J., Baehner, R. L., and Poplack, D. G. (1974). Lipid peroxidation in the killing of phagocytized pneumococci. *Infect. Immun.* **10**:1321.

48. Cochrane, C. G., and Koffler, D. (1973). Immune complex disease in experimental animals and man. *Adv. Immunol.* **16**:185.
49. Clark, R. A., and Klebanoff, S. J. (1975). Neutrophil-mediated tumor cell cytotoxicity: Role of the peroxidase system. *J. Exp. Med.* **141**:1442.
50. Sacks, R., Moldow, C. F., Craddock, P. R., Bowers, T. K., and Jacob, H. S. (1978). Oxygen radicals mediate endothelial cell damage by complement-stimulated granulocytes. An *in vitro* model of immune vascular damage. *J. Clin. Invest.* **61**:1161.
51. Salin, M. L., and McCord, J. M. (1975). Free radicals and inflammation. Protection of phagocytosing leukocytes by superoxide dismutase. *J. Clin. Invest.* **56**:1319.

DISCUSSION

FRIDOVICH: In the experiment by Johnston *et al.* [*J. Clin. Invest.* **55**:1357 (1975)], was the superoxide dismutase effective in protecting against bacterial killing by polymorphonuclear leucocytes when added to free solution, or was it necessary to use latex particles as a vehicle to carry the superoxide dismutase into the phagosome?

BABIOR: The latter.

JONES: In the studies of Johnston *et al.* that you quoted, were the catalase and bovine serum albumin preparations obtained from commercial sources? As you know, such commercial preparations contain superoxide dismutase.

BABIOR: The catalase, at least, was free of superoxide dismutase.

CUTLER: What happens to the intracellular level of superoxide dismutase after the neutrophils are stimulated to produce O_2^-? Is it increased to further protect the cell?

BABIOR: The work of McCord and Day [*FEBS Lett.* **86**:139 (1978)] has shown that there is no change.

SHEREMATA: In human chronic granulomatous disease, is the production of superoxide by macrophages normal?

BABIOR: Superoxide production by monocytes is probably absent in chronic granulomatous disease.

PIETTE: Did Dr. Johnston add iron to his methional reaction system? The generation of $HO^.$ is dependent on iron. It is not produced to any significant level with O_2^- and H_2O_2 alone.

BABIOR: No iron was added, but there was undoubtedly an adequate iron content in the cells.

MICHELSON: Your results indicate the production of 5×10^6 molecules of O_2^- per cell per second by activated neutrophils, but only 10^4 molecules of ethylene (as a reflection of HO·) in the presence of methional. That would be a yield of 0.2%. Would you comment on this?

BABIOR: Because of competing HO·-consuming reactions, it is not possible to estimate the stoichiometry of HO· generation from the rate of ethylene production.

FRIDOVICH: Was the methional level saturating with respect to ethylene production?

BABIOR: No, but it was not possible to increase the concentration because of potential damage to the cells.

BUETTNER: Can you estimate the amount of methional that would be present in the cell?

BABIOR: No.

DEMOPOULOS: Do lymphocytes under any conditions produce O_2^- radicals?

BABIOR: Not to my knowledge, but the possibility has not been fully tested.

MICHELSON: Human lymphocytes produce O_2^- when activated by phytohemagglutinin or by a serum elastogenic factor present in blood of patients with certain autoimmune diseases, such as lupus erythematosus, but very much less than that produced by activated polymorphonuclear leukocytes.

SHEREMATA: I would also like to comment on the superoxide anion production by lymphocytes. There are a significant number of lymphocyte subpopulations. A proportion of these cells bear myeloid membrane antigens and have some morphological characteristics resembling the "polymorphonuclear" series (Perleman *et al.*). The function of these cells is not clear, but they may act as "helper cells." Therefore, one should be cautious about ruling out a role for superoxide in lymphocyte function. It is also important that immunologically activated lymphocytes produce migration inhibitory factor, which induces macrophage activity, thereby introducing O_2^- as a tissue-destructive factor.

ŌYANAGUI: Have you examined the effects of various buffers on the stimulation of O_2^- production by neutrophils? I have observed an acceleration of O_2^- production by macrophages when tested in phosphate buffer.

BABIOR: We also noticed some stimulatory effect of our neutrophil preparations by phosphate buffer, but it was rather small. The only ion essential for O_2^- production was Ca^{2+}.

PETKAU: Does the time course of ethylene production closely match the respiratory burst?

BABIOR: It does not when methional is the reactant. This is possibly because of contaminants in the reagent.

McLENNAN:: Was there any effect on the resting and "activated" production of superoxide radical by the neutrophil plasma membrane when tested at oxygen concentrations of less than 20%?

BABIOR: No; O_2^- production was the same as in room air.

ŌYANAGUI: Are you using only the ferricytochrome c method for the detection of superoxide anion?

BABIOR: Yes.

ŌYANAGUI: Which reaction do you think kills the bacteria: the superoxide-oxidizing capacity or the superoxide-reducing capacity?

BABIOR: Superoxide itself, in my opinion, is not toxic. It serves as the source of H_2O_2 and hydroxyl radical (HO·), which are the real toxic agents.

Chapter *4*

The Stimulated Granulocyte as a Source of Toxic Oxygen Compounds in Tissue Injury

DALE E. HAMMERSCHMIDT AND HARRY S. JACOB

INTRODUCTION

The granulocyte is crucially important in host defenses against bacterial infections, a fact underscored by the striking incidence of infection in patients rendered neutropenic by disease or chemotherapy. The granulocyte carries out its protective function by engulfing opsonized microorganisms and destroying them. In order to accomplish this, it must first respond to a chemotactic stimulus, following a gradient to reach the site of infection. It then must recognize the invading organism and engulf it. Finally, it destroys the foreign organism by discharging toxic oxygen compounds and proteolytic enzymes into the phagocytic vacuole containing the organism.

The generation of toxic oxygen compounds is very important for the destruction of microbial invaders by granulocytes (1–5). Patients with defective oxidant-generating systems in their granulocytes, such as those with chronic granulomatous disease of childhood, have a great deal of difficulty with infections involving catalase-producing microorganisms (6).

Although the toxic oxygen compounds and proteolytic enzymes produced by the granulocyte may be highly effective in protecting the host

59

PATHOLOGY OF OXYGEN
Copyright © 1982 by Academic Press, Inc.

from bacterial invasion, these products are also capable of harming the tissues of the host, as first proposed by Metchnikoff almost a century ago (6–8). The most familiar example of this phenomenon is the "frustrated phagocytosis" model of immune tissue injury proposed by Hensen (9). In this circumstance, antibodies may be directed against a host tissue, or immune complexes containing other antigens may be deposited on a host tissue, including, for example, the glomerular basement membrane or the synovium in immune glomerulonephritis or arthritis. The plasma complement system is then activated, and chemotactic and opsonic fragments (most importantly C5a and C3b, respectively) are generated. Complement-derived anaphylatoxins—C3a, C4a, C5a—also alter local vascular permeability. The granulocyte is attracted to the coated tissue by the chemotaxins. Its approach is facilitated by altered vascular permeability, and the coating of the tissue with immunoglobulin and opsonic complement fragments makes the tissue attractive to engulf. Thus, the granulocyte attacks it as though it were an invading microbe. The granulocyte fails in this attempt since it is smaller than the tissue. The cell cannot form a phagosome around the tissue, and therefore the microbicidal products are discharged into an incompletely formed phagosome. The predictable result is that the toxic compounds gain access to the surrounding milieu, and tissue damage can result. This damage is amplified when granulocyte products activate the kinin system (10) and generate further chemotaxins (11–13) to recruit still more polymorphonuclear leukocytes (PMNs) to the scene.

INTRAVASCULAR PMN BEHAVIOR

In addition to this familiar model, evidence has accumulated that the *intravascular* behavior of the stimulated granulocyte may also be important in immune tissue injury. Briefly stated, the stimulated granulocyte has been shown to share with platelets the capacity to aggregate in response to a variety of stimuli and to damage endothelium, as well as basement membrane, by the release of toxic oxygen species (14).

Our interest in this problem dates back to the early 1960s, when neutropenia was noted in experimental animals undergoing hemodialysis. This was reported in human beings in 1968, at which time it was noted that the neutropenia was very sudden both in development and in resolution (15) (Fig. 1). It was initially thought that the granulocytes were sequestered in the dialyzer and then released, but this hypothesis became untenable when it was shown that plasma incubated in a dialyzer acquired the

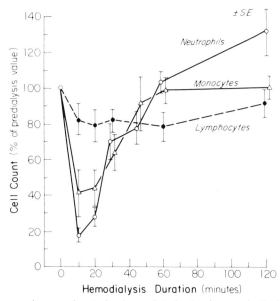

Fig. 1. Neutropenia occurring during hemodialysis. Our interest in the intravascular behavior of the stimulated granulocyte was spurred by the observation that transient and profound neutropenia occurred within the first half-hour in virtually all patients undergoing hemodialysis using cellophane membrane apparatus. As can be seen here, the neutropenia reversed and a rebound neutrophilia occurred within 2 hr. The monocyte count also fell, but lymphocytes and platelets remained approximately at predialysis levels. From Craddock *et al.* (17), with permission.

capacity to induce neutropenia (16). In a series of experiments, Dr. Craddock and Dr. Fehr of our section demonstrated that hemodialysis neutropenia was dependent on complement activation, which occurred via the alternative pathway when plasma contacted the cellophane membrane of the dialyzer; furthermore, neutropenia was reliably, and seemingly causally, associated with mild pulmonary dysfunction. In experimental animals, the pulmonary dysfunction was associated with histological evidence of microvascular leukostasis (Fig. 2), as well as perivascular edema and increased pulmonary lymph flow and lymph protein concentration. It seemed, therefore, that granulocytes were causing vascular injury, which was resulting in microvascular leakage of protein-rich fluid (17,18).

A mechanism for such pulmonary microvascular injury was suggested by other workers in our department. Dr. Sacks and Dr. Moldow grew human umbilical vein endothelial cells in tissue culture, labeled them with radioactive chromium, and subjected them to a variety of insults, measuring chromium release as an index of cytotoxicity (Fig. 3). When granulo-

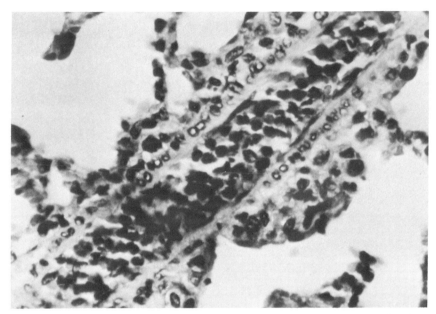

Fig. 2. Leukostasis in the lung during sham hemodialysis. When plasma that had been incubated with dialyzer cellophane was infused into experimental animals intravenously, leukostasis in small pulmonary vessels was prominent. This correlated with mild but readily demonstrable pulmonary dysfunction and with a rise in pulmonary lymph flow. The latter two events did not occur in animals that had been rendered granulocytopenic and in which leukostasis had thus been prevented. A probable cause-and-effect relationship was inferred; further studies indicated that leukostasis resulted from complement activation, which occurred when plasma contacted the cellophane membrane of the dialyzer. From Craddock *et al.* (17), with permission.

cytes were added to the incubation and were stimulated by endotoxin, the release of radiochromium increased, implying cell damage. When a source of activable complement was added to the incubation, this damage was markedly enhanced. The presence of superoxide dismutase and catalase in the incubation markedly inhibited the cytotoxicity, suggesting that it was mediated in large measure by the generation of toxic oxygen compounds (19). Harlan and co-workers (20) have shown, in addition, that the release of proteolytic enzymes from stimulated granulocytes may cause delamination of endothelial cells from their substratum, providing another mechanism for granulocyte-mediated microvascular injury. More recently, Weiss and co-workers (21) have shown that, when granulocytes are stimulated potently and for a long time, more extensive cytotoxicity results.

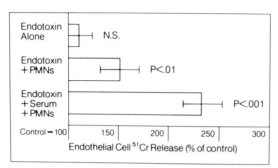

Fig. 3. Endothelial damage wrought by stimulated granulocytes. When cultured human endothelial cells were exposed to endotoxin (top bar), there was no increase in radiochromium release over that in control incubations (contrary to the conventional belief that endotoxin is bad for endothelium). The addition of granulocytes, which are known to be stimulated by endotoxin, to the incubation, however, resulted in a modest but highly statistically significant increase in radiochromium release, implying endothelial cell damage (middle bar). The addition of a source of activatable complement to the incubation markedly augmented radiochromium release (lower bar). The addition of platelets to the system caused a further enhancement of radiochromium release (not shown). The damage shown here was largely inhibited in the presence of superoxide dismutase and catalase, suggesting that it was inflicted in large measure by the generation of toxic oxygen compounds by the stimulated granulocytes.

In addition to the mechanism whereby granulocytes effect microvascular injury, our group was interested in what caused them to migrate to the pulmonary microvasculature in the first place. Investigating this question, Dr. Craddock and Dr. Hammerschmidt made the rather unexpected observation that granulocytes aggregate when stimulated and therefore have the potential to embolize to microvascular sites as clumps (22). Thus, when activated plasma complement is added to a stirred suspension of granulocytes in an aggregometer, there is an increasing wave of light transmission, which is reminiscent of a platelet aggregation wave and which can be documented microscopically to represent aggregation (Fig. 4). Furthermore, the possibility of this phenomenon occurring *in vivo* has been documented by intravital microscopy of capillary beds in experimental animals harboring fluorescent granulocytes and given infusions of activated complement (23).

This series of observations led us to conclude not only that the stimulated granulocyte is capable of doing damage in an inflammatory exudate, but also that its behavior is altered markedly when it is stimulated in the vascular space, and this altered behavior may have pathophysiological consequences.

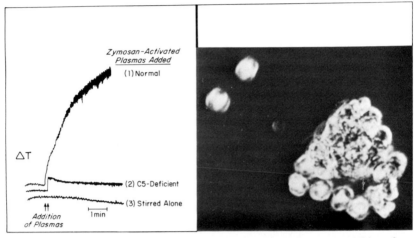

Fig. 4. Granulocytes aggregate in response to the addition of C5a. The addition of complement-activated plasma to a stirred suspension of granulocytes in an aggregometer results in an increasing wave of light transmission reminiscent of a platelet aggregation wave (left panel). That this indeed reflects aggregation can be demonstrated by examining via phase microscopy samples fixed during the peak of the wave; most of the granulocytes are then seen to be present in clumps rather than dispersed as singlets (right panel). The aggregating activity was shown to be complement dependent and the agent responsible to be of molecular weight and antigenic composition consistent with C5a or its desarginine derivative. Further evidence for the identity of the aggregant is the inability to generate aggregating activity in C5-deficient plasma when activated with cellophane or zymosan (left panel). From Greenberg *et al.* (23a), with permission.

INTRAVASCULAR GRANULOCYTE BEHAVIOR
IN THE ADULT RESPIRATORY
DISTRESS SYNDROME

Several clinical and pathological correlates suggested that the phenomena we were studying might play a role in the adult respiratory distress syndrome (ARDS), or "shock lung." First, the type of leukostasis that we observed in sham-dialyzed animals and in animals receiving infusions of activated complement is a prominent histological finding in the lungs of animals in shock or in the lungs of animals or patients early in the transition from shock to shock lung (24). Second, the clinical syndrome of shock lung most commonly occurs in situations involving activation of the complement system; these include most prominently sepsis, trauma, and acute pancreatitis (25). Third, in some experimental models, granulocyte or complement depletion leads to protection against the pulmonary manifestations of shock or the ultimate development of a syndrome similar to shock lung (26,27). We postulated, therefore, that the complement-stimulated granulocyte might play a role in triggering or amplifying pulmonary vascular damage in ARDS and sought evidence of this in patients with ARDS.

In a pilot study, a high proportion of patients with the clinical diagnosis of ARDS were found to have granulocyte-aggregating activity in their plasmas. When plasma from these patients was added to normal human granulocytes in an aggregometer, an aggregation wave occurred, much like that seen when activated complement was added. In fact, in these patients, the agent causing the granulocyte-aggregating activity was of molecular weight and antigenicity consistent with C5a. A prospective collaborative study was then undertaken in which the diagnostic criteria for ARDS were agreed on, the diagnosis of ARDS was made by physicians unaware of the complement studies in the patient, and the complement studies were performed by workers unaware of the clinical status of the patient. We were gratified that in these controlled studies a high and highly significant correlation was obtained between evidence of complement activation and the ultimate development of ARDS in patients at risk (28) (Table I). In some patients enough plasma samples were obtained to provide evidence that complement activation might be a useful predictor for the ultimate development of ARDS.

We continue to find attractive the hypothesis that the stimulated granulocyte may be an important effector organ in the development of ARDS. It is important, however, to note that several lines of evidence suggest a role for the platelet, the kinin system, and the coagulation system as well. It is likely that the pathophysiology of this syndrome is complex and that the stimulated granulocyte is not solely responsible for it. Our current

TABLE I

Association of Elevated Plasma C5a Levels (Presence of Granulocyte-Aggregating Activity in Plasma) with the Development of ARDS in Patients at Risk[a]

C5a level	All patients		Patients without sepsis	
	ARDS	No ARDS	ARDS	No ARDS
Elevated	31	5	18	3
Not elevated	2	23	1	23
	$\chi^2 = 36.3$		$\chi^2 = 31.9$	
	$p < .00001$		$p < .00001$	

[a] Modified from Hammerschmidt *et al.* (28), with permission.

working hypothesis is that the stimulated granulocyte causes cytotoxic damage and delamination of endothelial cells in the pulmonary microvasculature. This causes pulmonary edema; but perhaps more importantly, released granulocyte products activate the kinin and coagulation systems, and endothelial delamination allows for the deposition of platelets on the subendothelium. This process probably takes place in most patients who have a major complement-activating event. In some patients, however, the insult is prolonged or the body's defenses against the insult are imperfect; when this occurs, the damage is severe and full-blown ARDS develops.

ROLE OF THE GRANULOCYTE IN OTHER PULMONARY INJURY

Since the recognition of the predisposition to emphysema of patients lacking α1-antiprotease, the idea that emphysema may be caused by an imbalance between naturally occurring proteases and their naturally occurring inhibitors has gained popularity (29). In support of this concept, elastase is capable of inducing experimental lung injury, and one of the major physiological sources of this enzyme is the granulocyte (30). Granulocytes are recruited to the lung when tobacco is smoked, seemingly by the release of a non-complement-derived chemotaxin from alveolar macrophages (31–33). These recruited granulocytes, and the stimulated macrophages themselves (34), may then release elastase and cause tissue damage. It is becoming more widely accepted that an increase in the protease burden the lung must bear (for example, by recruiting granulocytes as just described) or a decrease in the capacity of the lung to withstand proteases (as in hereditary deficiency of any of the major protease inhibitors) leads to an imbalance which favors proteolytic damage to the lung.

In parallel with these observations, it has been noted that granulocytes recruited to the lung and stimulated by macrophage-derived chemotaxins also may produce and release toxic oxygen compounds. Studies by Fox and Repine of the Webb–Waring Institute (35,36) and others have shown that in some experimental situations the lung damage wrought by stimulated granulocytes can be inhibited by agents that detoxify oxygen compounds. It is becoming clear that protease balance is not the entire story and that toxic oxygen production is also important in granulocyte-mediated pulmonary injury. As an example, granulocyte release of toxic oxygen compounds seems important in hyperoxic lung damage; high oxygen

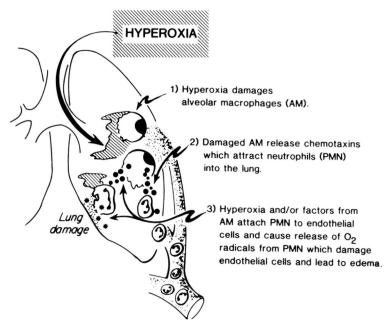

HYPEROXIA

1) Hyperoxia damages alveolar macrophages (AM).

2) Damaged AM release chemotaxins which attract neutrophils (PMN) into the lung.

3) Hyperoxia and/or factors from AM attach PMN to endothelial cells and cause release of O_2 radicals from PMN which damage endothelial cells and lead to edema.

Lung damage

Fig. 5. Schematic representation of the contribution of alveolar-macrophage-derived chemotaxin and of granulocyte toxic oxygen compounds to pulmonary injury in such states as hyperoxic lung injury. From Fox *et al.* (36a), with permission.

tensions lead to the release of macrophage-derived chemotaxins from lung tissue, recruiting granulocytes to the area and stimulating them as described above (36) (Fig. 5).

THE EOSINOPHIL: A SPECIAL CASE

The eosinophil has been reported to produce more superoxide on stimulation than does the neutrophil granulocyte (37), and it has been postulated that this enhanced production and release of superoxide is important for the damage of nonphagocytosable parasites by the cell (parasitic infestation being commonly associated with high eosinophil counts) (38). It is certainly plausible that the enhanced toxic oxygen production by the eosinophil is of clinical import in terms of damage to host as well protection against parasites. Thus, patients with prolonged extreme eosinophilia may have pulmonary infiltrates and may develop fibrosis of the endocardium. It is attractive to hypothesize that this fibrotic damage and some of the transient pulmonary findings may be the result of oxidant-mediated endothelial damage and its repair.

We have studied a number of patients with very high eosinophil counts and have prepared eosinophil-rich granulocyte preparations from patients with more modest eosinophilia due to allergy. In several such cases, a markedly augmented granulocyte aggregation response to activated complement has been seen (Fig. 6). The aggregates contain both eosinophils and neutrophils, suggesting that the presence of a large number of eosinophils may stimulate the granulocyte response to activated complement rather than indicating that eosinophils themselves merely aggregate better than granulocytes. This is supported by recent reports that superoxide may also enhance neutrophil locomotion (39). As can be imagined, the elucidation of this phenomenon is hampered by the infrequent appearance of appropriate patients for study.

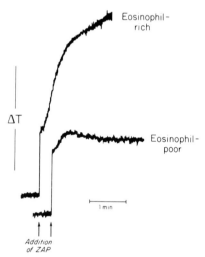

Fig. 6. Augmented granulocyte aggregation in eosinophilia. Eosinophils have been reported to produce more superoxide than do neutrophils, and superoxide has been reported to promote several granulocyte functions. In several, but not all patients studied with hypereosinophilia of diverse causes, there is a markedly augmented granulocyte aggregation response compared to that of normals. In patients with modest eosinophilia from allergy, it is possible on a density gradient to prepare an eosinophil-rich and an eosinophil-poor fraction and then compare their aggregation characteristics. The upper curve is the aggregation wave obtained in one such patient with the eosinophil-rich preparation (>70% eosinophils); it is of markedly higher amplitude and is irreversible compared with the wave of the eosinophil-poor preparation (<1% eosinophils) (lower curve). Aggregating stimulus: dilute zymosan-activated plasma complement (ZAP).

PHARMACOLOGICAL IMPLICATIONS

If the stimulated granulocyte causes tissue damage through the release of toxic oxygen compounds and proteolytic enzymes, agents that inhibit this activity should be of benefit in disease states in which the pathophysiological mechanism is operative. In ARDS, the clinical syndrome in which we are most actively interested, corticosteroids have been shown to be of benefit, but only when used very early in extremely high doses (40–42). If those who advocate the use of steroids are right, and if our hypothesis that the stimulated granulocyte is important in the genesis of ARDS is also correct, we should be able to demonstrate some specific effects of high concentrations of corticosteroids on granulocyte function. This is indeed the case. When granulocytes are exposed to an aggregating stimulus, corticosteroids inhibit the aggregation response in a dose-dependent fashion (43,44) (Fig. 7). Furthermore, in an interesting parallel to the clinical shock situation, the doses of corticosteroids required are considerably higher than conventional doses; with methylprednisolone, for example, 50% inhibition of aggregation occurs at about 0.6 mg/ml, very

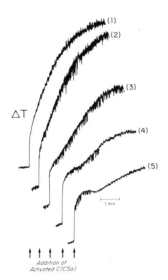

Fig. 7. Inhibition of granulocyte aggregation by corticosteroids. These granulocyte aggregation tracings were generated using a constant stimulus and a varied dose of methylprednisolone: (1) diluent alone; (2) 0.1 mg/ml methylprednisolone; (3) 0.25 mg/ml; (4) 0.5 mg/ml; (5) 1.0 mg/ml. Inhibition was not observed with modest doses but was observed with doses corresponding to the plasma levels seen in high intravenous bolus therapy as advocated in shock.

close to the expected plasma concentration shortly after a bolus dose of 30 mg/kg is given.

For a variety of reasons, high-dose corticosteroid therapy has not become routine in clinical situations, such as shock, in which it appears to be of some benefit (40–42). We have been interested in the possibility that inhibition of granulocyte function *in vitro* might be useful as an experimental model for testing drugs thought likely to be helpful in clinical situations in which activated granulocytes are having harmful effects. Thus, we have found that granulocyte aggregation is inhibited by several agents other than corticosteroids, including ibuprofen, betahistine, local anesthetics, nitroprusside, and calcium channel blockers. Furthermore, synergy exists among some of these agents in inhibiting granulocyte aggregation (45), and a lesser degree of synergy appears to be present in inhibiting toxic oxygen generation and lysosomal enzyme release by stimulated granulocytes. We have just begun to extrapolate these observations to animal models of shock and myocardial infarction, but preliminary results have been encouraging (45).

In addition to inhibiting the capacity of the granulocyte to produce and release toxic oxygen compounds, another obvious therapeutic strategem is to augment the capacity of the host to resist oxidative stress. Superoxide dismutase has had some application in veterinary practice; its short half-life limits its use, but it is possible in experimental animals to link it to Ficoll so that it can circulate for several hours. This agent might ultimately be prepared in a form that is useful in human systemic therapy. Dimethylthiourea, which has recently been used in experimental animals to block oxidative damage, shows low toxicity and considerable promise (46). Tocopherol and mannitol have been used experimentally for some time, and strategies for inducing the body's own oxidant protective enzymes are being explored. It seems reasonable to hope that, within a few years, it will be possible to combine synergistic inhibition of granulocyte function with techniques to enhance defenses against toxic oxygen compounds, such that tissue damage may be prevented very effectively with small and well-tolerated doses of several agents.

SUMMARY

The role of the stimulated granulocyte as an effector of tissue injury is becoming increasingly well recognized in a growing variety of clinical contexts. Although this has been most extensively studied in inflammatory exudates, it is becoming clear that the intravascular behavior of the granulocyte, with damage being inflicted on the microvasculature, is also important. It is also becoming apparent that much of the damage caused by stimulated granulocytes results from the production and release of toxic oxygen compounds. While these are interesting pathophysiological hypotheses for study in such syndromes as shock lung, they also open the door to exciting new possibilities in therapy, combining inhibition of granulocyte aggregation and production of toxic oxygen compounds with enhancement of host defenses against these compounds.

ACKNOWLEDGMENTS

This chapter reviews work that was done in our laboratory over several years, involving a number of researchers in addition to the authors. We would like particularly to give credit to Dr. Philip Craddock, Dr. Jorg Fehr, Dr. Timothy Bowers, Dr. Thomas Sacks, Dr. Charles Moldow, Dr. Joseph O'Flaherty, Dr. James G. White, and Dr. Agustin Dalmasso. This work has received grant support from several sources, including Variety Club of the Northwest, The Upjohn Company, and the National Institutes of Health (CA 15627, HL 19725, AM 15730, HL 25043, HL 26218).

REFERENCES

1. Babior, B. M., Kipnes, R. S., and Curnutte, J. T. (1973). Biological defense mechanisms: The production by leukocytes of superoxide, a potential bactericidal agent. *J. Clin. Invest.* **52:**741–744.
2. Babior, B. M. (1978). Oxygen-dependent microbial killing by phagocytes. *N. Engl. J. Med.* **298:**659–668.
3. Klebanoff, S. J. (1980). Oxygen metabolism and the toxic properties of phagocytes. *Ann. Intern. Med.* **93:**480–489.
4. Weiss, S. J., Rustagi, P. K., and LoBuglio, A. F. (1978). Human granulocyte generation of the hydroxyl radical. *J. Exp. Med.* **147:**316–323.
5. Weissmann, G., Smolen, J. E., and Korchak, H. M. (1980). Release of inflammatory mediators from stimulated neutrophils. *N. Engl. J. Med.* **303:**27–34.
6. Quie, P. G. (1975). Pathology of bactericidal power of neutrophils. *Semin. Haematol.* **12:**143–160.
7. Metchnikoff, E. (1887). Sur la lutte des cellules de l'organisme contre l'invasion des microbes. *Ann. Inst. Pasteur, Paris* **1:**321–336.
8. Metchnikoff, E. (1905). "Immunity in Infective Diseases." Cambridge Univ. Press, London and New York (reprinted by Johnson Reprint Corp. of New York, 1968).
9. Hensen, P. M. (1971). The immunological release of constituents from neutrophil leukocytes. *J. Immunol.* **107:**1535–1557.
10. Movat, H. Z., Habal, F. M., and MacMorine, D. R. L. (1976). Neutral proteases of human PMN leukocytes with kininogenase activity. *Int. Arch. Allergy Appl. Immunol.* **50:**257–281.
11. Ward, P. A., and Hill, J. H. (1970). C5 chemotactic fragments produced by an enzyme in lysosomal granules of neutrophils. *J. Immunol.* **104:**535–543.
12. Goldstein, I. M., and Weissman, G. (1974). Generation of C5-derived lysosomal enzyme releasing activity (C5a) by lysates of leukocyte lysosomes. *J. Immunol.* **113:**1583–1588.

13. Petrone, W. F., English, D. K., Wong, K., and McCord, J. M. (1980). Free radicals and inflammation: Superoxide-dependent activation of a neutrophil chemotactic factor in plasma. *Proc. Natl. Acad. Sci. U.S.A.* **77**:1159–1163.
14. Craddock, P. R., Hammerschmidt, D. E., Moldow, C. F., Yamada, O., and Jacob, H. S. (1979). Granulocyte aggregation as a manifestation of membrane interactions with complement: Possible role in leukocyte margination, microvascular occlusion and endothelial damage. *Semin. Haematol.* **16**:140–147.
15. Kaplow, L. S., and Goffinet, J. A. (1968). Profound neutropenia during the early phase of hemodialysis. *JAMA, J. Am. Med. Assoc.* **203**:1135–1137.
16. Jensen, D. P., Brubaker, L. H., Nolph, K. D., Johnson, C. A., and Nothum, R. J. (1973). Hemodialysis-coil induced transient neutropenia and overshoot neutrophilia in normal man. *Blood* **41**:399–408.
17. Craddock, P. R., Fehr, J., Dalmasso, A. P., Brigham, K. L., and Jacob, H. S. (1977). Hemodialysis leukopenia: Pulmonary vascular leukostasis resulting from complement activation by dialyzer cellophane membranes. *J. Clin. Invest.* **59**:879–888.
18. Craddock, P. R., Fehr, J., Brigham, K. L., Kronenberg, R. S., and Jacob, H. S. (1977). Complement and leukocyte-mediated pulmonary dysfunction in hemodialysis. *N. Engl. J. Med.* **296**:769–774.
19. Yamada, O., Moldow, C. F., Sacks, T., Craddock, P. R., Boogaerts, M. A., and Jacob, H. S. (1981). Deleterious effects of endotoxin on cultured endothelial cells: An *in-vitro* model of vascular injury. *Inflammation* **5**:115–126.
20. Harlan, J. M., Killen, P. D., Harker, L. A., Striker, G. E. and Wright, D. G. (1981). Neutrophil-mediated endothelial injury *in vitro*. Mechanisms of cell detachment. *J. Clin. Invest.* **68**:1394–1405.
21. Weiss, S. J., Young, J., LoBuglio, A. F., Slivka, A., and Nimeh, N. F. (1981). The role of hydrogen peroxide in neutrophil-mediated destruction of cultured endothelial cells. *J. Clin. Invest.* **68**:714–721.
22. Craddock, P. R., Hammerschmidt, D. E., White, J. G., Dalmasso, A. P., and Jacob, H. S. (1977). Complement (C5a)-induced granulocyte aggregation *in vitro:* A possible mechanism of complement-mediated leukostasis and leukopenia. *J. Clin. Invest.* **60**:261–264.
23. Hammerschmidt, D. E., Harris, P. D., Wayland, H., Craddock, P. R., and Jacob, H. S. (1981). Complement-induced granulocyte aggregation *in vivo. Am. J. Pathol.* **102**:146–150.
23a. Greenberg, Hammerschmidt, D. E., Craddock, P. R., and Jacob, H. S. (1979). Atheroma Cholesterol activates complement and aggregates granulocytes: possible role in ischemic manifestations of atherosclerosis. *Trans. Assoc. Amer. Phys.* **92**:130–135.
24. Redl, H. and Schlag, G. (1980). Morphologische Untersuchungen der Lunge im Schock. *Anaesthesiol. Intensivmed. (Erlangen, Fed. Repub. Ger.)* **25**:19–26.
25. Sandritter, W. C., Mittermayer, C., Riede, U. N., Freudenberg, N., and Grimm, H. (1978). Das Schocklungen-Syndrom (ein allgemeiner Überblick). *Beitr. Pathol.* **162**:7–23.
26. Heflin, A. C., and Brigham, K. L. (1981). Prevention by granulocyte depletion of increased vascular permeability of sheep lung following endotoxemia. *J. Clin. Invest.* **68**:1253–1260.
27. Hosea, S., Brown, E., Hammer, C., and Frank, M. (1980). Role of complement activation in a model of adult respiratory distress syndrome. *J. Clin. Invest.* **66**:375–382.
28. Hammerschmidt, D. E., Weaver, L. J., Hudson, L. D., Craddock, P. R., and Jacob, H. S. (1980). Association of complement activation and elevated plasma-C5a with adult respiratory distress syndrome: Pathophysiologic relevance and possible prognostic value. *Lancet* **1**:947–949.

29. Unsigned editorial (1980). Emphysema: Beginning of an understanding. *Br. Med. J.* **280**:961–962.
30. Janoff, A., Sloan, B., Weinbaum, G., Damiano, V., Sandhaus, R. A., Elias, J., and Kimbel, P. (1977). Experimental emphysema induced with purified human neutrophil elastase: Tissue localization of the instilled protease. *Am. Rev. Respir. Dis.* **115**:461–478.
31. Hunninghake, G. W., Gallin, J. I., and Fauci, A. S. (1978). Immunologic reactivity of the lung. The *in vivo* and *in vitro* generation of a neutrophil chemotactic factor by alveolar macrophages. *Am. Rev. Respir. Dis.* **117**:15–23.
32. Kramps, J. A., Bakker, W., and Dijkman, J. H. (1980). A matched-pair study of the leukocyte elastase-like activity in normal persons and in emphysematous patients with and without alpha-1-antitrypsin deficiencies. *Am. Rev. Respir. Dis.* **121**:253–262.
33. Gadek, J. E., Hunninghake, G. W., Zimmerman, R. L., and Crystal, R. G. (1980). Regulation of the release of alveolar macrophage-derived neutrophil chemotactic factor. *Am. Rev. Respir. Dis.* **121**:723–733.
34. Hinman, L. M., Stevens, C. A., Matthay, R. A., and Gee, B. L. (1980). Elastase and lysozyme activities in human alveolar macrophages: effects of cigarette smoking. *Am. Rev. Respir. Dis.* **121**:263–271.
35. Hoidal, J. R., Fox, R. B., LeMarbre, P. A., Perri, R., and Repine, J. E. (1981). Altered oxidative metabolic responses *in vitro* of alveolar macrophages from asymptomatic cigarette smokers. *Am. Rev. Respir. Dis.* **123**:85–89.
36. Fox, R. B., Hoidal, J. R., Brown, D. M., and Repine, J. E. (1981). Pulmonary inflammation caused by oxygen toxicity: Involvement of chemotactic factors and polymorphonuclear leukocytes. *Am. Rev. Respir. Dis.* **123**:521–523.
36a. Fox, R. B., Shasby, R. B., Harada, R. N., and Repine, J. E. (1981). A novel mechanism for pulmonary oxygen toxicity: Phagocyte-mediated lung injury. *Chest* **80S**:3S–4S.
37. Tauber, A. I., Goetzl, E. J., and Babior, B. M. (1979). Unique characteristics of superoxide production by human eosinophils in eosinophilic states. *Inflammation* **3**:261–270.
38. Bass, D. A., and Szeda, P. (1979). Mechanisms of killing of newborn larvae of *Trichinella spiralis* by neutrophils and eosinophils. *J. Clin. Invest.* **64**:1558–1564.
39. Suprunowicz, K., Lynch, R., Christensen, R., and Rothstein, G. (1981). Enhancement of neutrophil movement by superoxide anion. *Clin. Res.* **29**:349A.
40. Schumer, W. (1976). Steroids in the treatment of clinical septic shock. *Ann. Surg.* **184**:333–341.
41. Sladen, A. (1976). Methylprednisolone. Pharmacologic doses in shock lung syndrome. *J. Thorac. Cardiovasc. Surg.* **21**:800–805.
42. Wilson, J. W. (1972). Treatment or prevention of pulmonary cellular damage with pharmacologic doses of corticosteroids. *Surg., Gynecol. Obstet.* **134**:675–681.
43. Hammerschmidt, D. E., White, J. G., Craddock, P. R., and Jacob, H. S. (1979). Corticosteroids inhibit complement-mediated granulocyte aggregation: a possible mechanism for their efficacy in shock states. *J. Clin. Invest.* **63**:798–803.
44. Skubitz, K. M., Craddock, P. R., Hammerschmidt, D. E., and August, J. T. (1981). Corticosteroids block binding of chemotactic peptide to its receptor on granulocytes and cause disaggregation of granulocyte aggregates *in vitro. J. Clin. Invest.* **68**:13–20.
45. Hammerschmidt, D. E., Flynn, P. J., Vercellotti, G. M., Coppo, P. A., and Jacob, H. S. (1982). Synergy among agents inhibiting granulocyte aggregation. *Inflammation* **6**:169–176.
46. Fox, R. B., Tate, R. M., Bowman, C. M., Shasby, D. M., Harada, R. N., and Repine, J. E. (1981). Hydroxyl radical mediated pulmonary edema: The paradox of thiourea. *Clin. Res.* **29**:446A.

Chapter 5

A Mechanism for the Antiinflammatory Activity of Superoxide Dismutase

JOE M. McCORD, KENNETH WONG, STEVEN
H. STOKES, WILLIAM F. PETRONE, AND
DENIS ENGLISH

INTRODUCTION

The antiinflammatory activity of superoxide dismutase was empirically discovered more than a decade ago (1). For a number of years its mechanism of action was completely enigmatic. Even after its enzymatic function was discovered (2), a rational hypothesis could not be formulated to relate the two activities. At that time, almost nothing was known about the biological sources and roles of the superoxide radical. An important piece of information came in 1973 with the observation by Babior and coworkers (3) that phagocytosing granulocytes produce the superoxide radical and that a considerable fraction of the radical is released from these inflammatory cells into the suspending medium. The speculation that the radical was produced for bactericidal purposes was confirmed by Johnston *et al.* (4) shortly thereafter.

With these developments, a rational hypothesis for the mechanism of the enzyme's antiinflammatory activity was readily formulated (5): Any tissue that was invaded by a large number of metabolically activated inflammatory cells would be attacked by the superoxide radical produced

PATHOLOGY OF OXYGEN

by those cells; superoxide dismutase, if present in the extracellular fluid, could scavenge the cytotoxic radical and thereby prevent tissue damage, which would otherwise be manifested as inflammation. From the beginning it was understood that the cytotoxicity of the superoxide radical might be exerted directly, by superoxide per se, or indirectly, by species such as the hydroxyl radical generated secondarily from reactions of superoxide with other molecules.

In vitro studies lent support to the hypothesis. The generation of superoxide in synovial fluid in an amount comparable to that expected from the number of granulocytes commonly found in an inflamed joint resulted in a rapid decrease in the viscosity of the fluid (5). Such a breakdown of the properties of the fluid accompanies joint inflammation *in vivo*. A second study found that the suicidal behavior of granulocytes following phagocytosis was the result of the cytotoxic effects of their own superoxide production (6). The viability of phagocytosing granulocytes could be maintained equal to that of resting cells if superoxide dismutase were added to the medium. In both of these model studies, the damage that resulted was found not to be due to superoxide itself, but rather to the production of HO· via a reaction between superoxide and hydrogen peroxide:

$$O_2^- + H_2O_2 \rightarrow O_2 + OH^- + HO^·$$

In both systems the damage could be prevented by catalase as well as superoxide dismutase (either enzyme prevents the reaction by removing a reactant) or by mannitol (which scavenges the hydroxyl radical). The assumption was that this mechanism of toxicity was operative *in vivo*. The next logical step, therefore, was to test the hypothesis by probing the mechanism of inflammation *in vivo* with animal models.

TESTING THE HYPOTHESIS *IN VIVO*

Three models of induced inflammation in animals have now been studied in our laboratory (7,8): the reverse passive Arthus reaction in the rat, carrageenan-induced foot edema in the rat, and immune-complex-induced glomerulonephritis in the mouse. In the first two models, the sites of developing inflammatory lesions are the skin and foot, respectively. This presented a serious but solvable technical problem of pharmacokinetics — native bovine superoxide dismutase is cleared from the circulation with a half-life of about 6 min. Even though these models develop rapidly, requiring only about 3 hr, a single intravenous injection of the enzyme at time zero would undergo 30 half-lives by the time the inflammatory lesion reached its peak! Thus, it would appear to be difficult if not impossible to maintain a therapeutic dose level of native enzyme in the plasma and extracellular fluids of an animal. We have overcome this problem by the synthesis of chemically derivatized enzyme preparations that display greatly enhanced circulating lifetimes. By methods described elsewhere (7,9), we have covalently coupled such polymers as dextran, Ficoll, and polyethylene glycol to the enzyme, producing plasma half-lives of up to 35 hr. In the third animal model mentioned above (immune-complex-induced glomerulonephritis), rapid clearance of native enzyme worked to our advantage because, in this case, the kidney was both the site of the developing inflammatory lesion and the primary site of accumulation of enzyme removed from the circulation by glomerular filtration.

In all three models, treatment of the animal with an appropriate form and dosage of superoxide dismutase resulted in a dramatic prevention of the inflammatory lesion. In the first two models, the degree of inflammation was assessed by quantification of the edema produced (7). In the glomerulonephritis model, morphological damage was evaluated by light and electron microscopic examination of the kidney after 3, 6, and 12 days (8). At first glance, then, these data were consistent with the data obtained *in vitro* and supported the hypothesis of cytotoxicity mediated by superoxide and/or secondary products. Closer scrutiny of these and additional results from related experiments, however, led to some disquieting observations which could not be readily accommodated by the original hypothesis.

FOUR INCONGRUOUS OBSERVATIONS

It is well known, for example, that activated granulocytes possess a number of cytotoxic mechanisms including release of myeloperoxidase, neutral proteases, and other hydrolytic and digestive enzymes. Any cytotoxicity resulting from superoxide production should therefore represent but a fraction of the total tissue damage observed. In the reverse passive Arthus reaction, however, a long-lived derivative of superoxide dismutase produced essentially *total* (95%) inhibition of the edema (7). In the carrageenan model, the second phase of the reaction was likewise *totally* inhibited by a derivative of the enzyme (7). In the nephritis model, the morphological changes did not lend themselves to quantification (with one exception, mentioned below), but the degree of protection provided by the enzyme was striking (8). The first problem, then, was to explain the unexpectedly high efficacy of treatment with the enzyme. (Admittedly, this was not a *bad* problem, but nonetheless an explanation would be difficult to formulate on the basis of cytotoxicity.)

A second difficulty was presented by the studies carried out *in vivo*. Catalase (or derivatives thereof) and mannitol showed no antiinflammatory activity (7). The studies performed *in vitro* were equally sensitive to catalase and superoxide dismutase, presumably indicating that the actual cytotoxic or damaging species was the hydroxyl radical produced secondarily from superoxide as described earlier (5,6). In fact, much evidence suggests that the superoxide radical itself is relatively innocuous but that its primary destructive potential lies in its capacity to give rise to the powerfully oxidizing hydroxyl radical. However, we have no evidence at all that the tissue damage observed in our models *in vivo* in any way involves the hydroxyl radical. Our hypothesis must invoke a *superoxide-specific* mechanism.

The third observation was a very disturbing one. If granulocytes manifested their tissue-damaging effects by virtue of their superoxide production, then the intradermal injection of a superoxide-generating system other than granulocytes (e.g., xanthine oxidase and purine) ought to produce an edematous lesion similar to the Arthus reaction. It did not. No more edema was produced than in a saline-injected control. [There is a report in the literature that the injection of xanthine oxidase plus a substrate does produce edema and that superoxide dismutase partially inhibits the process (10). We have not been able to reproduce these findings.]

The fourth observation was equally disturbing and, ultimately, most enlightening. The working hypothesis predicted that the site of a potential inflammatory lesion in an animal treated with superoxide dismutase should contain a number of inflammatory cells equal to that in a lesion from an untreated animal. Tissue damage would be averted in the treated animals because the phagocyte-produced superoxide would be scavenged by superoxide dismutase in the extracellular fluid. Histological examination by light microscopy of (hematoxylin and eosin)-stained tissue sections from treated and untreated animals denied the prediction. In all three model systems the sites of potential lesions in animals treated with the enzyme were almost completely free of infiltration by inflammatory cells. *Clearly, the presence of superoxide dismutase in the extracellular fluid somehow prevented the influx of phagocytes to the site of the developing lesion.* This observation was certainly consistent with the first "problem" listed above. By preventing the accumulation of inflammatory cells, *all* granulocyte-mediated cytotoxicity would be eliminated, whether superoxide dependent or not; but how could superoxide dismutase prevent the accumulation of inflammatory cells?

A SUPEROXIDE-DEPENDENT
CHEMOTACTIC FACTOR

If a wandering granulocyte happens across a substance capable of causing an inflammatory response (immune complex or an opsonized bacterium, for example), that granulocyte will become metabolically activated. This, we believe, is the *primary* event in the development of an inflammatory lesion. The immediate objective of the granulocyte is to send out an alarm calling many more granulocytes to the site. The problem, then, is to communicate this information to other cells over a distance. To an outside observer (or another granulocyte), one of the few indications that the original cell is "turned on" is the production of superoxide on the outer surface of its plasma membrane. Could a gradient of superoxide serve as a chemotactic beacon for other cells to follow? Probably not. Because of its very short half-life and its reactivity, only a very steep gradient could result, covering a very short distance. Could the superoxide be translated into a stable chemotactic factor—for example, by reacting with an inactive plasma component to convert it to a stable, potent, chemotactic factor? This was certainly conceivable and also easily tested.

Normal human plasma was exposed to a source of superoxide production *in vitro* by incubation with xanthine oxidase and xanthine. The resulting plasma was powerfully chemotactic to normal human peripheral granulocytes when assessed by the Boyden chamber technique (11). The addition to the plasma of catalytic amounts of superoxide dismutase, but not catalase, totally prevented the development of the chemotactic factor. Heating the "activated" plasma to 56°C for 30 min destroyed the chemotactic activity; heating the plasma to 56°C for 30 min before exposure to superoxide prevented the formation of chemotactic activity. When activated plasma was subjected to gel filtration chromatography on Sephadex G-100, the chemotactic activity emerged just ahead of albumin, indicating a molecular weight of approximately 70,000. When resting granulocytes were incubated with activated plasma, the granulocytes were not metabolically activated; that is, the plasma factor is chemotactic but does not induce superoxide production by the attracted cells. This is a very important point, because it provides a self-quenching mechanism for the process. Chemotactic factor is produced only as long as metabolic stimulant is present. When all has been phagocytosed, the last wave of granulocytes to arrive will not be stimulated to make superoxide; no more chemotactic factor will be produced, and no more cells will be attracted. This point also explains why the injection of a superoxide-generating system did not cause inflammation. We would now predict that such an experiment would result in the attraction of granulocytes to the injection site, but without a metabolic stimulus the cells would remain resting and would not degranulate or release cytotoxic enzymes. The experiment was repeated, and again there were no grossly observable signs of inflammation. This time, however, a histological examination by light microscopy revealed a heavy infiltration of granulocytes, presumably due to the generation *in situ* of the chemotactic factor. Similarly, if plasma is treated with the superoxide-generating system *in vitro* and then injected intradermally in the rat, a heavy infiltration of granulocytes results without the formation of edema or hemorrhage.

CONCLUSION

We conclude from these studies that superoxide plays a key role in the initiation and perhaps also in the perpetuation of granulocyte-mediated inflammation. The mechanism appears to involve the reaction of superoxide with a plasma protein to form a potent chemotactic factor responsible for the initial accumulation of granulocytes at the site of the developing lesion. Superoxide dismutase, if present in the extracellular fluids, prevents the formation of the chemotactic factor, thereby preventing the infiltration of the tissue by inflammatory cells and likewise preventing the development of all granulocyte-mediated cytotoxic mechanisms that would otherwise ensue.

REFERENCES

1. Menander-Huber, K. B., and Huber, W. (1977). Orgotein, the drug version of bovine Cu-Zn superoxide dismutase. II. A summary account of clinical trials in man and animals. *In* "Superoxide and Superoxide Dismutases" (A. M. Michelson, J. M. McCord, and I. Fridovich, eds.), pp. 537–549. Academic Press, New York.
2. McCord, J. M., and Fridovich, I. (1969). Superoxide dismutase, an enzymatic function for erythrocuprein. *J. Biol. Chem.* **244**:6049–6055.
3. Babior, B. M., Kipnes, R. S., and Curnutte, J. T. (1973). Biological defense mechanisms. The production by leukocytes of superoxide, a potential bactericidal agent. *J. Clin. Invest.* **52**:741–744.
4. Johnston, R. B., Jr., Keele, B. B., Jr., Misra, H. P., Lehmeyer, J. E., Webb, L. S., Baehner, R. L., and Rajagopalan, K. V. (1975). The role of superoxide anion generation in phagocytic bacterial activity. Studies with normal and chronic granulomatous disease leukocytes. *J. Clin. Invest.* **55**:1357–1372.

5. McCord, J. M. (1974). Free radicals and inflammation: Protection of synovial fluid by superoxide dismutase. *Science* **185:**529–531.
6. Salin, M. L., and McCord, J. M. (1975). Free radicals and inflammation. Protection of phagocytosing leukocytes by superoxide dismutase. *J. Clin. Invest.* **56:**1319–1323.
7. McCord, J. M., and Wong, K. (1979). Phagocyte-produced free radicals: Roles in cytotoxicity and inflammation. *Ciba Found. Symp.* [N.S.] **65:**343–360.
8. McCord, J. M., Stokes, S. H., and Wong, K. (1979). Superoxide radical as a phagocyte-produced chemical mediator of inflammation. *Adv. Inflammation Res.* **1:**273–280.
9. Abuchowski, A., McCoy, J. R., Palczuk, N. D., van Es, T., and Davis, F. F. (1977). Effect of covalent attachment of polyethylene glycol of immunogenicity and circulating life of bovine liver catalase. *J. Biol. Chem.* **252:**3582–3586.
10. Ohmori, H., Komoriya, K., Azuma, A., Hashimoto, Y., and Kurozumi, S. (1978). Xanthine oxidase-induced foot-edema in rats: Involvement of oxygen radicals. *Biochem. Pharmacol.* **27:**1397–1400.
11. Boyden, S. (1962). The chemotactic effect of mixtures of antibody and antigens on polymorphonuclear leukocytes. *J. Exp. Med.* **115:**453–466.

DISCUSSION

PROCTOR: There is a system that may be similar to your use of xanthine oxidase to generate oxygen radicals. Copper ions, which have been reported to cause an analogous chemotactic response in granulocytes and fibroblasts, are thought to generate oxygen radicals. Do your results support this possibility? Also, are you aware of the possible role of oxygen radicals in the control of nucleotide cyclases?

McCORD: I am aware of the suggestion that redox-active radicals may modulate guanylate cyclase, but the data I have seen are not easily interpreted.

COHEN: Can you distinguish between chemotaxis and deformability in your Boyden chamber experiment?

McCORD: We have demonstrated the chemotactic activity of the factor using the "chemotaxis under agarose" technique in addition to the Boyden technique. I do not believe that an increase in deformability would lead to a positive result with the agarose method.

ŌYANAGUI: There are many chemotactants known to be involved in inflammation. What was the chemotactant used in your system?

McCORD: The chemotactant in all experiments performed *in vitro* was human plasma exposed to xanthine oxidase plus xanthine.

ŌYANAGUI: Is there any participation of prostaglandins in the process?

McCORD: At this point I can neither infer nor rule out participation by prostaglandins.

ŌYANAGUI: What was the route of administration of the superoxide dismutase you used in the Arthus reaction model?

McCORD: In all the animal models, superoxide dismutase or its derivatives were given intravenously.

SHAPIRO: Have you tested fractions of plasma isolated from Sephadex G-100 columns for their capacity to be "activated" by the xanthine–xanthine oxidase system in order to rule out the possibility of the formation of a low molecular weight activator that is subsequently bound to a protein, for example, to albumin?

McCORD: Yes, we have. The fractions are activable but with less efficiency than whole plasma. I can't give an unequivocal answer yet. If the factor is a complex of the type you describe, it is stable enough to survive gel filtration. This is possible, but I feel it is unlikely.

PIETRONIGRO: Have you tested the stability of your chemotactic factor toward glutathione peroxidase?

McCORD: No.

McLENNAN: The primary event in inflammation is increased capillary permeability. How does superoxide dismutase modify this?

McCORD: All we can say at this point is that superoxide dismutase prevents the influx of granulocytes and inhibits the formation of edema. I don't know what the effect is on capillary permeability before granulocyte involvement.

McLENNAN: What is the extravascular distribution of the superoxide dismutase, and does the intravascular compartmentalization of the catalase explain its lack of effect?

McCORD: We don't know how superoxide dismutase and the various derivatives are distributed among extravascular fluids. The lack of effect of catalase was also seen in its inability to prevent the formation of chemotactic factor *in vitro*. This could not be attributed to unfavorable pharmacokinetics.

SCHMIDT: Have you been able to demonstrate retention of normal renal function with the use of superoxide dismutase in the immune complex glomerular uptake model?

McCORD: In the model we used, the kidneys were not damaged severely enough to cease functioning. We are attempting to modify the model to attain renal impairment or failure.

SCHULTE: Dr. Ernest Willers, retired state veterinarian of Hawaii, successfully treated dogs with inflammatory conditions 20 years ago with a protein injection containing superoxide dismutase.

Chapter 6

Effect of Intraperitoneally Administered Superoxide Dismutase on Pulmonary Damage Resulting from Hyperoxia

GEOFFREY MCLENNAN AND
ANNE P. AUTOR

INTRODUCTION

Prolonged exposure to 95–100% oxygen at a pressure of 1 atmosphere causes progressive loss of pulmonary function accompanied by structural damage to the lungs in all mammalian species studied (1,2). The pulmonary damage resulting from hyperoxic exposure is generally believed to be caused by the production of oxygen-derived free radicals (3,4). Superoxide anion (O_2^-) hydrogen peroxide (H_2O_2) are produced in biological systems by the single-electron reduction of oxygen (5). By a mechanism that is yet to be clarified but is apparently nonenzymatically catalyzed by iron, O_2^- and H_2O_2 together can produce a highly reactive species resembling a hydroxyl radical ($HO^\cdot$) (6). It is this free-radical species that has been proposed to be the damaging agent in oxygen-induced cell lysis, membrane damage, and lipid peroxidation (7).

Superoxide dismutase, the enzyme that catalytically converts its substrate, O_2^-, to H_2O_2 and O_2 is present in mammalian cells in two forms. The manganese-containing enzyme is found in the mitochondrial matrix,

PATHOLOGY OF OXYGEN

and the copper/zinc-containing form is in the cytosol. There is a great deal of evidence that its function is to prevent the accumulation of cellular O_2^- (8). Hydrogen peroxide, which is produced by a number of biochemical reactions including the action of superoxide dismutase, is a substrate for catalase and glutathione peroxidase, enzymes that are both present in normal mammalian cells. The catalytic destruction of either the superoxide anion or hydrogen peroxide is therefore important in preventing the production of HO·.

Under normoxic conditions the endogenous cellular levels of superoxide dismutase, the glutathione peroxidase system, and catalase appear to be adequate for the control of the cellular flux of reactive oxygen metabolites. It has now been established that elevation of the levels of pulmonary catalase, glutathione peroxidase, and the superoxide dismutases through oxygen-mediated enzyme induction is an important factor in neonatal resistance to pulmonary oxygen toxicity (3,4,9).

Further evidence that these enzymes are an important part of the pulmonary defense mechanism against oxygen toxicity was provided by recent work showing that exogenously administered superoxide dismutase prevented the hyperoxic-induced depression of pulmonary serotonin clearance in the rat (10). Another study, in which superoxide dismutase was administered to rats by inhalation of aerosolized solution, failed to show any protective effect of the enzyme against hyperoxic exposure (11). Intermittent systemic administration of superoxide dismutase, however, is not entirely satisfactory as a means of testing the possible protective effects of the enzyme because of its very short half-life after administration resulting from rapid renal excretion (12–14). Continuous systemic administration could provide a more adequate means of testing the agent. The purpose of the study described here was to assess the effect of continuously administered superoxide dismutase in preventing or modifying pulmonary damage provoked by continuous exposure to normobaric hyperoxia.

METHODS

Adult male Sprague–Dawley rats (Biol-Lab, 175–200 g) were used for these studies. Animals to be exposed to hyperoxia were lightly anesthetized with ether, and a catheter was inserted through a small incision at the nape of the neck. The catheter was then passed subcutaneously to an intraperitoneal position and held in position with a silk suture. This catheter was then used for the continuous delivery of an intraperitoneal infusion, without the need to restrain the animal (Fig. 1). After waking, these animals were given either sterile normal saline or sterile normal saline with added superoxide dismutase (1500 units/ml; copper/zinc superoxide dismutase prepared from bovine liver, Truett Laboratories) as a slow intraperitoneal infusion (12–15 ml per 24 hr) using an infusion set (Venoset). The animals were exposed to a 95% oxygen atmosphere for 72 hr in a controlled-atmosphere chamber with continuous monitoring of oxygen, carbon dioxide, and water vapor pressure according to a previously described procedure (15).

Animal deaths were recorded at the end of the 72-hr exposure period. Surviving animals were lightly anesthetized with ether, and an arterial blood gas sample was drawn with a heparinized syringe from the abdominal aorta under direct vision. The arterial blood gas samples were placed immediately in ice water, and blood gas tension analysis was performed within 20 min (Instrumentation Laboratory Blood Gas Analyzer 713). The lungs were then removed *en bloc* and inflated to 25 cm of water pressure with 10% buffered formalin and fixed at this pressure. Lungs were sectioned and stained with hematoxylin and eosin. These tissue sections were evaluated histologically by a pathologist with no prior knowledge of the experimental protocol.

Another group of animals similarly fitted with intraperitoneal catheters

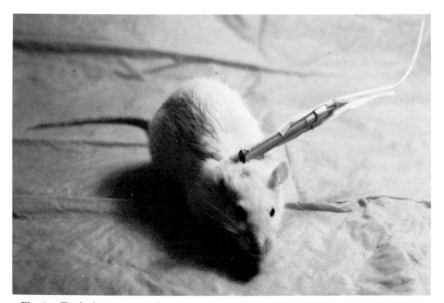

Fig. 1. Typical rat prepared for the continuous delivery of intraperitoneal infusion (saline or superoxide dismutase in saline). Animals were maintained without physical restraints.

received sterile normal saline with added superoxide dismutase, as previously described. The lungs of these animals were prepared for enzymatic analysis. After 24 hr, rats were anesthetized with ether, and a blood sample was collected by venepuncture. The blood sample was allowed to clot and the serum collected. The lungs of these animals were perfused *in situ* with 30 ml of ice-cold phosphate-buffered saline, pH 7.4, by injection into the right atrium. The lungs were removed *en bloc* from the animals, blotted dry, and excess tracheal and nonlung tissue was removed. The lungs were weighed and homogenized in sterile normal saline using a Sorvall Omnimixer. The homogenate was subjected to sonic disruption for 3 min. Superoxide dismutase activity was measured in this preparation. A group of control animals, which received an intraperitoneal infusion of normal saline only, were treated similarly.

Superoxide dismutase activity was measured by the method of McCord and Fridovich, modified by the addition of 5×10^{-5} M NaCN to the assay mixture (16). Total lung DNA was measured according to the method of Richards (17). Heme concentration was determined from the carbon monoxide difference spectra of blood, serum, and tissue homogenate samples (18). Superoxide dismutase activity attributable to contaminating blood in tissue samples was calculated from the known enzyme concentration in blood for all samples analyzed and was subtracted from the measured values.

RESULTS

Body fluids such as serum normally contain little or no superoxide dismutase (19). A very low level of activity was present in the serum of control rats receiving saline, possibly attributable to hemolysis during the preparation of the serum sample. However, the superoxide dismutase level in the serum of animals receiving the intraperitoneal infusion of superoxide dismutase was significantly greater than that of the control animals (Table I). Enzyme analysis of the homogenates of perfused lungs from the superoxide dismutase-treated animals demonstrated a significant increase in the enzyme level compared with the level in saline-treated rats (Table II).

The assessment of animal mortality showed that, whereas 42% of saline-treated animals died after 72 hr of continuous exposure to 95–100% oxygen at 1 atmosphere, only 20% of the superoxide dismutase-treated oxygen-exposed rats died (Table III). Postmortem examination of the animals that died during oxygen exposure showed dark hemorrhagic lungs

TABLE I

Superoxide Dismutase in Rat Serum[a]

Saline-treated rats (units of SOD/ml)	Superoxide dismutase-treated rats (units of SOD/ml)
3.8	11.0
2.5	10.7
4.0	12.3
4.5	

[a] Rats were given either saline or a total of $18–22.5 \times 10^3$ units of superoxide dismutase (SOD) (in saline) in a 24-hr period. Blood samples were taken and allowed to clot. Serum was removed and analyzed for enzyme activity as described in the text. Values are reported for each animal tested. The difference between the values for saline-treated and enzyme-treated animals is significant to $p < .001$.

and bilateral pleural effusions in both the saline-treated and superoxide dismutase-treated animals without any obvious difference (Table III).

In the surviving animals, arterial blood gas tension analysis demonstrated a significant difference between the saline-treated, oxygen-exposed animals and the superoxide dismutase-treated, oxygen-exposed rats in both arterial oxygen tension and blood pH ($p < .05$, Student t test). The PaO$_2$ of saline-treated, oxygen-exposed animals was 35 mm Hg, whereas that for the enzyme-treated animals was 55 mm Hg. The blood pH of the saline-treated group was 7.20, and that of the enzyme-

TABLE II

Superoxide Dismutase in Rat Lung Homogenates[a]

Saline-treated rats (units of SOD/μg DNA)	Superoxide dismutase-treated rats (units of SOD/μg DNA)
2.4	3.1
2.0	3.3
2.6	3.1
2.6	

[a] Rats were treated as described in Table I. Lung homogenate samples were obtained as described in the text. Values are reported for each animal tested. The difference between the values for saline- and enzyme-treated animals is significant to $p < .05$.

TABLE III

Mortality after 72 hr in a Controlled Atmosphere

Animals	Mortality	Gross pathological findings
Normal-air-exposed	0/4 (0%)	Normal
Saline-treated, O_2-exposed (95–100%)	5/12 (42%)	Hemorrhagic lungs[a]; bilateral effusions
Superoxide dismutase-treated, O_2-exposed (95–100%)	2/10 (20%)	Hemorrhagic lungs[a]; bilateral effusions

[a] Conducted only on animals that died during the exposure period and within 30 min of death.

treated group was 7.08. The arterial carbon dioxide tensions did not differ significantly.

For the purpose of histological comparison three major categories were used. Category I was assessed as minimal change (normal or nearly normal lungs) (Fig. 2). Category II included mild perivascular edema, focal

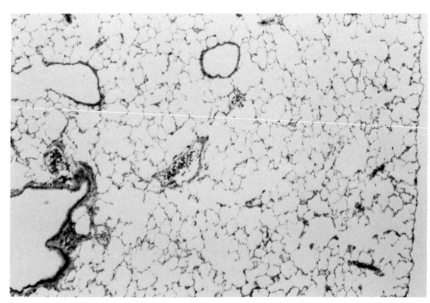

Fig. 2. Section of lung tissue of a rat maintained in air. This view is typical for rats in category I, defined as normal (see Table IV). × 40.

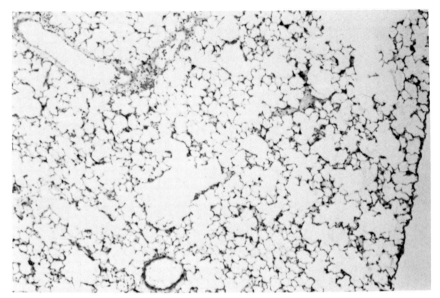

Fig. 3. Section of rat lung tissue typical for category II (see Table IV). Minimal level of pathological changes are present. × 40.

alveolar wall thickening, and focal areas of increased cellularity (Fig. 3). Category III was defined by severe perivascular edema, generalized alveolar wall thickening with increased alveolar infiltrate, hemorrhage, and well-developed hyaline membrane formation (Fig. 4). Histological evaluation demonstrated a difference between the lungs of oxygen-exposed, saline-treated rats and oxygen-exposed superoxide dismutase-treated rats. Whereas four of six saline-treated, oxygen-exposed animals showed severe lung damage (category III), only one of seven superoxide dismutase-treated rats showed similar damage (Table IV). In other studies it was shown that heat-inactivated superoxide dismutase provided no protection for lung cells subjected to toxic oxygen radicals (20).

A statistical analysis of these data was conducted by combining the results obtained from mortality assessment with the histopathological evaluation. Data from the two groups, category I and category II, were evaluated together. The extent of lung damage and the mortality rate were significantly higher in the rats subjected to 72 hr of continuous hyperoxic exposure and treated only with saline than in the oxygen-exposed animals treated with continuous superoxide dismutase (Fischer's Exact test, $p < .04$).

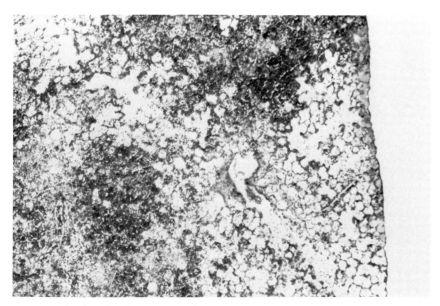

Fig. 4.   Section of rat lung tissue typical for category III (see Table IV). Extensive pathological findings are present in the lung. × 40.

TABLE IV

Histological Comparison of Saline- and Superoxide Dismutase-Treated Rats

Animals	Category I[a]	Category II[b]	Category III[c]	n
Normal	+ + +			3
O₂-Exposed with continuous infusion of saline		+ +	+ + + +	6
O₂-Exposed with continuous infusion of superoxide dismutase	+	+ + + + +	+	7

[a] Normal lungs.
[b] Mild perivascular edema, focal alveolar wall thickening, focal areas of hypercellularity.
[c] Severe perivascular edema, generalized alveolar wall thickening with alveolar infiltrate,
hemorrhage, well-developed hyaline membrane formation.

CONCLUSIONS

This study demonstrates that continuous intraperitoneal administration of superoxide dismutase provides protection against the pulmonary damage and mortality associated with normobaric, hyperoxic exposure of rats. Although significant, the protection was not complete, however.

Superoxide dismutase exerts a protective effect in bacteria exposed to hyperoxia (21) and to ionizing radiation (22–24), two sources of superoxide anion radical. This enzyme has also been shown to provide protection in isolated cell systems exposed to irradiation (20). Whole-animal studies have also demonstrated that superoxide dismutase provides protection from radiation damage to bone marrow cells (25). Superoxide dismutase appears to be a protective enzyme because of its catalytic removal of the superoxide anion-radical. Several lines of evidence support the interpretation that the superoxide anion-radical exerts its toxicity indirectly through its conversion to a more highly reduced entity, the hydroxyl radical.

Optimal protection against the toxic effects of oxygen may only be possible if superoxide dismutase is continuously present at the site of superoxide anion-radical generation. By the maintenance of a relatively constant serum level through continuous infusion, an equilibrium between blood and lung interstitial space can be established in a manner similar to that known to occur with plasma albumin. Albumin equilibration occurs in 3–5 hr in adult rodents (26,27). It is not known whether superoxide dismutase penetrates into the cytoplasm of the pulmonary endothelial or epithelial cells. Some cytoplasmic uptake of exogenous superoxide dismutase has been demonstrated in bone marrow cells, however. In addition, indirect evidence indicates some cellular accumulation of superoxide dismutase on *in vitro* incubation of pulmonary macrophages with the enzyme added to the medium (20). It is worth noting that cells may develop a compromised permeability barrier when exposed to prolonged hyperoxia *in situ*.

The site of lung damage after normobaric hyperoxic exposure in the adult rat, as well as the origin of the subsequent edema formation, is the pulmonary capillary endothelial cell. This has been demonstrated by sequential electron microscopy (28) and also by endothelial cell regeneration studies after oxygen exposure (29). However, edema formation occurs before any recognizable morphological change in the capillary endothelial cell (28). The precise mechanism by which oxygen exposure causes the initial pulmonary edema is unknown but may be related to damage to the fluid transport mechanism of the endothelial cells.

The effectiveness of superoxide dismutase in moderating the pulmonary damage occurring under normobaric, hyperoxic conditions is strong evidence that the superoxide anion-radical is involved in causing this damage. The superoxide anion-radical could be generated under hyperoxic conditions at a variety of intra- or extracellular sites in close association with endothelial cells. A potential source of oxygen radicals later in the process may be the polymorphonuclear leukocytes recruited to sites of chemically-induced injury. These cells constitute a significant source of biologically generated oxygen free radicals (30). Because superoxide dismutase probably does not cross the normal cell membrane to a great extent, it is likely that its effectiveness is related to removal of the superoxide radical at the plasma membrane of the endothelial cell. The protection afforded by the exogenous enzyme may be incomplete, therefore. In addition, one of the products of the catalytic activity of superoxide dismutase is hydrogen peroxide. The extracellular level of superoxide dismutase available from continuous infusion may remove some but not all O_2^- and thus contributes to the pool of H_2O_2. Under these conditions, therefore, in the presence of both reactants, which appear to generate $HO\cdot$, tissue damage will occur. By removing superoxide anion-radical, superoxide dismutase does reduce the potential for hydroxyl radical production and subsequent radical-initiated tissue damage via this mechanism.

REFERENCES

1. Haugaard, N. (1968). Cellular mechanisms of oxygen toxicity. *Physiol. Rev.* **48**:311.
2. Clark, J. M., and Lambertson, C. J. (1971). Pulmonary oxygen toxicity: A review. *Pharmacol. Rev.* **23**:37.
3. Stevens, J. B., and Autor, A. P. (1980). Proposed mechanism for neonatal rat tolerance to normobaric hyperoxia. *Federation Proc.* **39**:3138.
4. Autor, A. P., Fox, A. W., and Stevens, J. B. (1979). Effect of oxygen and related radicals on rat pulmonary cells. *In* "Biochemical and Clinical Aspects of Oxygen" (W. S. Caughey, ed.), pp. 767–783. Academic Press, New York.
5. Fridovich, I. (1976). Oxygen radicals, hydrogen peroxide, and oxygen toxicity. *In* "Free Radicals in Biology" (W. A. Pryor, ed.), Vol. 1, pp. 239–277. Academic Press, New York.
6. Groves, J. T., and McCluskey, G. A. (1979). Oxo- and peroxo-transition metal species in chemical and biochemical oxidations. *In* "Biochemical and Clinical Aspects of Oxygen" (W. S. Caughey, ed.), pp. 277–309. Academic Press, New York.

7. Willson, R. L. (1979). Hydroxyl radicals and biological damage *in vitro:* What relevance *in vivo? Ciba Found. Symp.* [N.S.] **65**:19–42.

8. Fridovich, I. (1979). Superoxide dismutase: Defense against endogenous superoxide radical. *Ciba Found. Symp.* [N.S.] **65**:77–93.

9. Frank, L., Bucher, J. R., and Roberts, R. J. (1978). Oxygen toxicity in neonatal and adult animals of various species. *J. Appl. Physiol.: Respir., Environ. Exercise Physiol.* **45**:699.

10. Block, E. R., and Fisher, A. B. (1977). Prevention of hyperoxic-induced depression of pulmonary seritonin clearance by pretreatment with superoxide dismutase. *Am. Rev. Respir. Dis.* **116**:441.

11. Crapo, J. D., DeLong, D. M., Sjöstrom, K., Hasler, G. R., and Drew, R. (1977). The failure of aerosolized superoxide dismutase to modify pulmonary oxygen toxicity. *Am. Rev. Respir. Dis.* **115**:1027.

12. Autor, A. P., and Brown, R. M. Unpublished observations.

13. Autor, A. P. (1974). Reduction of paraquat toxicity by superoxide dismutase. *Life Sci.* **14**:1309.

14. Petkau, A., Kelly, L., Chelak, W. S., Pleskach, S. D., Barefoot, D., and Meeker, B. E. (1975). Radioprotection of bone marrow stem cells by superoxide dismutase. *Biochem. Biophys. Res. Commun.* **67**:1167.

15. Stevens, J. B., and Autor, A. P. (1977). Oxygen-induced synthesis of superoxide dismutase and catalase in pulmonary macrophages of neonatal rats. *Lab. Invest.* **37**:470.

16. McCord, J. M., and Fridovich, I. (1969). Superoxide dismutase: An enzymic function for erythrocuprein (hemocuprein). *J. Biol. Chem.* **244**:6055.

17. Richards, G. M. (1974). Modifications of the diphenylamine reaction giving increased sensitivity and simplicity in the estimation of DNA. *Anal. Biochem.* **57**:369.

18. Estabrook, R. W., Peterson, J., Barm, J., and Hildebrandt, A. (1972). The spectrophotometric measurement of turbid suspensions of cytochromes associated with drug metabolism. *Methods Pharmacol.* **2**:321.

19. McCord, J. M. (1974). Free radicals and inflammation. Protection of synovial fluid by superoxide dismutase. *Science* **185**:529.

20. McLennan, G., Oberley, L. W., and Autor, A. P. (1980). The role of oxygen derived free radicals in radiation-induced damage and death of non-dividing eukaryotic cells. *Radiat. Res.* **84**:122.

21. Hassen, H. M., and Fridovich, I. (1977). Enzymatic defenses against the toxicity of oxygen and streptonigrin in *Escherichia coli. J. Bacteriol.* **129**:1574.

22. Oberley, L. W., Lindgren, A. L., Baker, S. A., and Stevens, R. H. (1976). Superoxide anion as the cause of the oxygen effect. *Radiat. Res.* **68**:320.

23. Misra, H. P., and Fridovich, I. (1976). Superoxide dismutase and the oxygen enhancement of radiation lethality. *Arch. Biochem. Biophys.* **176**:577.

24. Petkau, A., and Chelack, W. S. (1974). Protection of *Acholeplasma laidlawii* by superoxide dismutase. *Int. J. Radiat. Biol.* **26**:421.

25. Petkau, A., Chelack, W. S., and Pleskach, S. D. (1978). Protection by superoxide dismutase of white blood cells in X-irradiated mice. *Life Sci.* **22**:867.

26. Nicolaysen, G., and Staub, N. C. (1975). Time course of albumin equilibration in interstitium and lymph of normal mouse lung. *Microvasc. Res.* **9**:29.

27. Studer, R., and Potchen, J. (1971). The radioisotopic assessment of regional microvascular permeability to macromolecules. *Microvasc. Res.* **3**:35.

28. Weibel, E. R. (1971). Oxygen effect on lung cells. *Arch. Intern. Med.* **28:**54.
29. Evans, M. J., Hackney, J. D., and Bils, R. F. (1969). Effects of a high concentration of oxygen on cell renewal in the pulmonary alveoli. *Aerosp. Med.* **40:**1365.
30. Babior, B. M. (1978). Oxygen dependent microbial killing by phagocytes. *N. Engl. J. Med.* **298:**659, 721.

DISCUSSION

FRIDOVICH: You showed a large increase in CuZnSOD in lung lavage fluid. What were the changes in lung tissue upon hyperoxic exposure?

McLENNAN: We observe no change in the activity of CuZnSOD in lung tissue of adult rats upon hyperoxic exposure under the conditions described in these experiments.

MICHELSON: Indolamine dioxygenase activity should be measured during the time when hyperoxic-induced changes are occurring since Hayaishi and co-workers have shown that this enzyme is increased 20 to 40-fold during pulmonary inflammation (e.g., virus-induced). This enzyme not only metabolizes serotonin but also uses O_2^- as a substrate. Perhaps increased oxygen protection would be obtained by perfusion of both superoxide dismutase and indolamine dioxygenase.

McLENNAN: This is a good idea, but we have no experience with indolamine dioxygenase.

PROCTOR: There may be several different mechanisms of O_2 toxicity. For example, we have found that superoxide dismutase does not ameliorate hyperbaric, oxygen-induced convulsions but that catalase does.

McLENNAN: It is apparent that hyperbaric O_2 causes different damage than normobaric hyperoxia. However, whether the basic mechanism of damage is different is not known. We have been careful to ascertain that our administered superoxide dismutase is present in the lung as a statistically significant increase in lung enzyme activity. Superoxide dismutase does not appear to cross the blood–brain barrier in significant amounts. This may be one explanation for the failure of superoxide dismutase to modify hyperbaric O_2 toxicity in the central nervous system. We have not tried using catalase to ameliorate pulmonary O_2 toxicity, but certainly in neonatal rats this enzyme appears to be very important intracellularly.

RILEY: Did you perfuse the lungs of both control and experimental animals before analysis?

McLENNAN: The lungs prepared for superoxide dismutase analysis were perfused carefully and completely to remove blood. The lungs prepared for histology were not perfused.

Chapter 7

Macrophage-Generated Superoxide Radicals: Inflammation and Tumor Cell Growth

YOSHIHIKO ŌYANAGUI

INTRODUCTION

The superoxide radical O_2^- produced by granulocytes is partly responsible for killing engulfed microorganisms. In 1974, McCord demonstrated the involvement of superoxide in the degradation of synovial fluid (1). Influenced by this work, I proposed that an excessive production of superoxide radical might cause inflammation. To test this proposal I studied the process of inflammation using the carrageenan-induced paw edema model. This chapter is a summary of my research work in three related areas: the participation of superoxide radicals in rat paw edema induced by carrageenan (2), the screening method developed to test nonsteroidal antiinflammatory drugs (3–5), and the superoxide-scavenging effects of tumor ascites fluid and blood plasma.

CARRAGEENAN-INDUCED EDEMA

Paw swelling in normal rats was produced by the local injection of 1.5 mg of carrageenan (Fig. 1, curve A). Measurable swelling occurred

PATHOLOGY OF OXYGEN

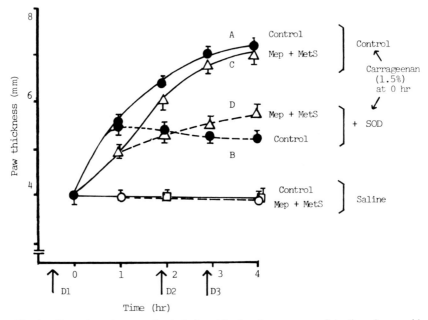

Fig. 1. Paw edema in normal rats induced by local carrageenan injection. Superoxide dismutase (SOD), 2 mg/kg, mepyramine (Mep), 10 mg/kg, and methysergide (MetS), 4 mg/kg, were administered (iv) at the times indicated (D1, D2, and D3). No suppression of carrageenan-induced paw swelling was seen with heat-inactivated superoxide dismutase (1– 2 mg/kg), catalase (2.4×10^5 units/kg), D-mannitol (400 mg/kg), sodium benzoate (160 mg/kg), or 1,3-diphenylisobenzofuran (5–20 mg/kg). The data are presented as the means ± standard error of 4–10 experiments.

immediately after a single injection and continued for 4 hr. When superoxide dismutase was administered (2 mg/kg, three times), no effect on swelling was seen until the first hour after carrageenan treatment (Fig. 1, curve B). It has been reported that this phase of carrageenan-induced swelling is provoked by histamine and serotonin (6). The prostaglandin (PG) phase of swelling, which began approximately 1 hr after carrageenan administration, was completely suppressed by superoxide dismutase (Fig. 1, curve B). Superoxide dismutase also suppressed swelling at 0.5 mg/kg but was less effective. Complete suppression of paw swelling was not achieved with superoxide dismutase at 2 mg/kg. Superoxide dismutase may be inactivated or lost rather rapidly from the bloodstream. Heat-inactivated superoxide dismutase, bovine liver catalase, and other oxygen radical scavengers (D-mannitol, benzoate, and 1,3-diphenylisobenzofuran) were ineffective as suppressors of paw swelling. Curve C represents the effect on paw swelling of the histamine antagonist mepyramine and the serotonin antagonist methysergide (injected three times intravenously). Only the first phase of swelling was inhibited. As might be expected, both phases of swelling were inhibited if superoxide dismutase (2 mg/kg) and the antagonists were given in combination (Fig. 1, curve D).

Identical experiments were conducted with agranulocytic rats (Fig. 2). DiRosa *et al.* (7) showed the importance of macrophages in carrageenan-induced paw edema. Agranulocytic rats were prepared by daily intraperitoneal injections of methotrexate for 3 days (8). Paw swelling in agranulocytic rats induced with carrageenan was similar to that in normal rats (Fig. 2, curves A and C), but swelling was suppressed to a greater extent by superoxide dismutase (Fig. 2, curve D). The first phase of paw swelling in agranulocytic rats may be associated with prostaglandin since it was inhibited by superoxide dismutase. In normal rats, the first-phase swelling induced by prostaglandin probably occurs but is masked by swelling induced by histamine and serotonin released by activated granulocytes.

Twenty percent of the total fatty acid esters in macrophages is found as arachidonate. Polymorphonuclear leukocytes, however, contain only 3% of the fatty acid esters as arachidonate (9). The high content of arachidon-

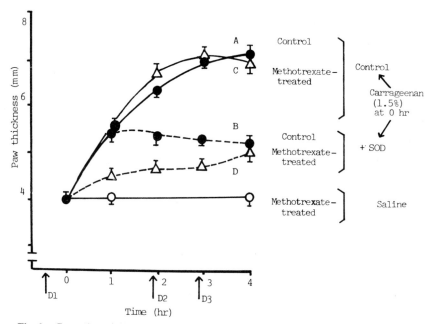

Fig. 2. Paw edema in agranulocytic rats. Edema was induced with carrageenan injection, and agranulocytosis was achieved by three daily ip injections of methotrexate, 2.5 mg/kg per day, in normal rats. Superoxide dismutase (SOD), 2 mg/kg, was administered (iv) at the times indicated (D1, D2, and D3).

ate may facilitate prostaglandin synthesis in macrophages. It is not certain whether prostaglandin is associated directly with the second phase of paw swelling or whether this phase is mediated by kinins, but the participation of superoxide anion is supported by these data. Some swelling in the absence of carrageenan was observed when superoxide dismutase was injected in rat plantar surface. The site of action of superoxide dismutase remains unknown.

MACROPHAGE PRODUCTION OF SUPEROXIDE RADICALS

Inhibition of Superoxide Radical Production in Isolated Macrophages by Antiinflammatory Drugs

A simple *in vitro* screening method for antiinflammatory drugs was developed using viable isolated guinea pig peritoneal macrophages by adopting a suitable method for the detection of superoxide (3). The assay for superoxide anion that depends on the reduction of ferricytochrome c (1) was unsuitable for this purpose for the following reasons:

1. Very low O_2^- production at the low pH (approximately 5–6) of inflamed tissue
2. The occurrence of complex, biphasic, time-dependent absorption changes at 340 nm caused by macrophage activity and the administered superoxide dismutase or antagonist drugs
3. Inhibition of the reaction by 0.1% dimethylformamide (DMF), which is used as a solvent for many antiinflammatory drugs
4. The occurrence of absorbence changes chemically induced by the drugs
5. The probability that cytochrome c may not act as an effective physiological oxygen radical scavenger on the cell surface

Many other assay methods require an alkaline pH at which macrophages cannot survive. The assay of Chan and Bielski (10) using lactate dehydrogenase (LDH)-bound NADH, therefore appeared to be the best choice. The two assay systems now in use are depicted in Fig. 3. Peritoneal macrophages were obtained from guinea pigs 3–5 days after injections of paraffin oil or thioglycollage broth. Macrophages from rats and mice, as well as nonstimulated guinea pig resident peritoneal cells, were obtained by the same procedure (4). All these cells produced superoxide anion. Used as the enzyme–NADH complex, pig heart LDH was more efficient for

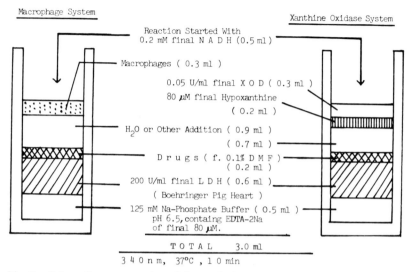

Fig. 3. Schematic representation of the methods used to detect superoxide anion. The macrophage system was designed to detect inhibition of the production of superoxide anion. The xanthine oxidase (XOD) system was designed to detect scavenging of formed superoxide anions.

detecting superoxide than the equivalent enzymatic units of rabbit muscle LDH, although most of the experiments employed rabbit muscle LDH (300 units/ml) (Fig. 4A). The optimum pH for superoxide production in this system was 6.5 (Fig. 4B). A high concentration of phosphate buffer (125 mM) was required for the macrophage assay system. N,N'-Dimethylformamide, used at a concentration of 0.1% to dissolve the non-water-soluble drugs, did not inhibit superoxide production at this concentration.

The effect of a number of nonsteroidal antiinflammatory drugs on the production of superoxide anion by macrophages is presented in Fig. 5. Dexamethasone and gold thiomalate were not inhibitory unless high concentrations were used, but nonsteroidal antiinflammatory drugs were inhibitory at comparatively low concentrations. To determine whether this inhibition was the result of blocking the production of superoxide radical or scavenging the radical once it was formed, the drugs were tested in the xanthine oxidase assay system. In general, nonsteroidal antiinflammatory drugs appeared to block the production of superoxide by macrophages but not to scavenge superoxide once it was produced by xanthine oxidase (Table I). Some of the metal ions had the same effect. A new nonsteroidal antiinflammatory drug, MK-447, had no effect on either system. Superoxide dismutase showed a positive action in both systems. Cytochalasin B, N-ethylmaleimide, and L-epinephrine, which inhibit superoxide pro-

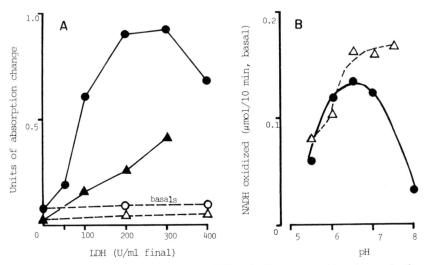

Fig. 4. Effect of lactate dehydrogenase (LDH) and pH on superoxide anion production by macrophages. (A) Effect of LDH on superoxide radical production by macrophages. Reactions were conducted in phosphate buffer (125 mM, pH 6.5). A macrophage density of 3.0×10^6 cells per milliliter was used. Data were recorded as units of absorption change at 340 nm per 10 min (ordinate of graph). ●, Pig heart LDH; ▲, rabbit muscle LDH; ○, △, basals. (B) Effect of pH on superoxide radical production by macrophages. Reactions were conducted in phosphate buffer (125 mM) and with 300 units/m rabbit muscle LDH. ●, Macrophages (2.7×10^6 per milliliter; △, xanthine oxidase (0.1 U/ml) plus hypoxanthine (80 μM).

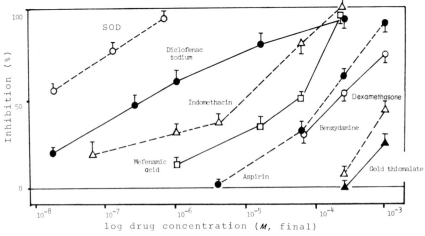

Fig. 5. Effect of various antiinflammatory drugs on superoxide radical production by peritoneal macrophages. From Ōyanagui (3) by permission.

TABLE I

Effect of Various Drugs on Superoxide Anion[a]

Drugs	Inhibitor of macrophage superoxide anion	Scavenger of superoxide anion
Antiinflammatory drugs		
Diclofenac sodium	+	−
Oxyphenbutazone	+	−
Indomethacin	+	±
Phenylbutazone	+	−
Mefenamic acid	+	−
Flufenamic acid	+	−
Colchicine	+	+
Aspirin	±	−
Benzydamine	±	−
MK-447	−	−
Superoxide dismutase	+	+
Dexamethasone	−	−
Gold thiomalate	−	−
Metal cation (chloride)		
Cu^{2+}	+	+
Mn^{2+}, Fe^{2+}, Hg^{2+}	+	±
Fe^{3+}, Ni^{2+}, Co^{2+}	±	−
Na^+, K^+, Ca^{2+}, Ba^{2+}	−	−
Cd^{2+}, Pb^{2+}, Pt^{4+}	−	−
Au^{3+}, Zn^{2+}	−	−

Drugs	Inhibitor of macrophage superoxide anion	Scavenger of superoxide anion
Nonantiinflammatory drugs		
Cytochalasin B	+	−
Pyrogallol	+	±
Ascorbate	+	+
N-Ethylmaleimide	+	−
L-Epinephrine	+	−
Chlorpromazine	±	±
Allopurinol	−	+
Catalase	−	
d-Mannitol	−	
1,3-Diphenylisobenzofuran	−	
Sodium azide	−	
Monoiodoacetate	−	
Penicillin	−	
Mitomycin C	−	
5-Fluorouracil	−	
Theophylline	−	
Nitroglycerin	−	
Cytochalasin A	−	

[a] The assay for detecting inhibition of superoxide anion production by peritoneal macrophages is illustrated in Fig. 3. The detection of superoxide anion scavenging depended on an assay employing xanthine oxidase and is illustrated in Fig. 3. Key: +, 50% inhibition by the test compound at a concentration equal to or less than $10^{-4}\ M$; ±, 50% inhibition by the test compound at a concentration between 10^{-4} and $10^{-3}\ M$; −, 50% inhibition by the test compound at a concentration equal to or greater than $10^{-3}\ M$.

duction, may act by altering the structure of the cell membrane or by inhibiting the superoxide-producing enzyme. Pyrogallol, ascorbate, and chlorpromazine may scavenge superoxide that is already produced. Allopurinol, a specific inhibitor for xanthine oxidase, was not inhibitory in the macrophage system. Catalase, other scavengers of active oxygen, and inhibitors of oxidative metabolism has no effect. Antibiotics, antitumor drugs, and various other drugs also had no effect. None of the drugs tested inhibited LDH activity.

Role of Anions in Activating Superoxide Radical Production by Macrophages and in Formation of Rat Paw Edema

It is known that superoxide production by macrophages is stimulated by certain anions contained in the assay medium measured by both the LDH–NADH method and the ferricytochrome c methods (5). Superoxide production by xanthine oxidase did not require the presence of these anions. The first group of stimulators tested included phosphate (P_i), pyrophosphate (PP_i), and sulfate (SO_4^{2-}), which were required in high concentrations (10^{-2} M) but which were effective, producing a two- to fivefold stimulation. The second group of stimulators of oxygen radical production included ATP, ADP, AMP, UTP, and ITP. The extent of stimulation was lower, but the effect was achieved at lower concentrations (10^{-3}–10^{-6} M). Many other anions tested, including Cl^-, NO_3^-, NO_2^-, SO_3^{2-}, SCN^-, and BO_4^{3-}, were ineffective. Only fluoride showed a twofold increase in superoxide production at 100 mM after a short time of incubation (5). The stimulatory effects of ATP, sulfate, and PP_i were additive but were suppressed with superoxide dismutase or Diclofenac (sodium). It is interesting that the anions found abundantly in areas of inflammation stimulated macrophage superoxide production. The level of PP_i is elevated in synovial fluids of osteoarthritis and pseudogout patients (11). The concentration of PP_i in extracellular fluid appears to be important in determining the quantity of calcium pyrophosphate crystals present in pseudogout inflammation (12). Phosphate can be produced by the decomposition of PP_i and ATP. Injections of PP_i or ATP into rats produce inflammation (13,14). It has been reported that ATP and ADP are potent stimulators of prostaglandin biosynthesis in various organs (15). Sulfate can be produced from hyaluronic acid by hydrolytic enzymes, the levels of which are elevated in synovial fluid of rheumatic patients (16). These stimulatory anions have the capacity to produce and maintain the inflammatory swelling of rat paws for up to 6 hr after intraplantar injection (5). Chloride and nitrate resulted in only temporary swelling, which diminished after 1 hr. This swelling may be caused by either osmotic shock or histamine release. Nevertheless, the stimulatory anions that produced superoxide anions maintained the swelling for up to 6 hr. Intravenous injection of superoxide dismutase produced partial inhibition (20–40%) of this chemically induced swelling at 6 hr. This inhibition is significant because in general the paw edema cannot be inhibited more than 60%.

Stimulatory Effect of Platinic Ion on the Production of Superoxide Radical by Xanthine Oxidase and Macrophages

Sodium platinic chloride (Na_2PtCl_6) and sodium gold chloride ($NaAuCl_4$) were found to be very effective stimulators in both the macrophage and xanthine oxidase test system (17). Platinic ion has long been known as a bactericidal agent. cis-Platinum(II, IV) diaminodichlorides are currently in use in clinical trials for cancer therapy (18). The stimulatory effect of platinic ion on the production of superoxide radical was observed in the range 0.1–1 mM and was inhibited by superoxide dismutase (17). Platinic ion may act by stabilizing superoxide radical or by generating more superoxide by a redox cycling similar to the action of paraquat (19) and streptonigrin (20). Antitumor agents, such as mitomycin C, bleomycin, and adriamycin, are presumed to act through their capacity to form active oxygen radicals (21–23).

The inflammatory effect in vivo of sodium platinic chloride (4 or 8 μmol per guinea pig paw) is illustrated in Fig. 6. The drug was injected into the plantar surface as an emulsion of 10% water and 90% olive oil, Figure 6A shows a typical paw 3 weeks after injection. Four weeks after injection the paw resembles a teratological deformity in which cartilage and bones are heavily damaged (Fig. 6B and C). Copper acetate, ferric chloride, lead chloride, and cadmium chloride, all administered at concentrations equimolar to sodium platinic chloride, do not produce similar damage.

SUPEROXIDE-SCAVENGING EFFECTS OF TUMOR ASCITES FLUIDS AND OF BLOOD PLASMA

Ehrlich and L-1210 ascites tumor cells from mice oxidized NADH in the absence of macrophages, yet the NADH oxidation was not inhibited by superoxide dismutase. Sarcoma 180 and P-388 tumor cells gave similar

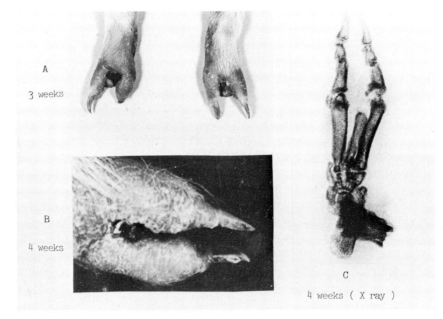

Fig. 6. Effect of sodium platinic chloride on guinea pig paw. Sodium platinic chloride (4 or 8 μmol) was injected into the plantar surface of guinea pig paw as an emulsion (0.2 ml containing 10% water and 90% olive oil).

results. Ehrlich ascites tumor cells did not scavenge superoxide radicals generated by xanthine oxidase, but the extracellular ascites fluid was effective (Fig. 7). This superoxide-scavenging effect could not be accounted for by contaminating erythrocytes or hemoglobin. Blood plasma from normal mice and Ehrlich-tumor-bearing mice at high protein concentration also scavenged superoxide radicals generated by xanthine and xanthine oxidase, with 50% inhibition in the assay system occurring at approximately 4 mg/ml protein. Bovine serum albumin (BSA) scavenged superoxide produced by xanthine oxidase at high concentrations, 5 mg/ml. It is probable that the scavenging effect of tumor ascites fluid derives from albumin-like protein in the fluid. The same oxygen-radical-scavenging effect of both BSA and ascites fluid was observed when oxygen radicals were produced by mouse peritoneal macrophages (Fig. 8). Tumor ascites fluid may therefore protect tumor cells from the attack of active oxygen radicals. It is also possible that blood plasma protects blood vessels from cytotoxic oxygen radicals. Of course, superoxide dismutase may be released from broken cells into these extracellular fluids, but there are no data on this point.

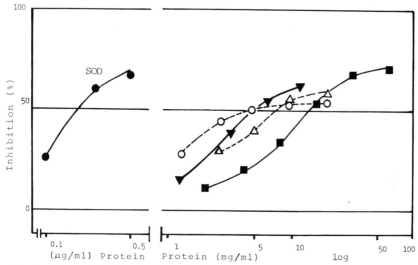

Fig. 7. Percent inhibition by various inhibitors of superoxide radicals generated by xanthine oxidase (0.05 U/ml) (average of two experiments). The assay was conducted according to the procedure described in Fig. 3. Key: ●, SOD; ○, Ehrlich ascites tumor-bearing mice blood plasma; △, BSA; ■, Ehrlich ascites fluid; ▲, normal mice blood plasma.

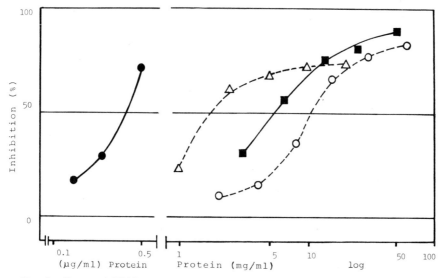

Fig. 8. Percent inhibition by various inhibitors of superoxide radicals generated by mouse macrophages (6–8 × 10⁵/ml) (average of two experiments). The assay was conducted according to the procedure described in Fig. 3. Key: ●, SOD; △, BSA; ■, Ehrlich ascites fluid; ○, sarcoma 180 ascites fluid.

CONCLUSIONS

Superoxide and other related active oxygen compounds produced by macrophages or granulocytes may work in many ways. My concept of the role of active oxygen in biological systems is shown in Fig. 9. Phagocytosis or cell contact with bacteria or immune complexes (24,25) may alter membrane structure or receptor(s) on macrophages and granulocytes, which activates NAD(P)H oxidase. This enzyme produces superoxide (26). Anions such as P_i, PP_i, and ATP stimulate this step (3,4). Superoxide may be released into phagocyte vacuoles and on the surface of the cell membrane. Bactericidal activity (27), inflammation (1,2), tumoricidal activity (28), and damage of cell components (29) by superoxide may be amplified by the existence of platinic ion, paraquat, or some type of antitumor agent. Several reports have demonstrated that superoxide regulates prostaglandin production (30,31). Rapid removal of the strongly inflammatory PGG_2 by a drug such as MK-447 is a way of moderating the development of inflammation (32). Thromboxane B_2 (TXB_2) and PGG_2 are reportedly chemotactic (33,34). The products of the synthetic process, PGE_2 and PGF_2, must serve as signals to terminate the inflammatory process through the suppression of lymphocyte transformation and the release of lymphokine migration inhibitory factor (MIF) (35–37). The concentration of PGG_2 (positively) and PGE_2 (negatively) may balance the activation and/or accumulation of macrophages at the site of inflammation. The exact role of prostacyclin (PGI_2) must still be clarified. It should

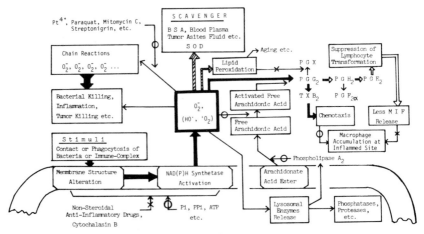

Fig. 9. Scheme depicting the possible biological role of superoxide radicals produced by macrophages (○, stimulation; X, inhibition).

be noted that lipid peroxides inhibit the formation of PGI$_2$ (38). Peroxidation of fatty acids other than arachidonic acid should be investigated for its role in the development of inflammation. It has been reported that hydroxyl radical (HO·) attacks lysosomal membranes (39), and the released enzymes may produce the inflammation. Phospholipase A$_2$ can be released from plasma membranes or lysosomes and can increase free arachidonic acid. Activation of free arachidonic acid by superoxide is reported to be necessary for efficient PG synthesis in platelets (40).

In conclusion, the importance of the site where superoxide-producing cells are operating should be emphasized, because not only superoxide dismutase but also blood plasma and tumor ascites fluid can scavenge superoxide. Furthermore, the stimulation of superoxide production of macrophages and granulocytes by P$_i$, PP$_i$, ATP, and related compounds must be considered.

REFERENCES

1. McCord, J. M. (1974). Free radicals and inflammation: Protection of synovial fluid by superoxide dismutase. *Science* **185**:529.
2. Ōyanagui, Y. (1976). Participation of superoxide anions at the prostaglandin phase of carrageenan foot-edema. *Biochem. Pharmacol.* **25**:1465.
3. Ōyanagui, Y. (1976). Inhibition of superoxide anion production in macrophages by anti-inflammatory drugs. *Biochem. Pharmacol.* **25**:1473.
4. Ōyanagui, Y. (1978). Inhibition of superoxide anion production in non-stimulated guinea pig peritoneal exudate cells by anti-inflammatory drugs. *Biochem. Pharmacol.* **27**:777.
5. Ōyanagui, Y. (1977). Role of phosphate, pyrophosphate, adenine nucleotides and sulfate in activating production of the superoxide radical by macrophages, and in formation of rat paw edema. *Agents Actions* **7**:125.
6. Vinegar, R., Schreiber, W., and Hugo, R. (1969). Biphasic development of carrageenin edema in rats. *J. Pharmacol. Exp. Ther.* **166**:96.
7. DiRosa, M., Giroud, J. P., and Willoughby, D. A. (1971). Studies on the mediators of the acute inflammatory response induced in rats in different sites by carrageenan and turpentine. *J. Pathol.* **104**:15.
8. DiRosa, M., Papadiumitroiou, J. M., and Willoughby, D. A. (1971). A histopathological and pharmacological analysis of the mode of action of nonsteroidal anti-inflammatory drugs. *J. Pathol.* **105**:239.
9. Mason, R. J., Stossel, T. P., and Vaughan, M. (1972). Lipids of alveolar macrophages, polymorphonuclear leukocytes, and their phagocytic vesicles. *J. Clin. Invest.* **51**:2399.
10. Chan, P. C., and Bielski, B. H. J. (1974). Enzyme-catalyzed free radical reactions with nicotinamide adenine nucleotides. II. Lactate dehydrogenase-catalyzed oxidation of reduced nicotinamide adenine dinucleotide by superoxide radicals generated by xanthine oxidase. *J. Biol. Chem.* **249**:1317.
11. Silcox, D. C., and McCarty, D. J. (1974). Elevated inorganic pyrophosphate concentrations in synovial fluids in osteoarthritis and pseudogout. *J. Lab. Clin. Med.* **83**:518.

12. Bennett, R. M., Lehr, J. R., and McCarty, D. J. (1975). Factors affecting the solubility of calcium pyrophosphate dihydrate crystals. *J. Clin. Invest.* **56**:1571.
13. Tomita, K., Ichikawa, A., and Hayashi, H. (1972). Effects of cyclic 3′,5′-adenosine monophosphate on inflammation induced by inorganic pyrophosphate, ATP and other phlogistins. *Jpn. J. Pharmacol.* **22**:8.
14. Willoughby, D. A., Dunn, C. J., Yamamoto, S., Capasso, F., Deporter, D. A., and Giroud, J. P. (1975). Calcium pyrophosphate-induced pleurisy in rats: A new model of acute inflammation. *Agents Actions* **5**:35.
15. Needleman, P., Minks, M. S., and Douglas, R., Jr. (1974). Stimulation of prostaglandin biosynthesis by adenine nucleotides. Profile of prostaglandin release by perfused organs. *Circ. Res.* **34**:455.
16. Ghosh, P., Stephens, R. W., and Taylor, T. K. F. (1975). The inhibition of synovial fluid polysaccharidases by gold sodium thiomalate. *Med. J. Aust.* **1**:317.
17. Ōyanagui, Y. (1977). Stimulatory effect of platinum (IV) ion on the production of superoxide radical from xanthine oxidase and macrophages. *Biochem. Pharmacol.* **26**:473.
18. Rosenberg, B., and VanCamp, L. (1970). The successful regression of large solid sarcoma 180 tumors by platinum compounds. *Cancer Res.* **30**:1799.
19. Autor, A. P. (1974). Reduction of paraquat toxicity by superoxide dismutase. *Life Sci.* **14**:1309.
20. Gregory, E. M., and Fridovich, I. (1973). Oxygen toxicity and the superoxide dismutase. *J. Bacteriol.* **114**:1193.
21. Ishida, R., and Takahashi, T. (1975). Increased DNA chain breakage by combined action of bleomycin and superoxide radical. *Biochem. Biophys. Res. Commun.* **66**:1432.
22. Handa, K., and Sato, S. (1975). Generation of free radicals of quinone group-containing anti-cancer chemicals in NADPH-microsome system as evidenced by initiation by sulfite oxidation. *Gann* **66**:43.
23. Fridovich, I. (1978). The biology of oxygen radicals. *Science* **201**:875.
24. Goldstein, I. M., Roos, D., Kaplan, H. B., and Weissmann, G. (1975). Complement and immunoglobins stimulate superoxide production by human leukocytes independently of phagocytes. *J. Clin. Invest.* **56**:1155.
25. Johnston, R. B., Jr., Lehmeyer, J. E., and Guthrie, L. A. (1976). Generation of superoxide anion and chemiluminescence by human monocytes during phagocytosis and on contact with surface-bound immunoglobin G. *J. Exp. Med.* **143**:1551.
26. Takanaka, K., and O'Brien, P. J. (1975). Mechanisms of H_2O_2 formation by leukocytes. Evidence for a plasma membrane location. *Arch. Biochem. Biophys.* **169**:428.
27. Curnutte, J. T., and Babior, B. M. (1975). Biological defense mechanisms. The effect of bacteria and serum on superoxide production by granulocytes. *J. Clin. Invest.* **53**:1662.
28. Edelson, P. J., and Cohn, Z. A. (1973). Peroxidase-mediated mammalian cell cytotoxicity. *J. Exp. Med.* **138**:318.
29. Lavelle, F., Michelson, A. M., and Dimetrijevic, L. (1973). Biological protection by superoxide dismutase. *Biochem. Biophys. Res. Commun.* **55**:350.
30. Rahimutula, A., and O'Brien, P. J. (1976). The possible involvement of singlet oxygen in prostaglandin biosynthesis. *Biochem. Biophys. Res. Commun.* **70**:893.
31. Zenser, T. V., Levitt, M. J., and Davis, B. B. (1977). Possible modulation of rat renal prostaglandin production by oxygen. *Am. J. Physiol.* **233**:F239.
32. Kuehl, F. A., Jr., Humes, J. L., Ham, R. W., Beveridge, G. C., and Van Arman, C. G. (1977). Role of prostaglandin endoperoxide PGG_2 in inflammatory processes. *Nature (London)* **265**:170.
33. Walker, J. R., Smith, M. G. H., and Ford-Hutchinson, A. W. (1976). Prostaglandins and leucotaxis. *J. Pharm. Pharmacol.* **28**:745.
34. Boot, J. R., Dawson, W., and Kitchen, E. A. (1976). The chemotactic activity of thromborane B_2: A possible role in inflammation. *J. Physiol. (London)* **257**:47P.

35. Gordon, D., Bray, M. A., and Morley, J. (1976). Control of lymphokine secretion by prostaglandins. *Nature* (*London*) **262**:401.
36. Goodwin, J. S., Bankhurst, A. D., and Messner, R. P. (1977). Suppression of human T-cell mitogenesis by prostaglandin. Existence of a prostaglandin-producing suppressor cell. *J. Exp. Med.* **146**:1719.
37. Webb, D. R., and Nowowiejski, I. (1977). The role of prostaglandins in the control of the primary 19S immune response to SRBC. *Cell. Immunol.* **33**:1.
38. Gryglewski, R. J., Bunting, S., Moncada, S., Flower, R. J., and Vane, R. (1976). Arterial walls are protected against deposition of platelet thrombi by a substance (prostaglandin *X*) which they make from prostaglandin endoperoxides. *Prostaglandins* **12**:685.
39. Fong, K.-L., McCay, P. B., Poyer, J. L., Keele, B. B., and Misra, H. (1973). Evidence that peroxidation of lysosomal membranes is initiated by hydroxyl free radicals produced during flavin enzyme activity. *J. Biol. Chem.* **248**:7792.
40. White, J. G., Rao, H. R., and Gerrad, J. M. (1977). Effects of nitroblue tetrazolium and Vitamin E on platelet untrastructure, aggregation, and secretion. *Am. J. Pathol.* **88**:387.

DISCUSSION

COHEN: In the detection system based on NADH oxidation, how do you distinguish between trapping superoxide and decreasing the chain of free-radical reactions?

ŌYANAGUI: It is impossible to distinguish between them, but trapping the initiating superoxide radical always resulted in decreased O_2^- production. The oxidation of NADH in my system was linear for at least 15 min and was suppressed completely with 4 μg/ml of superoxide dismutase. This was sufficient for my purpose, which was to check the inhibitory effects of drugs. The inhibited NADH oxidations were always linear and dose dependent.

BABIOR: What is the physiological significance of the tumor fluid effects on O_2^- production by macrophages?

ŌYANAGUI: Tumor cells may be protected from the attack of O_2^- on their growth and survival. I noted this phenomenon only recently, so I cannot say anything about the protecting component(s). It may be an albumin-like protein that is attracted to tumor cells.

ADDENDUM

The following new papers from this laboratory have been published and the observations, which are not included in this symposium report, are abstracted.

1. Ōyanagui, Y. (1980) Inflammation and superoxide production by macrophages. *Agents and Actions* **7**, Suppl. 174.

Nitroblue tetrazolium reduction by macrophages cultured with lymphocytes from BCG sensitized guinea pig and antigen (purified protein derivatives), was inhibited by superoxide dismutase ($10-100$ μg/ml) or D-mannitol ($10^{-4}-10^{-2}M$). Hydroxyl radical seemed to be involved in the cellular immunity.

2. Ōyanagui, Y. (1980) Superoxide and inflammation. *In* "Biological and Clinical Aspects of Superoxide and Superoxide Dismutase 11B." (W. H. Bannister and J. V. Bannister, eds.), p. 147. Elsevier/North-Holland, Amsterdam).

Inflammatory peritoneal fluids of rats induced by formalin (10 ml/kg) showed superoxide dismutase-like activities which began to increase at 4 hr. and reached 60% at 72 hr. Different molecular size substances in the fluid interact for this inhibitory activity and may work to limit the excessive development of acute inflammation.

3. Ōyanagui, Y. (1981) Steroid-like anti-inflammatory effect of superoxide dismutase in serotonin-, histamine- and kinin-induced edemata of mice: existence of vascular permeability regulating protein(s). *Biochem. Pharmacol.* **30:** 1791.

Subcutaneously administered superoxide dismutase (5 mg/kg) and dexamethasone (1 mg/kg) showed the maximum suppression of serotonin-induced paw edema of mice only after 2 hrs. of lag time. Prostaglandin inhibitor indomethacin (5–30 mg/kg) failed to suppress this model of inflammation. Cycloheximide, puromycin, or actinomycin treatment blocked the inhibitory effect of superoxide dismutase and dexamethasone and even increased the swelling of moderately inflamed paw edema. Superoxide dismutase may not stimulate adrenals and is postulated to diminish the degradation of the steroid-inducible unknown protein(s). This protein(s) may suppress the vascular permeability and have rapid turnover.

Chapter **8**

Oxygen Radicals, Hydrogen Peroxide, and Parkinson's Disease

GERALD COHEN

INTRODUCTION

Parkinson's disease is a disorder involving accelerated aging of the ni-grostriatal tract of the brain. The neurotransmitter in the nigrostriatal tract is dopamine, a catecholamine. Treatment of Parkinson's disease is directed toward supporting and/or supplementing neurotransmitter activity in order to restore control over motor function (namely, to ameliorate tremor and rigidity). This is accomplished most frequently with L-dopa, an amino acid precursor of dopamine. However, current evidence indicates that the underlying disease process continues during drug therapy, with progressive loss of dopamine-secreting neurons.

The experiments described here were undertaken to obtain an under-standing of the molecular mechanisms that may contribute to accelerated senescence or aging in catecholamine-secreting neurons. It is hoped that through such understanding will come the means to prevent or control the debilitating loss of neurons that is characteristic of Parkinson's disease and other neuronal disorders.

The experiments focused on several nerve cell toxins that selectively destroy monoamine neurons in experimental animals. The toxins are 6-hydroxydopamine (6-OHDA), 6-aminodopamine (6-ADA), and 5,7-dihy-droxytryptamine (5,7-DHT). Two of these neuronal toxins (6-OHDA and

115

PATHOLOGY OF OXYGEN
Copyright © 1982 by Academic Press, Inc.
All rights of reproduction in any form reserved.
ISBN 0-12-068620-1

6-ADA) spontaneously generate hydrogen peroxide (H_2O_2) and two free radicals, the superoxide radical and the hydroxyl radical, in aqueous solution. The third (5,7-DHT) generates H_2O_2 in an enzymatic reaction with monoamine oxidase; it is presumed, but has not been conclusively proved, that hydroxyl radicals are also generated. The neuronal toxins exert selective destructive effects in monoamine neurons *in vivo* because they are actively accumulated at the sites where damage takes place.

6-HYDROXYDOPAMINE AND 6-AMINODOPAMINE

In Vitro Observations (Superoxide Radicals)

6-Hydroxydopamine and 6-aminodopamine are analogs of dopamine (3,4-dihydroxyphenylethylamine) in which the 6 position is substituted with either a hydroxyl or an amino group. Unlike dopamine, these compounds are extremely unstable and are rapidly oxidized by molecular oxygen in less than 1 min at neutral pH to form quinoidal products and hydrogen peroxide (5). During this rapid autoxidation process, superoxide radicals are generated as intermediates and hydroxyl radicals are generated as by-products (2). The generation of the superoxide anion-radical is evident from the action of superoxide dismutase: Addition of superoxide dismutase markedly slows the formation of both H_2O_2 and quinoidal products (5). A proposed mechanism for the action of superoxide dismutase is similar to that put forth by Misra and Fridovich (7) for the autoxidation of epinephrine; namely, the first step [Eq. (1)] in the autoxidation reaction is relatively slow compared to later steps. Superoxide radicals (O_2^-) can oxidize 6-OHDA directly [Eq. (2)], bypassing the slow step and setting up a chain mechanism in which superoxide is regenerated [Eq. (3)] to function once again. Thus, in the presence of superoxide, the formation of H_2O_2 is catalyzed [reactions (2) and (3)]; the formation of quinone is also catalyzed by superoxide. The addition of superoxide dismutase inhibits reaction (2) and slows the overall rate of accumulation of H_2O_2 and quinone. It is assumed that, in this sequence, reaction (3) is also relatively fast and that the rate limitation exists at reaction (1).

$$6\text{-OHDA} + O_2 \rightarrow \text{semiquinone (SQ}^{\cdot}) + O_2^- + H^+ \qquad \text{slow} \qquad (1)$$

$$6\text{-OHDA} + O_2^- + H^+ \rightarrow SQ^{\cdot} + H_2O_2 \qquad \text{fast} \qquad (2)$$

$$SQ^{\cdot} + O_2 \rightarrow \text{quinone} + O_2^- + H^+ \qquad \text{fast} \qquad (3)$$

6-Aminodopamine behaves differently. Although the autoxidation rate at neutral pH is just as fast as that for 6-OHDA, and although superoxide is an intermediate and both H_2O_2 and quinones are products, the overall rate of reaction is *insensitive* to superoxide dismutase. It appears that, for 6-ADA, reaction (1) is fast and no rate limitation exists with regard to the reaction with oxygen. Thus, the catalysis of H_2O_2 production and quinone production from 6-OHDA by superoxide represents a basic difference between 6-OHDA and 6-ADA. This difference provides an experimental tool for *in vivo* studies.

In Vivo Studies (Superoxide Radicals)

In vivo experiments were designed to evaluate whether superoxide radicals play a critical role in the neurodegenerative action of 6-OHDA. Rats received iv injections of 6-OHDA or 6-ADA, and several hours later the integrity of the sympathetic (catecholamine) nerve plexus in the iris was studied with a tritium tracer method (8). Because catecholamines, in general, scavenge superoxide radicals (e.g., epinephrine oxidation by superoxide), it seemed probable that the endogenous catecholamine neurotransmitter (norepinephrine) in sympathetic nerves would be capable of competing with 6-OHDA for generated superoxide radicals. If this occurred, the formation of damaging quinones and H_2O_2 would be suppressed. Normal rats and rats whose neurons were depleted of norepinephrine by prior drug treatment (α-methyl-*p*-tyrosine) were tested. It had been shown previously (6) that rats depleted of norepinephrine were more sensitive to 6-OHDA. In our experiments, the norepinephrine content of one iris was restored to normal by intraocular injection of norepinephrine. Damage to neurons in the left versus right iris in the same rat was then compared. As a control, intraocular injection of octopamine was used. Octopamine is not a catechol (Fig. 1), and it does not scavenge su-

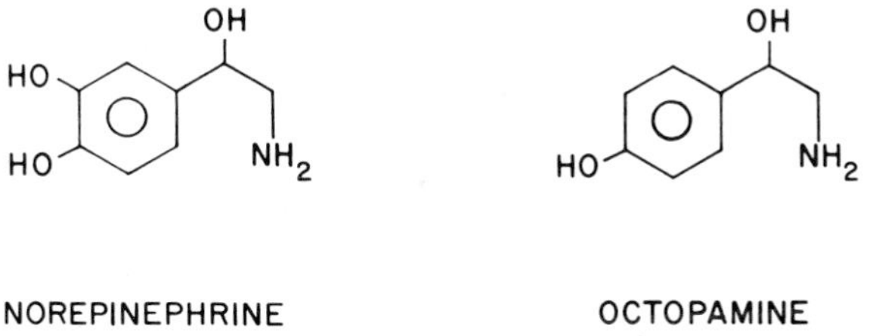

NOREPINEPHRINE   OCTOPAMINE

Fig. 1. Structures of norepinephrine and octopamine. Norepinephrine, the principal neurotransmitter in the sympathetic nervous system, reacts vigorously with superoxide radical. Octopamine is a "false neurotransmitter" which, like norepinephrine, is avidly taken up and concentrated by sympathetic nerve terminals. Octopamine does not react with superoxide radicals.

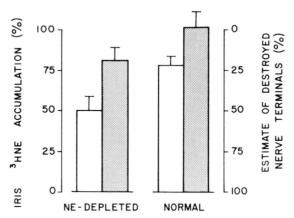

Fig. 2. The neurotoxicity of 6-OHDA and protection of the sympathetic nerve plexus in the iris by norepinephrine (NE). Normal rats and rats depleted of endogenous norepinephrine received intraocular injections of either saline (left eye, open bars) or 50 ng norepinephrine in saline (right eye, stippled bars) 1 hr before intravenous injection of 6-OHDA (5 mg/kg). Prior injection of norepinephrine protected the right iris. The measurement of [³H]norepinephrine uptake by isolated irides *in vitro* 4 hr after 6-OHDA injection served to estimate the degree of destruction of nerve terminals. In separate control experiments, it was shown that intraocular norepinephrine did not block the accumulation of 6-OHDA by nerve terminals in the iris. Data from Sachs *et al.* (8).

peroxide. However, both norepinephrine and octopamine are taken up and accumulated by sympathetic nerve endings in the iris.

We observed (8) that repletion of the norepinephrine content in the iris by means of an intraocular injection protected the iris against neuronal destruction (Fig. 2). Injection of octopamine, on the other hand, was without effect. When 6-ADA was used as a neurotoxin, no protective action was observed with either norepinephrine or with octopamine. These results (Table I) are as expected if superoxide radicals play an important role in regulating the toxicity of 6-OHDA but not 6-ADA.

In Vitro and *in Vivo* Studies (Hydroxyl Radicals)

Other studies focused on the potential toxic role of the hydroxyl radical (HO·), which can be generated as a by-product of H_2O_2, particularly when superoxide radicals are present. It was observed that both 6-OHDA and 6-ADA generate hydroxyl radicals *in vitro* during their respective rapid autoxidation (2). In chemical studies *in vitro*, the hydroxyl-radical-scavenging agent, 2-keto-4-thiomethyl butyrate, was used to assess HO· production. A product of the reaction is ethylene gas, which can be measured

TABLE I

Comparison of the Properties of 6-OHDA and 6-ADA

	Effect	
Condition	6-OHDA	6-ADA
Autoxidation *in vitro*		
Catalyzed by superoxide radicals	Yes	No
Slowed by norepinephrine	Yes	No
Slowed by octopamine	No	No
Neurotoxicity *in vivo*		
Diminished by norepinephrine	Yes	No
Enhanced by depletion of norepinephrine	Yes	No
Diminished by octopamine	No	No

by gas chromatography. Results shown in Table II indicate that hydroxyl radical production from 6-ADA is dependent on superoxide (inhibition by superoxide dismutase) and also on H_2O_2 (inhibition by catalase). Competitive scavengers of $HO^{\cdot}$, such as ethanol, benzoate, and thiourea, suppressed ethylene production (Table II). Urea, which is not an effective

TABLE II

Hydroxyl Radical Production by 6-ADA Measured by Formation of Ethylene Gas from 2-Keto-4-Thiomethylbutyric acid[a]

Addition	Amount added	$k(\cdot OH)$ (M^{-1} sec^{-1})	Ethylene[b] (% control level)
Control (no additions)	—		1.30 ± 0.08 nmol
Catalase	33 μg/ml		3.9 ± 0.1
Superoxide dismutase	50 μg/ml		51.3 ± 2.5
Ethanol	0.5 mM	1×10^9	90.1 ± 2.3
	5.0 mM		52.2 ± 1.5
Benzoate	0.5 mM	3×10^9	84.1 ± 3.7
Thiourea	0.5 mM	5×10^9	66.8 ± 1.8
	5.0 mM		15.5 ± 0.5
Methimazole	0.5 mM	Unknown	58.5 ± 2.0
PTTU	0.5 mM	Unknown	57.9 ± 3.0
Urea	0.5 mM	7×10^5	97.6 ± 2.4

[a] The reaction system contained 1 mM 2-keto-4-thiomethylbutyric acid, 1 mM H_2O_2, and 0.1 mM EDTA at pH 8.0. This elevated pH was required to solubilize 0.5 mM PTTU. The reaction was initiated by the addition of 6-ADA to 0.1 mM. Ethylene was measured at 6 min.

[b] Mean $\pm$ standard error with 7–10 samples. All results except urea were $p < .01$; for urea, $p > .4$. Data from Cohen *et al.* (4).

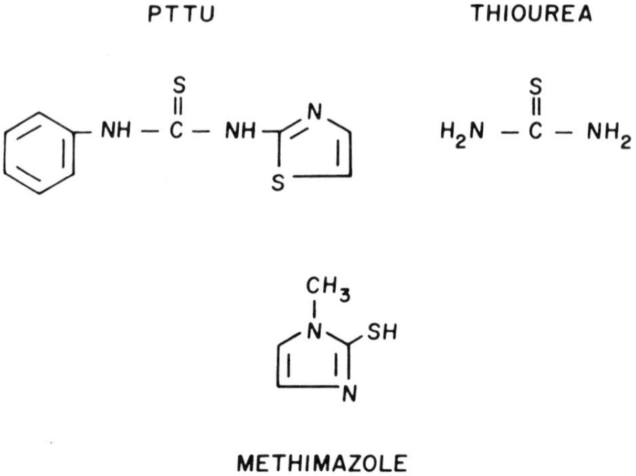

PTTU   THIOUREA

METHIMAZOLE

Fig. 3.   Structures of thiourea and two thiourea derivatives: methimazole and PTTU. The latter two can be taken up and concentrated by sympathetic neurons.

scavenger of HO·, was without significant action (Table II). In addition, two thiourea analogs, methimazole and 1-phenyl-3-(2-thiazolyl)-2-thiourea (PTTU) (Fig. 3), were also tested and were found to be effective scavengers of hydroxyl radicals. Methimazole and PTTU possess the special property of being accumulated *in vivo* in catecholamine neurons.

In vivo studies tested the efficacy of hydroxyl radical scavengers as protective agents against the neurotoxicity of 6-OHDA and 6-ADA (4). PTTU was a very effective protective agent (Table III). Methimazole was also effective. A small but significant protection was also observed with ethanol and 1-butanol (Table III). Therefore, it is apparent that hydroxyl radical scavengers can protect neurons against the destructive action of 6-OHDA or 6-ADA.

5,7-DIHYDROXYTRYPTAMINE

5,7-Dihydroxytryptamine is an unusual neuronal toxin. In peripheral sympathetic neurons, such as those in the heart or iris, 5,7-DHT exerts a destructive action that can be blocked by inhibitors of the enzyme monoamine oxidase. The enzymatic action of monoamine oxidase is shown in Eq. (4).

$$5,7\text{-DHT} + O_2 + H_2O \rightarrow 5,7\text{-dihydroxyphenylacetaldehyde} + H_2O_2 + NH_3 \quad (4)$$

Products of the reaction are an aldehyde and H_2O_2. Because H_2O_2 is a

TABLE III

Protection against the Neurodegenerative Action of 6-OHDA and 6-ADA by Hydroxyl Radical Scavengers[a]

Radical scavenger	Dose, g/kg	Neurotoxin	Dose, mg/kg	Nerve plexus, % control ± SEM (N)	
				− Scavenger	+ Scavenger
PTTU	0.2	6-ADA	10	31.8 ± 3.0 (22)	95.8 ± 5.6 (19)
PTTU	0.2	6-OHDA	7.5	21.6 ± 2.0 (22)	97.0 ± 3.3 (22)
PTTU	0.2	6-OHDA	10	17.3 ± 0.8 (109)	68.3 ± 4.5 (62)
Ethanol	4.0	6-OHDA	4	40.7 ± 3.8 (28)	58.7 ± 5.6 (26)
n-Butanol	0.8	6-OHDA	4	32.8 ± 2.9 (26)	49.7 ± 3.9 (27)
Methimazole	0.4	6-OHDA	4	28.4 ± 3.1 (18)	63.1 ± 6.2 (21)

[a] Drugs were administered intraperitoneally to male Swiss–Webster mice 1 hr before intravenous injection of 6-OHDA or 6-ADA. The doses of neurotoxin are expressed in terms of their acid salts, 6-OHDA · HBr and 6-ADA · 2HCl, respectively. After either 24 hr (PTTU experiments) or 4 hr (all other drugs), the left atria were removed, and the degree of neuronal damage was assessed. Measurement of the uptake of $[^3H]$norepinephrine served as an index of the integrity of the sympathetic nerve plexus in the left atrium. All p values with scavengers were less than .01 compared to the corresponding groups not pretreated with scavengers. Data from Cohen *et al.* (4).

product, it seemed reasonable to expect the formation of hydroxyl radicals. Experiments with HO· scavengers revealed that PTTU and ethanol were good protective agents against the toxicity of 5,7-DHT (Table IV). Therefore, it appears that 5,7-DHT may exert its toxic action in sympathetic nerves via the generation of hydroxyl radicals, promoted by monoamine oxidase.

A WORKING HYPOTHESIS FOR PARKINSON'S DISEASE

On the basis of the foregoing experiments, it is possible to formulate a working hypothesis about accelerated senescence of catecholamine neurons in Parkinson's disease (3). Let us suppose that H_2O_2 is generated in neurons via normal pathways of metabolism such as by monoamine oxidase and other enzymes. In catecholamine neurons, high levels of substrate (catecholamine) for monoamine oxidase are present. The catecholamine is mainly bound in vesicles, but a considerable quantity is also free in the cytoplasm. Therefore, the continuous oxidative deamination of ca-

TABLE IV

Protection against the Neurodegenerative Action of 5,7-DHT by Hydroxyl Radical Scavengers (PTTU, Ethanol) and an Inhibitor of Monoamine Oxidase (Nialamide)[a]

			Nerve plexus integrity, % control ± SEM (N)	
Protective agent	Dose, mg/kg	5,7-DHT, mg/kg	− Protective agent	+ Protective agent
PTTU	200	40	62.2 ± 6.9 (16)	102.8 ± 5.3 (12)
Nialamide	50	40	62.2 ± 6.9 (16)	95.6 ± 5.7 (5)
PTTU	200	60	34.9 ± 3.4 (35)	60.3 ± 5.4 (23)
Ethanol	4 g/kg	60	34.9 ± 3.4 (35)	72.5 ± 4.9 (13)
Nialamide	50	60	34.9 ± 3.4 (35)	81.4 ± 6.8 (9)

[a] PTTU and ethanol were administered intraperitoneally to male Swiss–Webster mice 1 hr before intravenous injection of 5,7-DHT. Nialamide was given intraperitoneally 2 hr before intravenous injection of 5,7-DHT. Twenty-four hours later, the left atria were removed, and the degree of neuronal damage was assessed. Measurement of the uptake of [³H]norepinephrine served as an index of the integrity of the nerve plexus. All p values with protective agents were less than .005 compared to control mice not receiving protective agents. Data from Allis and Cohen (1).

techolamine under steady-state conditions could represent a source of oxidative stress within these neurons. If a precipitating factor were present, the oxidative stress might be amplified to provoke an unusually high rate of senescence. Precipitating factors could fall into two classes: (a) defects in the usual mechanisms for detoxifying H_2O_2 or (b) a defect in catecholamine storage, resulting in the oxidative deamination of a larger than usual amount of catecholamines. It is known that the level of monoamine oxidase increases with age; therefore, an age-related activity change could be an important ancillary factor bringing out the expression of the disease in later life. If either (a) or (b) exists, a consequence would be increased cellular levels of both H_2O_2 and reactive oxygen free radicals. This could result in a biological pressure toward oxidative damage and accelerated aging.

An important factor to be considered is the simultaneous protective role of dopamine within the neurons of the nigrostriatal tract. As discussed earlier, dopamine and other catecholamines are good scavengers of superoxide. Therefore, the high dopamine levels in neurons could contribute to the scavenging of superoxide in neurons along with superoxide dismutase. This action of catecholamines could be beneficial to the neuron. Therefore, when catecholamine levels begin to fall, as in the earlier stages of Parkinson's disease,* the neuron may become increasingly disposed to an acceleration in senescence rate.†

This mechanism for deterioration of the nigrostriatal tract in Parkinson's disease is similar to but very much slower than that proposed for the destruction of neurons by 6-OHDA and 6-ADA. Essentially, H_2O_2 and oxygen radicals promote oxidative damage and accelerate the aging process. The natural characteristic of affected neurons (i.e., their catecholamine content) provides a reason for the relative specificity of the brain lesion.

H_2O_2 PRODUCTION IN BRAIN *IN VIVO*

Experiments were designed to detect H_2O_2 production in rat brain *in vivo* by a special reaction of catalase. The reaction involves aminotriazole, which inhibits catalase irreversibly only when H_2O_2 is present, as shown in reactions (5) and (6):

$$\text{Catalase} + H_2O_2 \rightarrow \text{compound I (catalase–}H_2O_2) \qquad (5)$$

$$\text{Compound I} + \text{aminotriazole} \rightarrow \text{inhibited catalase} \qquad (6)$$

Therefore, when inhibition of brain catalase by aminotriazole is observed, it can be inferred that H_2O_2 is present. When aminotriazole is injected into rats (9), the catalase in the brain parenchyma of the striatum is progressively inhibited (Table V). When ethanol is injected before aminotriazole, the catalase is protected. Ethanol is a substrate for the peroxidatic activity of catalase [Eq. (7)].

$$\text{Compound I} + \text{ethanol} \rightarrow \text{free catalase} + \text{acetaldehyde} \qquad (7)$$

Protection by ethanol is the result of reaction (7), which is competitive with reaction (6). These results with ethanol confirm that the aminotriazole method measures H_2O_2 production by brain. In these experiments, the catalase of erythrocytes and capillaries was carefully excluded.

---

* It is generally considered that the fall in dopamine levels in Parkinson's disease reflects a loss of dopamine-secreting neurons. However, this is by no means established. In this chapter, an alternative possibility is considered, namely, that endogenous dopamine levels may fall before overt neuronal senescence.

† Another assumption is required: The fall in dopamine levels has greater impact as a loss in superoxide-scavenging activity than as a loss in monoamine oxidase-related, H_2O_2-generating activity. Actually, this seems reasonable because monoamine oxidase levels increase with age, because an accentuation of a vesicular "storage defect" for dopamine could maintain or increase dopamine turnover, and because there are sources of H_2O_2 other than monoamine oxidase.

TABLE V

***In Vivo* Inhibition of Rat Brain Catalase by Injection of 3-Amino-1,2,4-Triazole**

Tissue[a]	Catalase, units/g (N)[b]		
	Control	1 hr	5 hr
Striatum	4.6 ± 0.8 (16)	2.5 ± 0.4 (12) (−45%)	0.8 ± 0.4 (4) (−82%)
Prefrontal/Cortex	5.7 ± 0.7 (12)	2.6 ± 0.7 (8) (−55%)	0.9 ± 0.3 (4) (−84%)

[a] The tissue supernatant was prepared by a careful, slow homogenization procedure. It was essentially free of contamination by catalase from either erythrocytes or capillaries.

[b] Units are the mean ± standard deviation. Control rats received ip saline in place of ip aminotriazole (1 g/kg). All values at 1 and 5 hr are $p < .001$ compared to controls. Data from Sinet *et al.* (9).

CONCLUSIONS

These experiments demonstrate that several nerve cell toxins exert their destructive actions on monoamine neurons via the generation of superoxide radicals, hydroxyl radicals, and H_2O_2. Sympathetic nerves are protected, in part, by endogenous catecholamines, which act as superoxide-scavenging agents. Strong protection is observed when scavengers of hydroxyl radicals are administered. In ancillary experiments, H_2O_2 production was observed in rat brain *in vivo*. An attempt has been made to integrate these observations into a working hypothesis concerning the accelerated senescence of catecholamine neurons seen in Parkinson's disease.

ACKNOWLEDGMENT

These studies were supported by USPHS Grant NS-11631, "Clinical Center for the Study of Parkinson's and Allied Diseases."

REFERENCES

1. Allis, B., and Cohen, G. (1977). The neurotoxicity of 5,7-dihydroxy-tryptamine in the mouse atrium: Protection by 1-phenyl-3-(2-thiazolyl)-2-thiourea and by ethanol. *Eur. J. Pharmacol.* **43**:269.

2. Cohen, G., and Heikkila, R. E. (1974). The generation of hydrogen peroxide, superoxide radical, and hydroxyl radical by 6-hydroxydopamine, dialuric acid and related cytotoxic agents. *J. Biol. Chem.* **249**:2447.
3. Cohen, G., Dembiec, D., Mytilineou, C., and Heikkila, R. E. (1976). Oxygen radicals and the integrity of the nigrostriatal tract. *In* "Advances in Parkinsonism. Biochemistry, Physiology, Treatment" (W. Birkmayer and O. Hornykiewicz, eds.), p. 251. Editiones Roche, Basle.
4. Cohen, G., Heikkila, R. E., Allis, B., Cabbat, F., Dembiec, D., MacNamee, D., Mytilineou, C., and Winston, B. (1976). Destruction of sympathetic nerve terminals by 6-hydroxydopamine: Protection by 1-phenyl-3-(2-thiazolyl)-2-thiourea, diethyldithiocarbamate, methimazole, cysteamine, ethanol and n-butanol. *J. Pharmacol. Exp. Ther.* **199**:336.
5. Heikkila, R. E., and Cohen, G. (1973). 6-Hydroxydopamine: Evidence for superoxide radical as an oxidative intermediate. *Science* **181**:456.
6. Jonsson, G., and Sachs, C. (1973). Effect of tyrosine hydroxylase inhibition on the action of 6-hydroxydopamine. *Res. Commun. Chem. Pathol. Pharmacol.* **5**:287.
7. Misra, H. P., and Fridovich, I. (1972). The role of the superoxide anion in the autoxidation of epinephrine and a simple assay for superoxide dismutase. *J. Biol. Chem.* **247**:3170.
8. Sachs, C., Jonsson, G., Heikkila, R., and Cohen, G. (1975). Control of the neurotoxicity of 6-hydroxydopamine by intraneuronal noradrenaline in rat iris. *Acta Physiol. Scand.* **93**:345.
9. Sinet, P. M., Heikkila, R. E., and Cohen, G. (1980). Hydrogen peroxide production by rat brain in vivo. *J. Neurochem.* **34**:1421.

DISCUSSION

OBERLEY: Why aren't there superoxide dismutases and catalases present to inhibit the type of damage you have described?

COHEN: We do not rule out cellular superoxide dismutase activity as a protective mechanism, but we also rule *in* superoxide scavenging by cellular catecholamines in high concentrations as a significant contributory mechanism. Catalase is present in a very small amount and is packaged (or compartmentalized) in small vesicles, the microperoxisomes. There is no catalase in mitochondria. Glutathione peroxidase is present, in a small amount, in both mitochondria and cell cytoplasm and probably contributes significantly as a protective factor.

SHEREMATA: If the primary defect in Parkinson's disease is one of storage, one would expect an accelerated rate of deterioration in patients treated with L-dopa. This presumes that L-dopa administration results in increased dopamine production, which is generally assumed. Parkinsonian patients do not deteriorate more rapidly, however, Also, would you please comment on the use of deprenyl (the B-monoamine oxidase inhibitor), which has recently come into use in the treatment of this clinical disorder? One might expect either acceleration or slowing of the clinical course. However, in the Oxford studies neither was seen, although the "on–off" phenomenon was significantly ameliorated.

COHEN: L-Dopa would be expected to have three actions: (a) Conversion to dopamine is beneficial because it facilitates neurotransmission; (b) deamination of dopamine is damaging because it produces H_2O_2; and (c) L-dopa itself is beneficial because it is a catechol and, as such, can contribute to O_2^- scavenging. It is difficult to predict if (b) and (c), on balance, would result in increased damage or increased protection. However, it is known that the progressive deterioration of the nigrostriatal tract continues during L-dopa therapy. Deprenyl is of special interest to us because its action as a monoamine oxidase inhibitor may result in diminished senescence of dopamine neurons. No data are available as yet on its potential action.

CUTLER: How does the superoxide dismutase level in the brain tissue of patients with Parkinson's disease compare with that of the normal population?

COHEN: A small number of analyses performed by Dick Heikkila have not revealed any difference between the level in brain tissue of patients with Parkinson's disease and normal brain (autopsy specimens). However, it would still be of interest to look more closely by immunofluorescent techniques at the subcellular distribution of superoxide dismutase (particularly in the mitochondria) and at the various cell types (e.g., neurons versus glia).

Chapter 9

Oxygen Free Radicals in Central Nervous System Ischemia and Trauma

HARRY B. DEMOPOULOS, EUGENE FLAMM,
MYRON SELIGMAN, AND
DENNIS D. PIETRONIGRO

INTRODUCTION

Ischemic or traumatic injuries to the brain or spinal cord result in more extensive tissue damage, more easily, than do equivalent insults to other organs. This quantitative difference in response to injury appears to result from rapidly proliferating pathological free-radical reactions, initiated by oxygen-related species, which spread quite readily throughout the heavily lipoidal membranes of the central nervous system (CNS) (6,15). The following factors may also facilitate pathological radical reactions in the CNS:

1. Molecular oxygen is seven to eight times more soluble in nonpolar environments, such as the hydrophobic midzone of cell membranes, than in aqueous cell compartments (6).

2. Membrane lipids, such as cholesterol and the polyunsaturated phospholipids, can be attacked by oxygen noncatalytically, unless sufficient antioxidants and protective enzymes are present (6,15,41).

3. The brain and spinal cord tissues and cells contain extensive membrane systems including a large number of cristae-rich mitochondria and

PATHOLOGY OF OXYGEN
Copyright © 1982 by Academic Press, Inc.
ISBN 0-12-068620-1

myelin. The latter insulates nerve fibers and is composed of multiple lamellar wrappings of the plasma membrane from glial supporting cells (the oligodendrogliocytes).

4. Because of the extensive cellular demands for ATP, neuronal cells are rich in the components of electron transport and oxidative phosphorylation, such as the ubiquinones [coenzyme Q (CoQ)]. This group of compounds, when reduced, readily autoxidize to produce superoxide O_2^-. It is possible, therefore, that the abundance of CoQ in the CNS may be a liability under some circumstances (5,15).

5. Neurons contain a large number of lysosomes, the membranes of which may be subject to radical-initiated damage, resulting in the release of lysosomal hydrolytic enzymes into the cytoplasm of the neuron.

6. The blood vessels of the brain and spinal cord, particularly in the microcirculation, have frail support and are easily torn. This produces extravasation of blood, resulting in the release into tissues of two catalysts of free-radical generation, iron and copper.

7. There is a high concentration of ascorbic acid in the gray and white matter of the CNS (43). The concentration is second only to the level found in the adrenal glands. The brain has a specific active transport system for ascorbic acid in the choroid plexus which elevates the concentration of ascorbate in the cerebrospinal fluid 10-fold above the plasma level. Furthermore, neural tissue cells have a second transport system that concentrates intracellular ascorbate an additional 10-fold. The result is that the cells have 100 times more ascorbic acid than the blood plasma. Whereas ascorbic acid is an antioxidant when present alone in high concentrations, in the presence of copper and iron released by the extravasation of blood, as occurs in trauma and ischemia, ascorbic acid produces large quantities of O_2^- and H_2O_2. In CNS injury, therefore, the high levels of ascorbic acid may be a liability (38).

INITIATION AND PROPAGATION OF PATHOLOGICAL FREE-RADICAL REACTIONS IN CNS ISCHEMIA AND TRAUMA

The biomolecules that comprise the lipoidal framework of cell membranes are among the macromolecules most susceptible to pathological free-radical action. The reasons for this may be (a) the preferential solubility of oxygen and of ferroorganic complexes in the hydrophobic milieu of cell membranes and (b) the formation from membrane lipids of metastable, intermediate free-radical products, which may create a slow free-radical propagation process leading to oxidative breakdown of the macromolecules (6). Examples of these reactions are shown in Table I.

Membrane damage, induced by uncontrolled lipid free-radical reactions, can result in poorly functioning cells that are still viable and perhaps repairable. Conversely, there can be outright cell death or states of functional loss intermediate between these two states depending on the rates of propagation of radical reactions. The mechanism by which damage to membranes may be initiated by pathological radical reactions is depicted schematically in Figs. 1 and 2. If the rate of damage exceeds the repair capacity of the cell, permanent cell changes may result. The repair processes of the cell require intact endoplasmic reticulum (ER) and mitochondria, both membranous structures susceptible to free-radical injury (18). These organelles are the sites of the largest number of normally occurring free-radical reactions (15,36). Normal reactions in the ER apparently involving free-radical generation include hydroxylation reactions (4), which require phospholipids (16), reductases, cofactors, and cytochrome P-450. In the mitochondria (36) these reactions include oxidative phosphorylation, which is dependent on the easily autoxidized CoQ and FAD molecules. If these radical-generating reactions are decontrolled, the related subcellular organelle may become impaired. Such an event can render the cell vulnerable to free-radical attack at lower rates of radical generation and may explain the synergistic effects that are commonly seen in free-radical pathology. For example, carbon tetrachloride and ethanol, each present in concentrations too low to cause damage alone, can result in fatal hepatic necrosis when combined. Carbon tetrachloride is known to attack the ER, and ethanol is known to attack mitochondria (10,44).

In considering the initiation of pathological free-radical reactions as in cell membrane lipids, it must be remembered that, under free-radical stress, aerobic organisms are continuously associated with ambient molecular oxygen (24). Oxygen is lethal to organisms that have not evolved cellular protective agents such as the superoxide dismutases and catalase. Oxygen is involved in free-radical reactions, as illustrated in Table I.

The mechanism whereby regional cerebral ischemia initiates and propagates free-radical membrane pathology may involve the decontrol of coenzyme Q (the ubiquinones) (5,15). Cerebral ischemia is not total, as is the case with most pathological interruptions of blood flow. There is a low flow from collateral branches that bring in a small amount of O_2, estimated to be about 20% of normal (12). At this concentration, the O_2 is limiting for cytochrome oxidase activity, and the components of the electron transport chain become reduced. However, CoQ, being lipid soluble, may autoxidize in its reduced state and produce O_2^-, H_2O_2, and HO⋅ (1,2).

TABLE I
Lipid Free-Radical Damage

Initiation and formation of metastable intermediary products

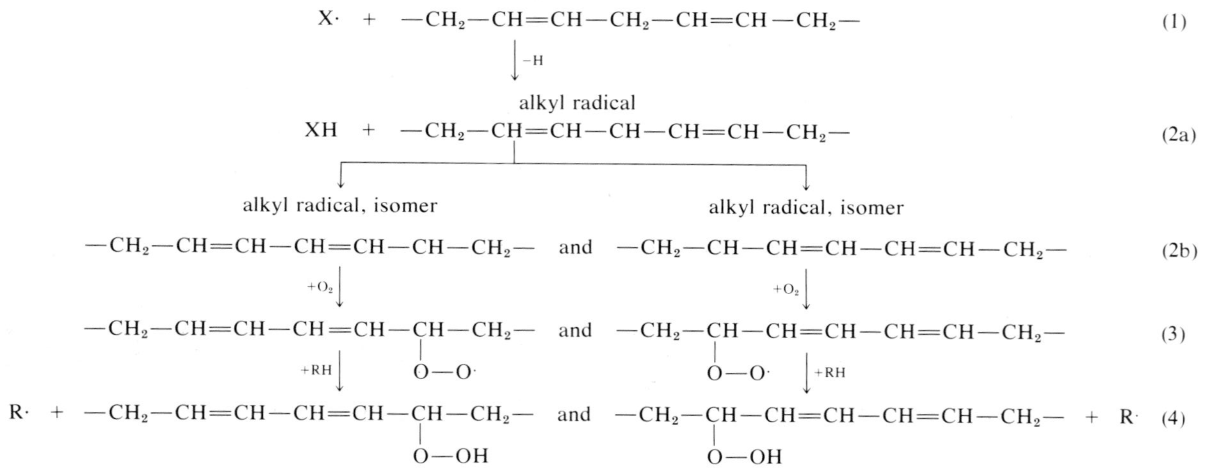

$$X\cdot \; + \; -CH_2-CH=CH-CH_2-CH=CH-CH_2- \qquad (1)$$

$$\xrightarrow{-H}$$

alkyl radical

$$XH \; + \; -CH_2-CH=CH-CH-CH=CH-CH_2- \qquad (2a)$$

alkyl radical, isomer

alkyl radical, isomer

$$-CH_2-CH=CH-CH-CH=CH-CH_2- \quad \text{and} \quad -CH_2-CH-CH=CH-CH=CH-CH_2- \qquad (2b)$$

$$\xrightarrow{+O_2} \qquad\qquad\qquad\qquad \xrightarrow{+O_2}$$

$$-CH_2-CH=CH-CH-CH=CH-CH_2- \quad \text{and} \quad -CH_2-CH-CH=CH-CH=CH-CH_2- \qquad (3)$$
$$O-O\cdot \qquad\qquad O-O\cdot$$

$$\downarrow +RH \qquad\qquad\qquad\qquad \downarrow +RH$$

$$R\cdot \; + \; -CH_2-CH=CH-CH-CH=CH-CH_2- \quad \text{and} \quad -CH_2-CH-CH=CH-CH=CH-CH_2- \; + \; R\cdot \qquad (4)$$
$$O-OH \qquad\qquad O-OH$$

Eq. (1): Part of a fatty acid chain with two unsaturated bonds; however, identical reactions occur in fatty acids with one unsaturation and in cholesterol. Here $X\cdot$ is a free radical (a substance with a lone electron) and most often represents molecular O_2 (a diradical) or the hydroxyl radical ($\cdot$OH).

Eq. (2a): A radical center is located on the carbon that is adjacent to carbons with double bonds and is now referred to as an alkyl radical. The original free radical ($X\cdot$) has abstracted a hydrogen to this lipid and is now no longer a radical (XH).

Eq. (2b): Several configurational changes occur almost immediately. There are massive electron shifts which (a) result in the lone electron being shifted to other carbon atoms, (b) cause the double bonds to move closer together and thus form conjugated unsaturations, which can be detected spectrophotometrically as an index of early radical damage, (c) cause some of the double bonds to change from the bent (cis) configuration that characterizes normal unsaturated fatty acids to the straight (trans) configuration.

Eq. (3): Oxygen adds by free-radical reactions to form peroxy radicals.

Eq. (4): The peroxy radicals have abstracted hydrogen from nearby molecules (other unsaturated lipids, proteins, antioxidants, nucleic acids, represented as RH) and have become metastable lipid hydroperoxides; metastable means that the product is only transiently stable.

Catalysis and propagation

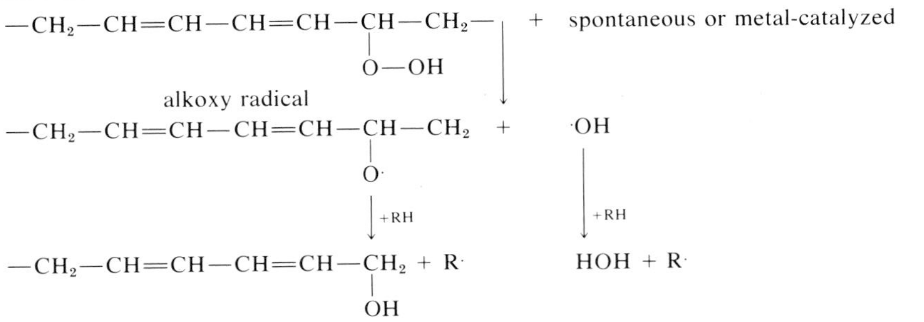

$$-CH_2-CH=CH-CH=CH-CH-CH_2- \longrightarrow \quad + \quad \text{spontaneous or metal-catalyzed} \qquad (5)$$
$$\underset{O-OH}{|}$$

alkoxy radical

$$-CH_2-CH=CH-CH=CH-CH-CH_2- \quad + \qquad \cdot OH \qquad (6)$$
$$\underset{O\cdot}{|} \xrightarrow{+RH}$$

$$-CH_2-CH=CH-CH=CH-CH-CH_2 + R\cdot \qquad \xrightarrow{+RH} \qquad HOH + R\cdot \qquad (7)$$
$$\underset{OH}{|}$$

Eqs. (5) and (6): A hydroperoxide can break up spontaneously to form hydroxyl radicals and oxygen-centered radicals on the lipid which are termed alkoxy radicals. Metals produce alkoxy and peroxy radicals with hydroxy or hydrogen ions.

Eq. (7): Abstracting hydrogens from adjacent molecules, RH, the alkoxy and hydroxyl radicals are terminated, but additional radicals form in the molecules from which hydrogen was abstracted (2R).

(continued)

TABLE I (*Continued*)

Fragmentation and termination

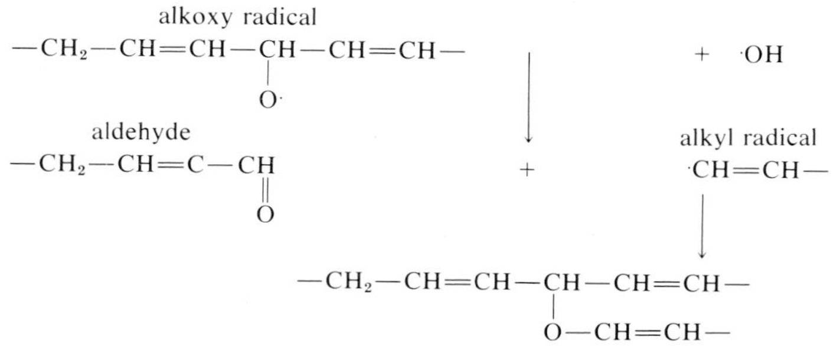

alkoxy radical

$$-CH_2-CH=CH-CH-CH=CH- \quad \longrightarrow$$
$$\underset{O\cdot}{|}$$

$$+ \quad \cdot OH \qquad (8)$$

aldehyde

$$-CH_2-CH=C-CH \quad + \quad$$
$$\underset{O}{\overset{|}{}}$$

alkyl radical

$$\cdot CH=CH-$$

$$-CH_2-CH=CH-CH-CH=CH- \quad \longrightarrow$$
$$\underset{O-CH=CH-}{|} \qquad (9)$$

Eq. (8): An alkoxy radical can be further oxidized and fragmented as a result of continued radical attacks on other carbons that are adjacent to the double bonds, resulting in the formation of bishydroperoxides (i.e., two —OOH groups form on one fatty acid). The fatty acid then fragments to form aldehydes and alkyl radical fragments.

Eq. (9): The alkyl radicals can react with other surrounding radicals, e.g., other alkoxy radicals, and terminate to form an oxygen-linked bridge.

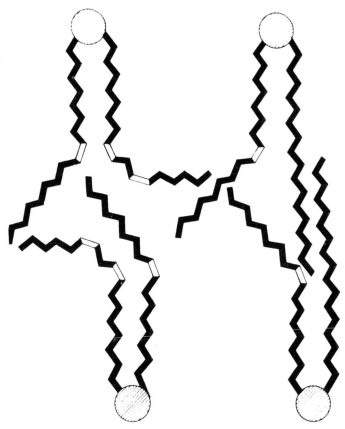

Fig. 1. Schematic representation of bimolecular leaflet of phospholipid molecules forming the structure of a plasma membrane. The circles are the glycerophosphate head groups, which are polar, whereas the fatty acid tails extend into the hydrophobic midzone. Unsaturated bonds are bent at an angle of 123°, in the cis isomeric configuration in the fatty acid tails. In the normal membrane, there is a saturated carbon separating the two carbons that have unsaturated bonds. This saturated carbon is partly activated and can lose one of its hydrogens quite readily. Note the spaces between the phospholipids. These are the archways wherein cholesterol and other sterol-like compounds may intercalate. From Demopoulos *et al.* (7).

These radicals have the potential to initiate membrane free-radical pathology. The residual blood flow in models of regional cerebral ischemia ensures sufficient O_2 levels to maintain CoQ autoxidation and to yield oxygen-related radicals. The rate of H_2O_2 generation by normal mitochondrial preparations is directly related to O_2 tension under specific conditions (1). Little H_2O_2 is produced by mitochondria at low O_2 tension. However, *in vivo*, during ischemia, there is still a significant concentration of O_2 from

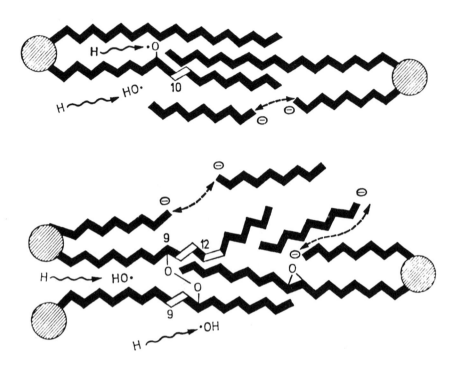

Fig. 2. Schematic summary of free-radical peroxidative damage to fatty acids that form the hydrophobic midzone seen in Fig. 1. The double bonds are now largely in the nonbent trans configuration; a saturated carbon no longer separates the carbons with unsaturated bonds. Alkoxy radicals (RO·) are present and can react to form peroxides (ROOR) or to join two adjacent fatty acids in an abnormal bond. Reactive HO$^\infty$ radicals are shown as abstracted, possibly from adjacent lipid and protein molecules. Abstracted hydrogens react with hydroxyls to form water in the hydrophobic midzone. Fragmentation of fatty acid tails is shown with the eventual production of negatively charged carboxylic acid groups, represented by an encircled minus sign. The numerals, 9, 10, and 12 signify the carbon atom number in the carbon chain that makes up the fatty acid. From Demopoulos et al. (7).

collateral flow, and small quantities of H_2O_2 may initiate damaging chain reactions in membrane lipids. Experimental work in radiation biology indicates that free-radical reactions with a pathological potential can occur at low oxygen tension (Fig. 3) (19).

Coenzyme Q autoxidative cycling may be responsible for initiating the tissue damage seen with regional cerebral ischemia (5,15). The CoQ free radical (CoQ·), which is intermediate between the fully oxidized and fully

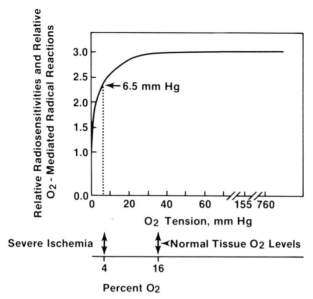

Fig. 3. An idealized illustration of the dependence of radiosensitivity and of free-radical reactions on oxygen concentration. The oxygen-mediated enhancement of radiation damage in biological systems is due to the increased production of free radicals resulting from the participation of oxygen in the radical reactions. Oxygen helps to propagate geometrically spreading free-radical chain reactions and does so at relatively low tissue oxygen concentrations. Hence, the curve in this figure, which relates O_2 tension and enhanced radiosensitivity, also relates O_2 tension and oxygen-mediated free-radical reactions. If radiosensitivity and free-radical reactions are arbitrarily assigned a value of unity, the radiosensitivity and the increased degree of free-radical reactions are about 3 under normally oxygenated conditions, i.e., a 300% increase. The O_2 tension of most normal tissues is in the range of 20–40 mm Hg. If O_2 tension falls to 20–30% of the normal values, as occurs after an experimental middle cerebral artery occlusion or following spinal cord impact, the tissue O_2 tension may drop to a range of 4–8 mm Hg. At this range, there is marked stimulation of glycolytic pathways, increased lactic acid production, and decreased ATP synthesis. If we use an average figure of 6 mm Hg, there is still sufficient oxygen tension to support oxygen-mediated radical reactions to a degree that is almost the same as that under conditions of full oxygenation (enhancement by a factor of 2.5 compared to a factor of 3). Hence, decreases in O_2 tension to levels that are 20–30% of normal values caused no significant change in radiosensitivity or in oxygen-mediated free-radical reactions. Even at O_2 tensions of 1–2 mm Hg, there is still a 50% enhancement of radical reactions (factor is 1.5 at 1–2 mm Hg).

reduced forms, is scavenged immediately by a rapidly acting barbiturate, methohexital. This and other "fast-acting" barbiturates produce remarkable protection against ischemia (15), and the formation of a charge-transfer complex between these barbiturates and coenzyme Q may be, in part, the mechanism of barbiturate protection (5). (Fig. 4) Coenzyme Q is not unique in having a free-radical intermediate between its fully reduced and

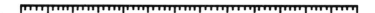

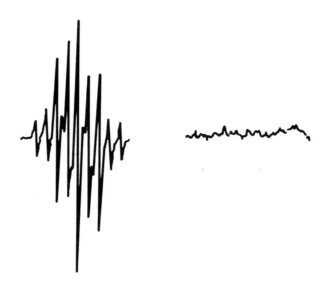

Fig. 4.   Left: The EPR spectrum of the coenzyme Q free radical. Normal decay time in this solution (alkaline ethanol with tetrahydrofuran and DMSO) is 45 min. Right: The addition of equimolar methohexital, a highly lipid soluble barbiturate, immediately abolishes the EPR signal of CoQ in a preparation whose remaining decay time is 40 min. From Demopoulos *et al*. (5).

fully oxidized states and, further, with O_2^- generated during oxidation. A similar reaction takes place with ascorbic acid. The semidehydro form of ascorbic acid is produced regularly in tissues as the ascorbyl radical and results in the synthesis of O_2^-. The ascorbyl radical (Fig. 5) has proved helpful in the semiquantitation of the rates of pathological free-radical reactions in tissues, as described in a later section.

Initiation and propagation of destructive free-radical reactions in the spinal cord injury model are associated with petechial hemorrhages in the central gray matter. Polyunsaturated fatty acids are abundant in the central gray matter, which contains organelle-rich neurons. The extravasation of blood introduces organic as well as inorganic forms of both iron and copper (33), which catalyze lipid peroxidation (6). The radical prod-

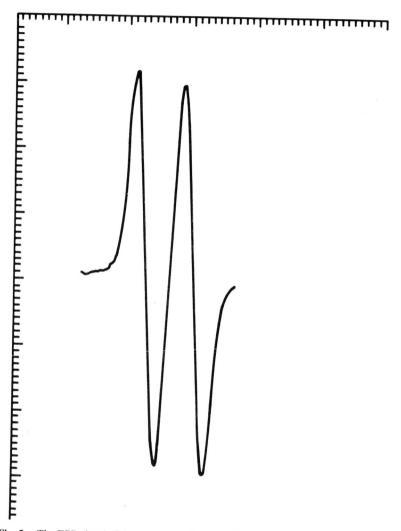

Fig. 5. The EPR signal of the ascorbyl radical, obtained as follows. Machine parameters: scan range, 0.5×10^2 G; field set, 3400 G; time constant, 1 sec; scan time, 4 min; modulation amplitude, 0.5×1 G; receiver gain, 2×10^5; microwave power, 10 mW; microwave frequency, 9.535 Hz. Signal characteristics: g value, 2.0052; splitting,1.70 G. From Demopoulos *et al.* (7).

ucts can cause a decrease in blood flow by (a) decreasing the activity of adenylate cyclase, which is phospholipid dependent (16), and (b) inhibiting PGI_2 formation in the endothelium (17,22,27). If adenylate cyclase is inhibited, cyclic AMP levels decrease. When this occurs in vascular smooth muscle cells, muscle spasm occurs (14). If PGI_2 is inhibited, platelets adhere and aggregate, causing coagulation of blood (17,22,27). Lipid peroxides inhibit PGI_2 synthesis, which is crucial for preventing the aggregation of platelets (17,22,27). The sequence of events following ischemia involving the CoQ cycle described above and the propagation of free-radical reactions may explain the extensive dissolution of spinal cord structure at the site of physical trauma (33,37) (Figs. 6–13).

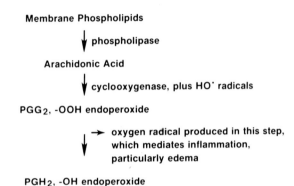

Membrane Phospholipids

↓ phospholipase

Arachidonic Acid

↓ cyclooxygenase, plus HO˙ radicals

PGG₂, -OOH endoperoxide

→ oxygen radical produced in this step,
↓ which mediates inflammation,
    particularly edema

PGH₂, -OH endoperoxide

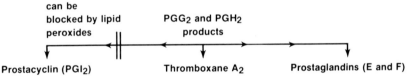

can be
blocked by lipid   PGG2 and PGH2
peroxides   products

Prostacyclin (PGI₂)   Thromboxane A₂   Prostaglandins (E and F)

Fig. 6. Prostanoid cascade. Possibly one of the most strategically located cell membranes is the plasma membrane of the endothelial cell, which provides the inner surface lining of blood vessels. This surface must be smooth and continually provide prostacyclin (PGI_2) to keep blood platelets from aggregating and sticking to the inner vessel. Platelets are rich in arachidonic acid, a 20-carbon-long fatty acid that has four unsaturated bonds. Arachidonic acid, via closely controlled free-radical reactions, is converted to prostaglandins (key regulatory substances for cells and tissues) and also to thromboxane A_2 (TxA_2). Platelets produce large quantities of the latter factor, which fosters platelet adhesiveness. This must be countered by a balanced production of PGI_2 in endothelial lining cells. When these two factors are in balance, blood flow is normal. When there is injury, pathological radical reactions impair PGI_2 synthesis (27) and platelets aggregate under the action of TxA_2. When bleeding must stop, this action of TxA_2 is desirable. However, in other situations, the pathology may be amplified. For example, in the acute CNS free-radical models described here, it has been demonstrated by the use of topological scanning electron microscopy that free-radical reactions result in occlusions of the microcirculation. This decrease in blood flow produces further ischemia, with further free-radical injury. The delivery via the circulation of antioxidants that could control the radical reactions is therefore impaired (refer to Figs. 7–13).

TISSUE FREE-RADICAL PATHOLOGY: DETECTION OF DAMAGE, ASSESSMENT OF BIOMOLECULES AFFECTED, AND DETERMINATION OF RATES OF ASSOCIATED REACTIONS

Pathological radical reactions in tissues can rarely be detected by direct means, such as electron paramagnetic resonance (EPR) spectrometry, because the steady-state concentration of any specifically defined radical is not sufficiently high (6,32). Determining the content of altered biomolecules resulting from the reaction with free radicals is one means of detecting pathological free radicals in tissue.

Cellular unsaturated lipids are susceptible to free-radical damage through the process of lipid peroxidation, which produces malonaldehyde, an end product of oxidative cleavage of lipids (40). Malonaldehyde, however, is a reactive molecule and has the potential to combine with proteins, nucleic acids, and other substances (40). In certain biological systems, therefore, it can be unreliable as a measure of lipid peroxidation. Other methods have been used to quantitate lipid peroxidation, including the determination of fluorescent complexes of malonaldehyde with cellular macromolecules, but these methods are also rather nonspecific (40).

Determining the loss of polyunsaturated fatty acids from membrane phospholipids is a reliable method, as is quantifying the loss of extractable cholesterol (15). Model studies have been conducted with liposomes that have undergone limited free-radical damage. These well-defined, pure membrane lipid systems have provided information useful for studying the losses of susceptible lipids in complex biological membrane systems as a measure of free-radical damage (29,31,39). In the CNS, this approach is particularly valuable since brain mitochondria do not oxidize fatty acids in the oxidative phosphorylation system. Furthermore, there are no enzymes in brain mitochondria that metabolize cholesterol. The loss of polyunsaturated compounds and cholesterol, therefore, cannot be explained by normal metabolism. Furthermore, the selective loss of the highly polyunsaturated fatty acids (22:6 docosohexanoic acid and 20:4 arachidonic acid), compared to minor or no losses of the mono- and diunsaturated fatty acids, provides another indication of free-radical damage since the highly unsaturated lipids are much more susceptible to radical reactions (15).

Measuring the appearance of stable free-radical products produced by oxidative reactions with polyunsaturated fatty acids is difficult because so many products may be formed, e.g., a variety of short-chain fatty acids, carbonyl compounds, and branched-chain fatty acids. By contrast, studying the radical products of cholesterol is somewhat easier since fewer products are formed (41). In addition, analysis of cholesterol oxidation products provides the means of determining the molecular nature of oxygen or the active oxygen species involved (23,41).

The rate of consumption of endogenous antioxidants has proved to be helpful in approximating the rate of free-radical damage in tissues (7,13,34). In particular, measuring the rate of loss of ascorbic acid as the reduced species (the antioxidant state) is a rapid, reliable, and versatile method for studying CNS free-radical damage (7,13). It is analogous to measuring the decrease in the amount of reduced glutathione (GSH) in tissues in which free-radical damage has occurred (34). The assay of the reduced form of ascorbic acid involves extracting it from tissue completely and initiating its controlled oxidation to produce the ascorbyl radical intermediate, which is then determined by EPR spectrometry (7,13). Dimethyl sulfoxide (DMSO) is a very suitable extracting agent since it both removes and oxidizes the ascorbic acid. It also stabilizes the semidehydroascorbyl radical intermediate so that the steady-state concentration is sufficiently high to be reliably measured by EPR spectrometry. The lifetime of the radical and its decay span is 10–15 min. which allows sufficient time for EPR measurement.

The assay is performed as follows, with attention to precise timing and concentration: To 100 mg wet weight of tissue, 0.5 ml DMSO is added, and the tissue is minced within 15 sec. The mince is incubated without shaking at room temperature for 5 min, and the supernatant solution is placed into a flat quartz cell for analysis in a Varian E-3 EPR spectrometer. The curves generated by spectral analysis relate the logarithm of the amplitude of the signal to the logarithm of the concentration of ascorbyl radical. This assay has proved to be a highly sensitive indicator of free-radical pathological reactions in tissues of precise timing and tissue processing are observed.

The EPR spectrometric assay of ascorbic acid was evaluated in liposomes subjected to controlled lipid free-radical reactions in the presence of calibrated concentrations of ascorbic acid (7). The assay has been used extensively in the two model systems of regional cerebral ischemia and spinal cord impact (7,13,15). By this means it has been found that ascorbic acid in the CNS is directly correlated with the other evidence of lipid free-radical damage. Antioxidants that ameliorate free-radical tissue damage preserve the normal level of tissue ascorbic acid (see Table III).

ANIMAL MODELS FOR CEREBRAL DAMAGE

Two types of feline model systems were used: regional cerebral ische-mia and spinal cord impact. The ischemia model resembles the most com-mon human disorders, that is, "stroke" and cerebral palsy (15). In these conditions the blood level is decreased only in specific regions of the brain. To produce this model of regional cerebral ischemia, the middle cerebral artery of anesthetized (25 mg/kg pentobarbital) adult cats (3 kg) was unilaterally occluded through a retroorbital approach using an operat-ing microscope (15). The cats were maintained under anesthesia and killed at specific time intervals after occlusion (1, 3, and 5 hr). The spinal cord impact model was designed to reproduce the pathological changes occurring in human beings who become quadriplegic or paraplegic as a result of injuries such as those associated with automobile, skiing, and horseback riding accidents (33). In the overwhelming majority of human spinal cord injuries, the cord tissue itself is not grossly or severely dam-

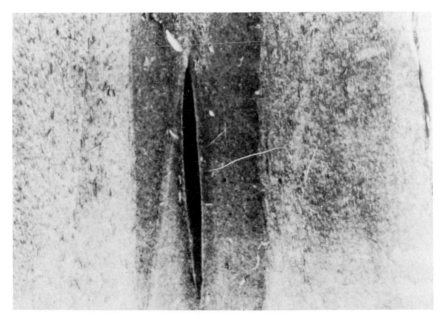

Fig. 7. Topological scanning electron micrograph of obliquely cut spinal cord observed at low magnification. The central canal and the gray matter are well delineated. Normal adult cat. × 28.

aged. Rather, the cord is subjected to a combination of severe bending and/or twisting, coupled with extensive jarring (33). Few cases involve actual transection, either partial or complete. It has never been understood why the cord degenerates so completely at the site of injury. Experimentally, the most satisfactory model involves performing a laminectomy on an anesthetized cat at the level of the ninth or tenth thoracic vertebra and inflicting a controlled impact by dropping a specific weight for a specific distance onto the intact dura (33). This model is widely used and mimics the microscopic pathological changes seen in most human cord injuries that lead to paralysis (33). A 20-g weight dropped 20 cm through a tube held perpendicular to the cord produces a 400 g-cm force, which permanently paralyzes 90% of adult cats. By contrast, a 10-g weight dropped 20 cm causes a 200 g-cm impact and results only in transient paresis (weakness) (33).

Views of normal cat spinal cord are shown in Figs. 7–9. Views of the spinal cord in the impact model are shown in Figs. 10–13. No significant structural changes are seen shortly after impact (33). There are a few, minute petechial hemorrhages in the central gray matter in the first 5 min after impact, but there is no structural shearing of neural fibers seen even on examination by electron microscopy. Approximately 3 hr are needed

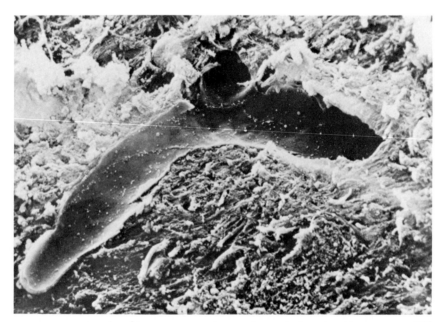

Fig. 8. Normal capillary in a control, nonimpacted cat spinal cord. White matter. × 4900.

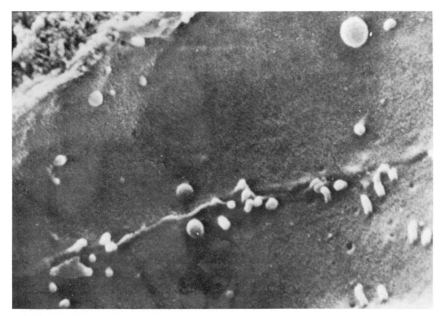

Fig. 9. Higher magnification of Fig. 8 showing normal endothelial cell junctions, villi, and openings of pinocytic vesicles. × 12,600.

to produce irreversible changes. In this period there is a steady increase in the amount of bleeding in the central gray matter. In terms of the pathological response, this is the most dramatic. Four hours after impact, about 25% of the myelinated fibers in the long tracts show serious damage and there is periaxonal swelling (11). For the next few hours the structure of the cord at the impact site undergoes progressive dissolution, leaving a structural and functional gap in the continuity of the long tracts.

Histological examination reveals that the regional cerebral ischemia model leads to swelling of the mitochondria, including the cristae, as well as the ER within 15–30 min after occlusion. These represent the first structural changes. Functionally, the regional blood flow promptly decreases to 20% of normal (i.e., a decrease of 80%), and the cortex becomes electrically silent within a few minutes of occlusion (12). Progressive ischemic changes occur in the neurons; these become irreversible after 3 hr, as in the spinal cord impact model. If reperfusion is allowed before this time, no permanent tissue damage occurs. Experimental evidence shows that the series of events leading to neuronal death require approximately 3 hr (13).

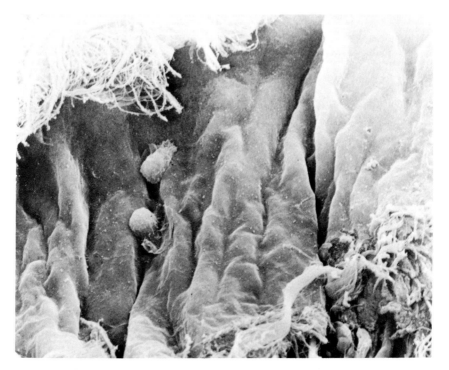

Fig. 10. One hour after impact an arteriole in the white matter shows adhering white blood cells. On the right a pathological crater is seen, and just below that an adhering group of platelets. The arteriole has an undulating appearance from contraction of the arteriole smooth muscle cells caused by the perfusing fixative. × 3710.

EVIDENCE FOR PATHOLOGICAL
FREE-RADICAL REACTIONS AND THEIR
CONTROL IN THE CNS

Table II contains a summary of the evidence for free-radical reactions in the CNS during ischemia or trauma. In the regional cerebral ischemia model, the amelioration of damage by certain barbiturates is virtually complete (Table III). This effect is not related to the sedative properties of barbiturates or to their metabolism. Barbiturates at the usual anesthetic doses of 25 mg/kg do not protect. If additional doses of 25 mg/kg per hour are given, protection occurs (15). At such high doses, supportive treatment is necessary to prevent collapse of the cardiovascular and respiratory systems and death of the treated animals. After several hours, the

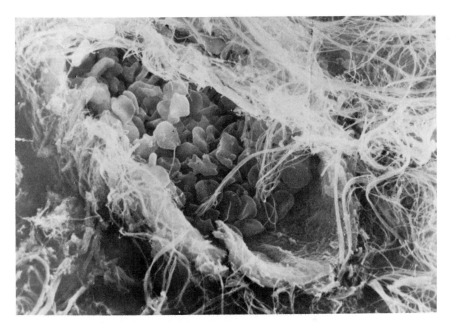

Fig. 11. Two hours after impact a white matter arteriole shows occlusion. This is not seen earlier. Site of impact. ×2800.

barbiturate administration can be discontinued (20). Apparently, collaterals are able to maintain the tissue when the acute phase of pathological free-radical reactions is completed. It should be noted that other anesthetic agents and other substances that lower the cerebral metabolic rate of O_2 consumption do not protect against cerebral ischemia. In an *in vitro* system consisting of liposomes peroxidized by ultraviolet light, such barbiturates as thiopental and methohexital are excellent antioxidants (Table IV).

The antioxidant properties of barbiturates were studied employing a system of iron-catalyzed peroxidation of liposomes. Only thiopental was observed to be effective (35,42). In this peroxidation system there is also an apparent requirement for the antioxidant to act as an iron chelator. In some systems, such as the spinal cord impact model, extensive hemorrhage occurs, and subsequent radical damage appears to be catalyzed by iron and copper (33). In the spinal cord impact models barbiturates have no ameliorative effect. D-Penicillamine, a major chelator of tissue iron and copper, provides some protection, however (21).

Methohexital treatment considerably reduces the loss of specific tissue components induced by oxidative damage, i.e., (a) the polyunsaturated

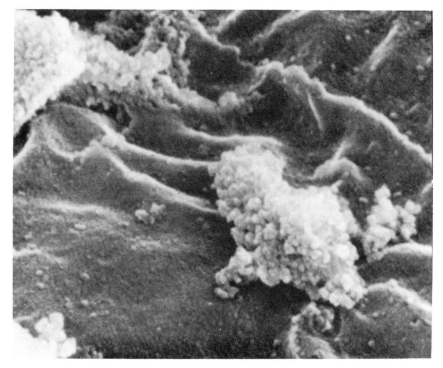

Fig. 12.   Two hours after impact there is increasing platelet aggregation and adherence to vessel walls. White matter arteriole from Fig. 11 at higher magnification. × 42,400.

fatty acids (22:6 and 20:9) in membrane phospholipids, (b) the cholesterol in the membranes, and (c) ascorbic acid (15) (Table III). Cells of the cerebral cortex contain a large amount of coenzyme Q, which may be the source of cellularly generated oxygen radicals. Since CoQ is a membrane lipid, lipophilic barbiturates may reach the intracellular site of CoQ and thus more easily quench the generated free radicals. Barbiturates are protective only in regional cerebral ischemia. If ischemia is complete, as with cardiac arrest or bilateral occlusion of the carotids, barbiturates do not provide protection (26). In such instances of profound cerebral ischemia, complete loss of blood flow results in a lack of nutrients as well as an accumulation of metabolic waste products in the affected tissues, which culminates in tissue necrosis.

Regional cerebral ischemia, as seen in "strokes" and cerebral palsy, is common in human beings. In these cases, only certain parts of the brain are affected and are partially ischemic. Acute ischemic reactions cause microocclusions in the microcirculation, leading to tissue damage. If the

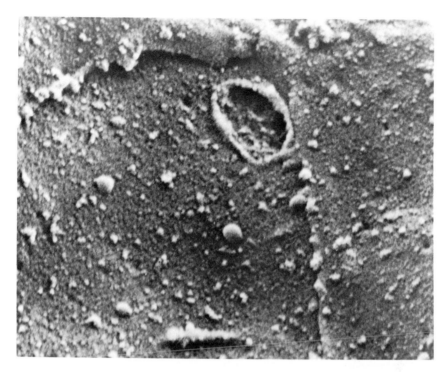

Fig. 13. Two hours after impact the endothelial cells show overriding, larger craters and adherence of particulate cell debris, which most likely represents fragments of adhering platelets that were washed away during perfusion fixation.

initial acute reactions can be ameliorated in the first 1–3 hr, then the existing collateral blood flow can supply the cerebral tissue even though the primary source of blood has been compromised (20). Such microocclusions are the result of platelet adherence and aggregation and occur in the absence of prostaglandin PGI_2, causing the initiation of the coagulation process. (Figs. 6–13). The synthesis of PGI_2 in endothelium is inhibited by lipid peroxides (17,22,27). Large doses of methohexital protect the microcirculation in regional cerebral ischemia models (9). Acting as antioxidants, barbiturates could prevent the formation of lipid peroxides and the inhibition of PGI_2 synthesis. The net result of methohexital treatment, however, is that the microcirculation, as studied by scanning electron microscopy (8), remains patent and maintains the collateral blood flow after induced ischemia (9).

Preliminary studies have been conducted using CuZnSOD (2 mg/kg) in animal models of acute regional cerebral ischemia. Superoxide dismutase

TABLE II

Systems that Induce Free-Radical Lipid Damage in the Central Nervous System[a]

Spinal cord impact injury model in cats
    Potentiation of trauma by ethanol
    Appearance of increased levels of malonaldehyde
    Appearance of increasing levels of lipid-soluble fluorescence, representing addition
        products of malonaldehyde
    Destructive loss of extractable cholesterol
    Consumption of a major CNS antioxidant, ascorbic acid
Focal CNS cold trauma in cats and rats
    Amelioration of cerebral edema with diphenyl-p-phenylenediamine, an antioxidant
    Destructive loss of polyunsaturated fatty acids from gray and white matter
    Destructive loss of extractable cholesterol from gray and white matter
    Consumption of a major CNS antioxidant, ascorbic acid, from gray and white matter
    Amelioration of all free-radical pathology parameters with synthetic corticosteroids,
        which also have antioxidant properties in model membrane systems undergoing
        free-radical damage
    Increased production of malonaldehyde
    Loss of thiols
Regional CNS ischemia in cats
    Destructive loss of polyunsaturated fatty acids from the gray matter
    Destructive loss of extractable cholesterol from the white matter
    Consumption of a major CNS antioxidant, ascorbic acid, from gray and white matter
    Amelioration of all of the above with barbiturates, which have lipid antioxidant proper-
        ties in model membrane systems undergoing free-radical damage
Hypoxia, brain
    Loss of thiols
Biogenic amines
    6-OH-Dopamine is concentrated in sympathetic fibers, which results in the destruction
        of these fibers, apparently by free-radical reactions
Deficiency states
    α-Tocopherol deficiency leads to encephalomalacia

[a] Details are given by Ransohoff (33).

gives approximately 50% of the protection afforded by barbiturates. Ascorbic acid levels fall by about 20% with superoxide dismutase treatment compared with a 44% decrease without treatment. With barbiturate therapy the ascorbic acid level falls by only 4% (Table III). Superoxide dismutase would not be expected to offer complete protection since the enzyme may not be able to penetrate the cell in sufficient concentration to quench intracellular sources of O_2^- (5,15). It is conceivable that higher doses of superoxide dismutase and prolonged treatment, possibly with the addition of catalase to catalytically remove H_2O_2, would provide more protection. The cardiotoxicity of adriamycin was ameliorated by this combination of enzymes, indicating that such an approach is feasible (25).

TABLE III

**Reduction in Membrane Lipids and Antioxidants Following
Middle Cerebral Artery Occlusion for 5 hr**

Compound	Control (% loss)	Treated[a] (% loss)
Phospholipids		
Palmitic acid (16:0)	9	<3
Stearic acid (18:0)	11	<3
Arachidonic acid (20:4)	37	<5
Docosahexanoic acid (22:6)	27	<5
Cholesterol	23	0
Ascorbic acid	44	4

[a] Animals were treated with methohexital, 25 mg/kg per hour, intravenously, starting at the time of occlusion and continuously thereafter for 5 hr.

Adriamycin readily forms free radicals, which can be observed by EPR spectrometry (30). Because there are similarities between CoQ-mediated damage in regional cerebral ischemia and adriamycin-mediated cardiotoxicity, it is reasonable to expect that a combination of superoxide dismu-

TABLE IV

Effects of Barbiturates on the Peroxidation of Liposomes[a]

Time (min)	% decrease in lipid peroxidation compared to control liposomes[b]		
	Thiopental A	Methohexital B	Barbital A
0	9	6	0
15	51	36	22
30	61	42	7
60	63	45	4
90	56	51	0

[a] Liposomes were prepared from phosphatidylcholine and irradiated in UV light as described in previous work (41). Lipid peroxidation was determined by spectrophotometric analysis of the malonaldehyde–thiobarbituric acid (TBA) complex at 532 nm. Control liposomes without barbiturates were irradiated, and the production of TBA-reactive product measured at the times indicated.

[b] Two concentrations of the barbiturates were used (A, $1.08 \times 10^{-2} M$; B, $1.08 \times 10^{-3} M$). The values shown are the percent *decreases* in the production of lipid peroxidation compared to the control liposomes irradiated at the same time interval. Each number represents triplicate determinations.

tase and catalase might provide a defense against tissue necrosis resulting from regional cerebral ischemia.

Control of pathological free radicals in the spinal cord impact models is very difficult for the following reasons. (a) Iron and copper are released in large quantities from hemolyzed erythrocytes as a result of multiple hemorrhages in the central gray matter (33), and (b) progressive occlusion of the microcirculation occurs (8), which causes ischemia (37). As previously explained, this could stimulate the generation of oxygen free radicals from CoQ, similar to the model of regional cerebral ischemia. Thus, attempts have been made to control hemorrhage in the central gray matter by chelation of the iron and copper (21).

Bleeding in the central gray matter is progressive over a period of several hours after impact; therefore, the more rapidly it is controlled, the better are the chances for survival. The cause of the continuous low rate of hemorrhage is not known but is thought to be, at least in part, abnormal vasospasm in the microcirculation (33). That is, if there is considerable spasm of venules, the increase in hydrostatic pressure in the capillaries may result in a loss of structural integrity. Another explanation may be that excessive arteriolar spasm may result in capillary endothelium ischemia with free-radical damage to the capillary and microocclusions that can compromise the capillary bed and lead to permeability of the arteriolar system.

The most successful treatment used in the spinal cord impact model has been the administration of a combination of aminophylline and Isuprel (33), which increases vascular and tissue cAMP and prevents both vasospasm and platelet aggregation (14,33). With this drug combination, blood flow, as measured with [14C]antipyrine autoradiographs, is maintained at a normal rate following impact and does not decline, as it does 2 hr after injury in untreated animals (28,37). Furthermore, as seen by histological examination, there is far less hemorrhage in the central gray matter when the injured animal is treated with aminophylline and Isuprel. The degree of improvement observed histologically is equivalent to that seen following treatment with Amicar (ε-aminocaproic acid) and steroids (methylprednisolone) (Figs. 14 and 15). Amicar prevents the destruction of occlusions by fibrinolysin and thereby helps to stop hemorrhage (3). It does not, however, maintain normal blood flow as does aminophylline and Isuprel. Amicar- and steroid-treated animals show less tissue damage on histological examination, although this is deceptive since blood flow is not improved. The basic difference between aminophylline/Isuprel treatment and Amicar/steroid treatment is that aminophylline/Isuprel therapy prevents permanent paralysis, whereas treatment with Amicar/steroids does not (3,33). Although Amicar stops bleeding, it also stops blood flow. The

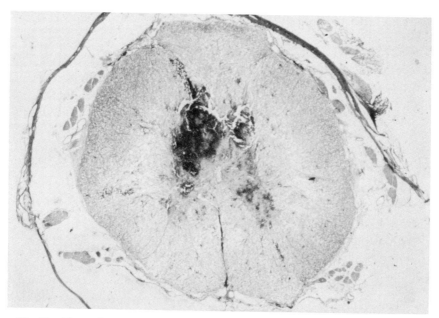

Fig. 14. Hemorrhage in the central gray matter 5 hr after impact in the feline model system with no treatment. × 21.

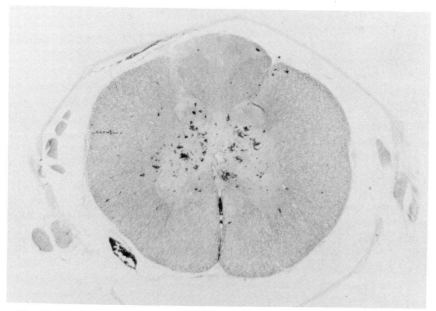

Fig. 15. Marked decrease in the hemorrhage of the central gray matter 5 hr after impact when treated with Amicar and steroids. Compare with Fig. 14. × 21.

choice of steroids in the combination regimen was based on their putative membrane-stabilizing effects. Seligman has shown that these steroids are excellent antioxidants (41). Despite the use of steroids with the expectation of an antioxidant action, this regimen did not provide sufficient protection. This may have been the case because not all cellular sources of O_2^- were controlled, e.g., iron/copper catalysis and ischemia with the generation of O_2^- from CoQ.

CONCLUSION

The spinal cord impact model illustrates the fact that a complete understanding of all the pathological mechanisms is necessary in order to use antioxidants or other agents successfully. With the spinal cord impact model there is bleeding and spasm in the cord following impact, which produces elevated tissue levels of metal ions from lysis of erythrocytes. This and the autoxidation of CoQ are sources of oxygen radicals. Both reactions must be controlled by the maintenance of normal blood flow, which can be accomplished with aminophylline and Isuprel (33). The results show that two approaches to the amelioration of ischemic injury can be taken: the use of antioxidants or control of the primary causes of the free-radical pathology.

REFERENCES

1. Boveris, A. (1977). Mitochondrial production of superoxide radical and hydrogen peroxide. *Adv. Exp. Med. Biol.* **78**:67–75.
2. Boveris, A., Cadenas, E., and Stoppani, A. O. M. (1976). Role of ubiquinone in the mitochondrial generation of hydrogen peroxide. *Biochem. J.* **156**:435–440.
3. Campbell, P., DeCrescito, V., Tomasula, J. J., Demopoulos, H. B., Flamm, E. S., and Ortega, B. D. (1974). Effects of antifibrinolytic and steroid therapy on the contused spinal cord in cats. *J. Neurosurg.* **40**:726–730.
4. Coon, M. J. (1978). Oxygen activation in the metabolism of lipids, drugs, and carcinogens. *Nutr. Rev.* **36**:319–328.
5. Demopoulos, H. B., Flamm, E. S., Seligman, M. L., Jorgensen, E., and Ransohoff, J. (1977). Antioxidant effect of barbiturates in model membranes undergoing free radical damage. *Acta Neurol. Scand.* **56** (Suppl.):152–153.
6. Demopoulos, H. B., Flamm, E. S., Seligman, M. L., Mitamura, J. A., and Ransohoff, J. (1979). Membrane perturbations in central nervous system injury: Theoretical basis for free radical damage and a review of the experimental data. *In* "Neural Trauma" (A. J. Popp, R. S. Bourke, L. R. Nelson, and H. K. Kimelberg, eds.) pp. 63–78. Raven, New York.
7. Demopoulos, H. B., Flamm, E. S., Seligman, M. L., Poser, R., Pietronigro, D. D., and

Ransohoff, J. (1977). Molecular pathology of lipids in CNS membranes. *In* "Oxygen and Physiological Function" (F. F. Jöbsis, ed.), pp. 491–508. P.I.L., Dallas.

8. Demopoulos, H. B., Yoder, M., Gutman, E. G., Seligman, M. L., Flamm, E. S., and Ransohoff, J. (1978). The fine structure of endothelial surfaces in the microcirculation of experimentally injured feline spinal cords. *Scanning Electron Microsc.* Vol. 2, pp. 667–682.

9. Demopoulos, T. R., Flamm, E. S., Yoder, M., Kaley, G., and Demopoulos, H. B. (1983). The ischemic cerebral cortical microcirculation and the effects of barbiturates. *Scanning Electron Microsc.* (in press).

10. Di Luzio, N. R., Stege, T. E., and Hoffman, E. O. (1973). Antioxidants lipid peroxidation, and chemical-induced liver injury. *Fed. Proc., Fed. Am. Soc. Exp. Biol.* **32**:1875–1881.

11. Dohrman, G. J., Wagner, F. C., and Bucy, P. C. (1972). Transitory traumatic paraplegia: Electron microcopy of early alterations in myelinated nerve fibers. *J. Neurosurg.* **36**:407–415.

12. Flamm, E. S., Demopoulos, H. B., Seligman, M. L., Mitamura, J. A., and Ransohoff, J. (1979). Barbiturates and free radicals. *In* "Neural Trauma" (A. J. Popp, R. S. Bourke, L. R. Nelson, and H. K. Kimelberg, eds.), pp. 289–296. Raven, New York.

13. Flamm, E. S., Demopoulos, H. B., Seligman, M. L., Poser, R. G., and Ransohoff, J. (1978). Free radicals in cerebral ischemia. *Stroke* **9**:445–447.

14. Flamm, E. S., Schiffer, J., Viau, A. T., and Naftchi, N. E. (1978). Alterations of cyclic adenosine monophosphate in cerebral ischemia. *Stroke* **9**:400–402.

15. Flamm, E. S., Seligman, M. L., and Demopoulos, H. B. (1980). Barbiturate protection of the ischemic brain. *In* "Anesthesia and Neurosurgery" (J. E. Cottrell and H. Turndorf, eds.), pp. 248–266. Mosby, St. Louis, Missouri.

16. Fourcans, B., and Jain, M. H. (1974). Role of phospholipids in transport and enzymic reactions. *Adv. Lipid Res.* **12**:147–226.

17. Gryglewski, R. J., Bunting, S., Moncada, S., Flower, R. J., and Vane, J. R. (1976). Arterial walls are protected against deposition of platelet thrombi by a substance (prostaglandin X) which they make from prostaglandin endoperoxides. *Prostaglandins* **12**:685–690.

18. Hahn, H. K., Tuma, D. J., Barak, A. J., and Sorrell, M. F. (1976). Effect of phenobarbital on lipid peroxidation in the liver. *Biochem. Pharmacol.* **25**:769–772.

19. Hall, E. T. (1973). The oxygen effect. *In* "Radiology for the Radiologist" (E. T. Hall, ed.), pp. 48–50. Harper, New York.

20. Hoff, J. T., Pitts, L. H., Spetzler, R., and Wilson, C. B. (1977), Barbiturates for protection from cerebral ischemia in aneurysm surgery. *Acta Neurol. Scand.* **56** (Suppl.):158–159.

21. Hourani, B. T., and Demopoulos, H. B. (1969). Inhibition of S-91 mouse melanoma metastasis and growth by D-penicillamine. *Lab. Invest.* **21**:434–439.

22. Kuehl, F. A., Ham, E. A., Egan, R. W., Doughey, H. W., Bonney, R. J., and Humes, J. L. Studies on a destructive oxidant released in the enzymatic reduction of prostaglandin G_2 and other hydroperoxy acids. This volume.

23. Lamola, A. A., Yamane, T., and Trozzola, A. M. (1973). Cholesterol hydroperoxide formation in red blood cell membranes and photohemolysis in erythropoietic protoporphyria. *Science* **179**:1131–1133.

24. Masterton, W. L., and Slowinski, E. (1977). "Chemical Principles," p. 203 and Plate 5. Saunders, Philadelphia, Pennsylvania.

25. McGinness, J. E., Proctor, P. H., Demopoulos, H. B., Hokanson, J. A., and Van, N. T. In vivo evidence for superoxide and peroxide production by adriamycin and cis-platinum. This volume.

26. Michenfelder, J. D. (1979). Barbiturates and cerebral ischemia. *Jt. Conf. Stroke Cerebral Circ., 4th,* February 9, 1979, Phoenix, Arizona.
27. Moncada, S., Gryglewski, R. J., Bunting, S., and Vane, J. R. (1976). A lipid peroxide inhibits the enzyme in blood vessel microsomes that generates from prostaglandin endoperoxides the substance (prostaglandin x) which prevents platelet aggregation. *Prostaglandins* **12:**715–720.
28. Nelson, E., Gertz, S. D., Rennels, M. L., Ducker, T. B., and Balumanis, O. R. (1977). Spinal cord injury: The role of vascular damage in the pathogenesis of central hemorrhagic necrosis. *Arch. Neurol. (Chicago)* **34:**332–333.
29. Pietronigro, D. D., Jones, W. G. B., Kalty, K., and Demopoulos, H. B. (1978). Interaction of DNA and liposomes as a model for membrane-mediated DNA damage. *Nature (London)* **267:**78–79.
30. Pietronigro, D. D., McGinness, J. E., Koren, M. J., Crippa, R., Seligman, M. L., and Demopoulos, H. B. (1979). Spontaneous generation of adriamycin semiquinone radicals at physiologic pH. *Physiol. Chem. Phys.* **11:**405–414.
31. Pietronigro, D. D., Seligman, M. L., Jones, W. B. G., and Demopoulos, H. B. (1976). Retarding effects of DNA on the autoxidation of liposomal suspensions. *Lipids* **11:**808–813.
32. Pryor, W. A., ed. (1976). "Free Radicals in Biology." Academic Press, New York.
33. Ransohoff, J., Flamm, E. S., and Demopoulos, H. B. (1980). Mechanisms, and treatment of acute spinal cord trauma. *In* "Anesthesia and Neurosurgery" (J. E. Cottrell and H. Turndorf, eds.), pp. 361–386. Mosby, St. Louis, Missouri.
34. Rap, Z. M., and Wideman, J. (1976). Changes in sulfhydryl group level and influence of exogenous glutathione on dynamics of vasobrain edema. *In* "Dynamics of Cerebral Edema" (H. M. Pappius and W. Feindel, eds.), pp. 164–168. Springer-Verlag, Berlin and New York.
35. Rehncrona, S., Smith, D. S., Akesson, B., Westerberg, E., and Siesjö, B. K. (1980). Peroxidative changes in brain cortical fatty acids and phospholipids, as characterized during Fe^{++}—and ascorbic acid-stimulated lipid peroxidation in vitro. *Anesthesiology* (in press).
36. Ruzica, F. J., Beinert, H., Schepler, K. L., Dunham, W. R., and Sands, R. H. (1975). Interaction of ubisemiquinone with a paramagnetic component in heart tissue. *Proc. Natl. Acad. Sci. U.S.A.* **72:**2886–2890.
37. Sandler, A. N., and Tator, C. H. (1976). Effect of acute spinal cord compression injury on regional spinal cord blood flow in primates. *J. Neurosurg.* **45:**660–676.
38. Schaefer, A., Kumlos, M., and Seregi, A. (1975). Lipid peroxidation as the cause of the ascorbic acid induced decrease of ATPase activities of rat brain microsomes and its inhibition by biogenic amines and psychotropic drugs. *Biochem. Pharmacol.* **24:**1781–1787.
39. Seligman, M. L., and Demopoulos, H. B. (1973). Spin-probe analysis of membrane perturbations produced by chemical and physical agents. *Ann. N.Y. Acad. Sci.* **222:**640–667.
40. Seligman, M. L., Flamm, E. S., Goldstein, B., Poser, R. G., Demopoulos, H. B., and Ransohoff, J. (1977). Spectrofluorescent detection of malonaldehyde in response to ethanol potentiation of spinal cord trauma. *Lipids* **12:**945–950.
41. Seligman, M. L., Mitamura, J., Shera, N., and Demopoulos, H. B. (1979). Corticosteroid (methylprednisolone) modulation of photoperoxidation by ultraviolet light in liposomes. *Photochem. Photobiol.* **29:**549–558.
42. Smith, D. S., Rehncrona, S., and Siesjö, B. K. (1980). Inhibitory effects of different barbiturates on lipid peroxidation in brain tissue in vitro. Comparison with the effects of promethazine and chlorpromazine. *Anesthesiology* (in press).

43. Spector, R. (1977). Vitamin homeostasis in the central nervous system. *N. Engl. J. Med.* **296**:1393–1398.
44. Wei, E., Wong, L. C. K., and Hine, C. H. (1971). Selective potentiation of carbon tetrachloride hepatotoxicity by ethanol. *Arch. Int. Pharmacodyn. Ther.* **189**:5–11.

DISCUSSION

SHEREMATA: The production of ischemia results in hypoxia or anoxia, but pure anoxia has been produced and is a different model. The structural integrity of the CNS, as determined by electron microscopy, is maintained if perfusion with saline is performed for periods of up to 20 min. Have you looked at functional differences (other than electroencephalogram analysis) in such a model? these decade-old observations suggest to me that either structural distortion or the effect of some intravascular material (such as O_2^-, $HO^{\cdot}$, H_2O_2, or other radicals) initiates structural changes. It will be important to study the latter model in the elegant way in which you have studied the ischemic model.

DEMOPOULOS: I think your idea that saline perfusion may "wash away" toxic radicals and radical intermediates, such as hydroperoxides, is an excellent one. We should test such models.

KUEHL: In stressing the importance of prostacyclin (PGI_2) in preventing platelet aggregation, I believe that you are referring to the report by Vane *et al.* that 15-hydroperoxyarachidonic acid (15-HPETE) inhibits PGI_2 synthase. We have recently found this not to be the case. Our data indicate that the depressed synthesis of PGI is brought about by the reaction of 15-HPETE with a peroxidase, a reaction that liberates a destructive oxidizing species, which deactivates PGI_2 synthase. The resulting depression of PGI_2 formation can be prevented by including a radical scavenger in the incubation mixture.

DEMOPOULOS: I was not aware of these new details on PGI_2 inhibition. The *net* result, however, is that pathological radicals hinder PGI_2 production and that antioxidants may help to preserve PGI_2 production.

Chapter 10

Free Radicals and Microvascular Permeability

ROLANDO F. DEL MAESTRO, JACOB BJÖRK,
AND KARL E. ARFORS

INTRODUCTION

On exposure to bacteria and other stimuli, polymorphonuclear leukocytes, macrophages, and monocytes undergo a respiratory burst (1–3). An important component of this activity is the univalent enzymatic reduction of O_2 to the superoxide anion-radical O_2^- (4,5). A proportion of the O_2^- generated is released into the extracellular space (6), where spontaneous dismutation can occur [Eq. (1)] with the formation of H_2O_2 and O_2. Some of the O_2 produced may be in the singlet state $O_2(^1\Delta_g)$ (7).

$$O_2^- + O_2^- + 2H^+ \rightarrow H_2O_2 + O_2 \tag{1}$$

The simultaneous presence of O_2^-, H_2O_2, and metal catalyst(s) in the extracellular space results in the O_2^--mediated reduction of the metal catalyst(s) [Eq. (2)], which can then react with H_2O_2 to form the hydroxyl radical (HO·) via a Fenton-type reaction [Eq. (3)] (8–12).

$$O_2^- + Me^{n+} \rightarrow O_2 + Me^{(n-1)+} \tag{2}$$

$$Me^{(n-1)+} + H_2O_2 \rightarrow OH^- + HO· + Me^{n+} \tag{3}$$

Kellogg and Fridovich (13) have suggested that the O_2 released in this reaction sequence may be $O_2(^1\Delta_g)$. Singlet oxygen may also be released by the myeloperoxidase reaction associated with phagocytizing polymor-

PATHOLOGY OF OXYGEN

phonuclear leukocytes (14). Although these reactive molecular species may aid in bacterial killing (15–17), they may also cause lipid peroxidation damage to cellular membranes (13,18) and depolymerize essential biopolymers (19–21).

It was therefore considered important to study the influence of the extracellular generation of these radical species on an *in vivo* microvascular preparation to learn more about their respective roles in the inflammatory process. The hamster cheek pouch microvasculature has been extensively used (22–25) to study the influence of various agents on microvascular permeability and was employed in this study. The oxidation of hypoxanthine to uric acid by xanthine oxidase results in the univalent reduction of O_2 to O_2^-, the formation of H_2O_2, and the subsequent generation of $HO^.$ and possibly $O_2(^1\Delta_g)$ (8,26). This enzyme system was used to generate these active oxygen species both *in vitro* and on the surface of the cheek pouch, and changes in the underlying microvasculature were continually assessed by *in vivo* microscopy.

MATERIALS AND METHODS

Preparation of Animals

Male golden hamsters weighing 70–120 g (Stockholm Biologiska Laboratorium) were anesthetized with 60 mg (per gram) ip sodium pentobarbital (Nembutal, Abbott, Chicago). A tracheotomy was performed and a P_{10} (Portex) catheter placed into a femoral vein for administration of supplemental doses of anesthetic and tracer substance. The cheek pouch was everted and prepared according to Duling (22) with modifications (25) for intravital microscopy of macromolecular permeability. The hamster with prepared pouch was transferred to the stage of a Leitz Ortholux microscope, where the cheek pouch could be continuously superfused, and the body temperature monitored and maintained at 37°C. FITC-Dextran 150 (fluorescein-labeled dextran, $\bar{M}_w$ 150,000, Pharmacia, Uppsala, Sweden) was administered intravenously (25 mg per 100 gm) in a 5% solution in 0.9% NaCl.

Microscopy

The cheek pouch was viewed through a Leitz Ortholux microscope, transilluminated with a 100-W mercury dc lamp (Irem Model EIXH5 P/L) with observations carried out at 35× magnification. Micrographs were taken of regions assessed.

Enzymes

Xanthine oxidase (grade 1), catalase, superoxide dismutase (SOD), and cytochrome (type VI) were obtained from the Sigma Chemical Co., St. Louis. The superoxide dismutase showed a specific activity of 1700 units per milligram protein when assayed by the method of Crapo *et al.* (27).

Chemicals

Hypoxanthine was obtained from Sigma Chemical Co., and uric acid, L-methionine, and the buffer salts were from E. Merck, Darmstadt, West Germany. Dimethyl sulfoxide (DMSO) was a gift from Dr. Stanley Jacob.

Solutions

The cheek pouch superfusion fluid was a bicarbonate-buffered saline solution with the following composition (mM): NaCl, 131.9; KCl, 4.7; CaCl$_2$, MgSO$_4$, 1.2; and NaHCO$_3$, 18. All solutions used for either *in vivo* or *in vitro* studies were prepared in the bicarbonate buffer purged with 5% CO$_2$ and 95% N$_2$ to maintain the pO$_2$ between 2 and 4 kPa, pH 7.35, and were warmed to 37°C.

PERMEABILITY STUDIES

The cheek pouch was observed for a 60-min equilibration period following injection of FITC-dextran 150. The macromolecular leakage sites (23) were counted at 10-min intervals before application of the solutions. These applications were carried out using standardized procedures.

Group 1: The superfusion was discontinued, and the solution was removed from the microscopic stage reservoir. This was replaced by 10 ml of freshly prepared solutions of either (a) bicarbonate buffer, (b) 0.96 mM hypoxanthine, or (c) 0.96 mM uric acid.

Group 2: Superfusion was discontinued, and either a 1.0-ml solution of denatured xanthine oxidase (20 min at 100°C) or 1.0 ml of active xanthine oxidase was added to the surface of the cheek pouch to give a final concentration in the reservoir of 0.05 unit/ml enzyme.

Group 3: Superfusion was stopped and the reservoir pool replaced with

0.96 mM hypoxanthine solution to which was added 1.0 ml of active xanthine oxidase solution.

In all experiments the solution(s) were left in contact with the cheek pouch for 1 min and then removed by commencing the superfusion. The cheek pouch area was scanned and leakage sites counted at 5, 10, and 15 min and thereafter at 10-min intervals for a total experimental observation time of 85 min.

The results of these experiments were clarified by additional experiments in which the reservoir solution was replaced with one containing either a scavenger substance or catalase to which active xanthine oxidase was added (final reservoir concentration 0.05 unit/ml) for 1 min and changes were followed as previously described. Control experiments were performed by adding the active enzyme to the reservoir solution in the absence of any test substances.

ASSAY OF SUPEROXIDE GENERATION

The reduction of ferricytochrome c by O_2^- was assayed in an *in vitro* system composed of 0.96 mM hypoxanthine and 50 μM ferricytochrome c in bicarbonate buffer to which xanthine oxidase was added at a concentration of 0.05 unit/ml. The increase in absorbance at 550 nm was monitored at 37°C with a double-beam spectrophotometer (model 124, Hitachi, Perkin Elmer, Connecticut) equipped with 1-cm thermostated curvettes ($\Delta E^M_{1cm} = 21{,}000$) (28).

Tissue homogenates were prepared from eight control cheek pouches, which, after freeze-drying (mini-Fast, model 1700, Edwards, Sussex, England), were suspended in bicarbonate buffer (0.5 ml buffer per 10 mg freeze-dried pouch). The supernatant was obtained after centrifuging for 20 min at 2000 rpm. Superoxide radical generation was assessed in a solution containing 50 μM ferricytochrome c and 1.2 ml of supernatant with and without 0.05 unit/ml of xanthine oxidase in a total volume of 2.5 ml.

ASSAY OF URIC ACID PRODUCTION

The uric acid produced from hypoxanthine by xanthine oxidase was determined in the system described for O_2^- generation by assaying the absorbance increase at 290 nM ($\Delta E^M_{1cm} = 14{,}000$).

STATISTICAL METHODS

Measurements quoted are mean values ± standard error. Statistical significance was calculated using the Student t test for *in vitro* experiments and the Rank-sum test (29) for the cheek pouch data.

RESULTS

FITC-Dextran 150 appeared in all cheek pouch preparations within 8–20 sec after intravenous administration and was seen in the entire microvascular bed within 35 sec. Fluorescent microscopy clearly demonstrated the hamster cheek pouch microvascular architecture (Fig. 1A). The number of leakage sites per square centimeter observed during the 60-min equilibration period varied among individual preparations, but no statisti-

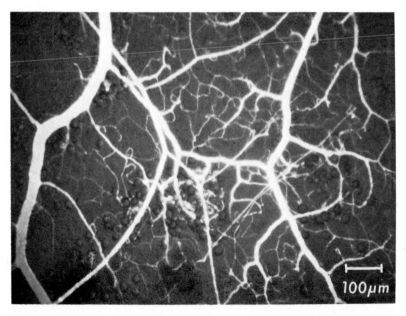

Fig. 1. (A) Micrograph of cheek pouch microvasculature taken in fluorescent light at ×35 magnification before application of 0.96 m*M* hypoxanthine and xanthine oxidase (0.05 unit/ml). (B) Same region 15 min following application of substrate and enzyme demonstrating FITC-dextran 150 extravasation from postcapillary venules. (C) Same area demonstrating clearing of postcapillary venular leakage 40 min following application.

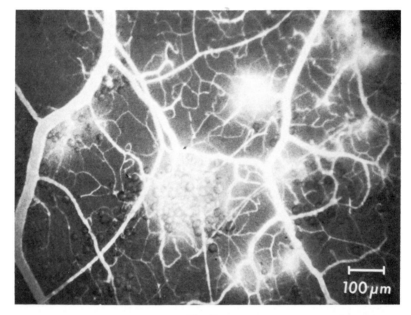

Fig. 1b.

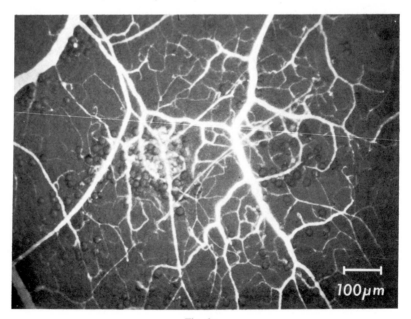

Fig. 1c.

cal differences were found among the different groups before test substance application (Table I).

No significant alteration in the number of leakage sites per square centimeter was observed after application of 0.96 mM hypoxanthine, 0.96 mM uric acid, or denatured enzyme as compared to bicarbonate buffer (Table I). The application of active xanthine oxidase or 0.96 mM hypoxanthine and active xanthine oxidase (Fig. 1B) was associated with a marked increase in the number of leakage sites, which reached a maximum 10 min after application and then decreased (Table I, Fig. 1C). The majority of leakage sites observed were associated with postcapillary venules (Fig. 1B). However, macromolecular leakage also occurred from large veins (Fig. 2), and in two of six cheek pouches in which hypoxanthine and active enzyme were added petechial hemorrhages (Fig. 3) were seen at 50 and 80 min. Arteriolar vasoconstriction and leukocyte rolling and adhesion were also observed only after topical application of active enzyme alone or combined with substrate. The causes of these changes are presently under investigation.

Since neither hypoxanthine (the substrate of the aerobic oxidation by xanthine oxidase) nor uric acid (the product of the reaction) resulted in increased permeability, it was hypothesized that the changes seen may be

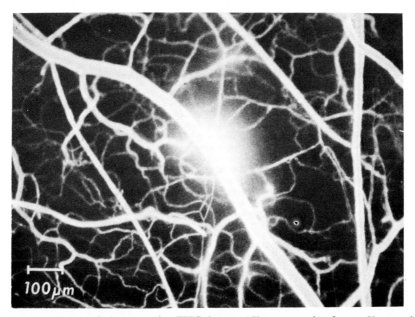

Fig. 2. Micrograph demonstrating FITC-dextran 150 extravasation from a 50-μm vein 15 min after application of xanthine oxidase (0.05) units/ml).

TABLE I

Effect of Topical Application of Test Solution(s) on Macromolecular Leakage Sites[a]

Test solutions(s)	Preapplication	Time after topical application (min)				
		5	10	25	45	85
Bicarbonate buffer	1.5 ± 0.9	2.5 ± 1.6	1.7 ± 1.1	2.0 ± 1.1	1.7 ± 1.0	4.7 ± 3.8
Hypoxanthine (0.96 mM)	3.2 ± 2.7	4.8 ± 2.8	5.7 ± 3.3	10.3 ± 7.5	6.6 ± 4.3	6.6 ± 4.3
Uric acid (0.96 mM)	3.4 ± 1.6	4.9 ± 2.0	5.1 ± 2.8	3.7 ± 2.2	4.7 ± 2.8	8.8 ± 5.9
Xanthine oxidase, denatured (0.05 unit/ml)	0.0 ± 0.0	0.7 ± 0.5	1.0 ± 0.6	0.0 ± 0.0	0.7 ± 0.5	2.5 ± 1.7
Xanthine oxidase (0.05 unit/ml)	1.5 ± 1.2	107.9 ± 38.2*	265.4 ± 36.7*	127.5 ± 52.2*	80.4 ± 39.4*	38.7 ± 15.2
Hypoxanthine (0.96 mM) and xanthine oxidase (0.05 unit/ml)	2.2 ± 1.1	207.9 ± 64.0*	295.6 ± 37.0*	164.0 ± 44.8*	93.7 ± 28.5*	89.7 ± 40.8*

[a] Values are mean number of leakage sites per square centimeter ± standard error (SE) for six hamsters in each group. Leakage site values were compared at each time period against bicarbonate buffer as a control using the Rank-sum test. Significant difference is indicated (*) when $\alpha < 0.025$ (29).

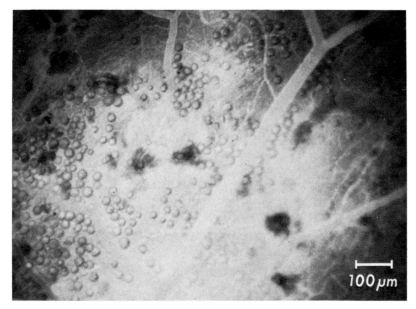

Fig. 3. Marked extravasation of FITC-dextran 150 and multiple petechial hemorrhages seen 50 min after application of 0.96 mM hypoxanthine and xanthine oxidase (0.05 unit/ml).

related to the associated free-radical flux. Xanthine oxidase oxidizes a wide variety of compounds (30), and therefore intrinsic cheek pouch substances could provide the substrates needed for generation of a free-radical flux when extrinsic substrate was omitted. To test this concept xanthine oxidase was added to cheek pouch tissue homogenates, and this was associated with an O_2^- flux of 4.3 ± 0.7 nmol/min ml ($n = 8$) compared to an O_2^- flux of 0.3 ± 0.06 nmol/min ml ($n = 8$) in its absence. This confirms that intrinsic substrates are available in the cheek pouch that can result in O_2^- generation on addition of active enzyme.

The substrate–xanthine oxidase system is also associated with the production of H_2O_2, HO·, and possibly $O_2(^1\Delta_g)$ (8,26). In an attempt to ascertain which of these reactive species may be involved in the permeability changes seen, scavengers and catalase were used. However, since an inhibition of enzyme function would also result in a decreased radical flux *in vitro,* experiments were carried out to rule out this mechanism as the primary one for the compounds tested. No decrease in uric acid formation was observed with any of the substances used (Table II). However, L-methionine significantly increased the rate of uric acid formation. L-Methionine did not significantly alter O_2^- generation (Table II), which was significantly lowered only by superoxide dismutase [catalyst for reaction (1)

TABLE II

Rate of *in Vitro* O_2^- and Uric Acid Formation[a]

Test compound	O_2^- formation (nmol/min ml)	Uric acid formation (nmol/min ml)
Controls	12.0 ± 0.5	12.9 ± 0.7
SOD (10 μg/ml)	$4.9 \pm 0.3^*$	12.8 ± 0.2
SOD (50 μg/ml)	$3.3 \pm 0.1^*$	13.1 ± 0.2
Catalase (50 μg/ml)	10.5 ± 0.5	12.7 ± 0.4
DMSO (10 mM)	10.4 ± 0.7	13.7 ± 0.3
L-Methionine (10 mM)	11.0 ± 0.3	$16.3 \pm 0.3^*$

[a] The assay mixtures contained 0.96 mM hypoxanthine plus 50 μM (cytochrome c)$^{3+}$ in bicarbonate buffer (ph 7.35) to which xanthine oxidase (0.05 unit/ml) was added. To this control mixture was added the test compounds in the concentrations indicated. Values represent means $\pm$ SE for six experiments in each case, and O_2^- and uric acid generation rates were calculated as described in the section on materials and methods. Statistical significance from control values was calculated using the Student t test. Significant difference is indicated (*) when $p < .05$.

(31)], suggesting that although L-methionine increased uric acid formation the total O_2^- flux remained unaltered in its presence.

The addition of superoxide dismutase (50 μg/ml) to the reservoir was associated with a significant decrease in the number of leakage sites observed (Fig. 4). Some decrease was also seen with superoxide dismutase (10 μg/ml), although this was not statistically significant. Catalase (50 μg/ml), which catalytically removes H_2O_2 by reducing it to H_2O, was also associated with a significant decrease in leakage sites (Fig. 5). These results suggest that neither H_2O_2, which would increase when O_2^- was catalytically scavenged by superoxide dismutase, nor O_2^-, which would be unaltered by the removal of H_2O_2 by catalase, is the primary reactive species responsible for the permeability changes seen (Fig. 6). Both of these substances appear to be necessary to produce the active agent. Superoxide anion may reduce metal complexes present in the cheek pouch or buffer [Eq. (2)], and H_2O_2 could react with these complexes to generate and HO· and possibly $O_2(^1\Delta_g)$ [Eq. (3)]. These reactive molecules could be instrumental in the production of the macromolecular permeability increases observed. This was further clarified by the use of DMSO (10 mM), an HO· scavenger (32) that was also found to decrease the number of leakage sites significantly. L-Methionine (10 mM), which reacts with both HO· (32) and $O_2(^1\Delta_g)$ (33), appeared to be even more effective in this regard (Fig. 7).

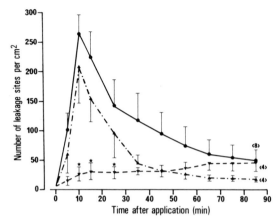

Fig. 4. Mean number ($\pm$ SE) of FITC-dextran 150 leakage sites per square centimeter after addition of 10 (—·—) and 50 μg/ml superoxide dismutase (---) to the reservoir before application of xanthine oxidase (0.05 unit/ml), compared to controls (—), in which no superoxide dismutase was added. Numbers in parentheses represent number of animals in each group. Leakage site values for the superoxide dismutase groups are compared with those for the group administered xanthine oxidase alone for each time period using the Rank-sum test. Significant difference is indicated (*) when $\alpha < 0.025$.

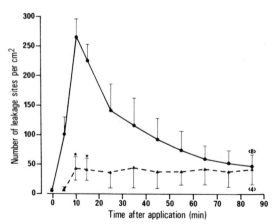

Fig. 5. Values are means $\pm$ SE of leakage sites per square centimeter with (---) and without (—) addition of 50 μg/ml catalase to the reservoir before addition of active enzyme (0.5 unit/ml). Numbers in parentheses represent number of animals. Leakage site values for the catalase group are compared with those for the group administered xanthine oxidase alone for each time period using the Rank-sum test, and significant difference is indicated (*) when $\alpha < 0.025$.

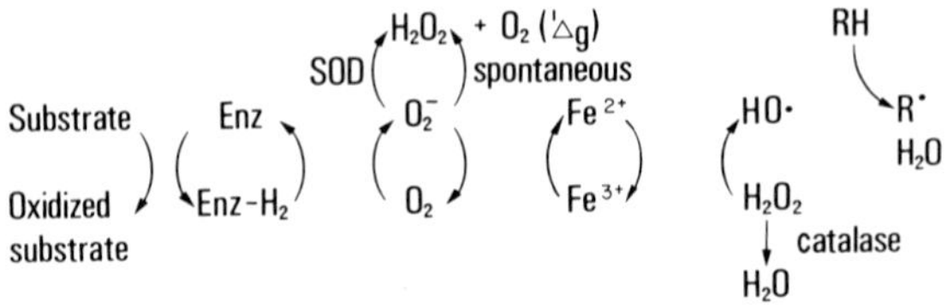

Fig. 6. Proposed scheme for the electron flow in the enzyme system studied. The electron flux is from the substrate (extrinsic and/or intrinsic) to the enzyme xanthine oxidase (Enz-H_2), which then reduces O_2 to O_2^-. Superoxide anion-radical can then reduce Fe^{3+} to Fe^{2+}, which reacts with H_2O_2 by the Fenton reaction to generate the HO· radical. The HO· radical can react with a wide variety of compounds such as biopolymers and lipids to generate other damaging radicals (R·). The generated O_2^- can undergo spontaneous dismutation [with the production of some $O_2(^1\Delta_g)$] but can be catalytically converted to H_2O_2 by superoxide dismutase. The mechanism of superoxide dismutase protection would be to remove O_2^- catalytically and prevent the O_2^--mediated reduction of Fe^{3+} and other metals. Since less Fe^{2+} would be available to react with H_2O_2 to form HO·, less tissue injury would result. Catalase catalytically decomposes H_2O_2 to H_2O and would prevent the production of HO. This would decrease the amount of HO· available to react with other cellular components.

DISCUSSION

The topical application of active xanthine oxidase and extrinsic substrate hypoxanthine to the hamster cheek pouch resulted in a spectrum of changes in macromolecular permeability, which ranged from leakage in postcapillary venules to large venular leakage to late petechial hemorrhage. Active xanthine oxidase application was associated with less macromolecular leakage, and petechial hemorrhages were not observed. Arteriolar vasoconstriction and leukocyte endothelial adhesion were also seen in both these groups.

It was hypothesized that these changes were associated with the free-radical flux induced by the aerobic oxidation of either extrinsic or intrinsic substrates by xanthine oxidase. Since both superoxide dismutase (50 μg/ml) and catalase (50 μg/ml) added to the reservoir decreased the expected macromolecular extravasation, HO· and possibly $O_2(^1\Delta_g)$ appeared to be the major species involved in initiating these changes. Both DMSO (10 mM) and L-methionine (10 mM) decreased the macromolecular leakage; therefore, it appears that HO· radical was involved. Using these scavengers, one cannot assess the role of $O_2(^1\Delta_g)$, although if produced it could certainly play a part in causing the changes observed.

Tissue injury and infection are associated with an alteration in the vascular endothelial cells, which results in a flux of H_2O and albumin into the extracellular space. The resultant edema is an important component of

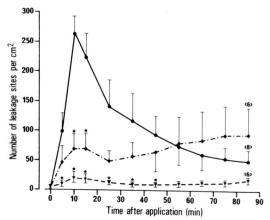

Fig. 7. Values are means ± SE of leakage sites per square centimeter after addition of 10 mM DMSO (—·—) and 10 mM L-methionine (---) to the reservoir before addition of active enzyme (0.05 unit/ml). Numbers in parentheses represent number of animals. Leakage site values for these groups are compared with the group administered xanthine oxidase alone (—) for each time period using the Rank-sum test, and significant difference is indicated (*) when $\alpha < 0.025$.

the inflammatory response. Histamine (24), bradykinin (23), and prostaglandins PGE_1, PGE_2, and $PGF_{2\alpha}$ (23) were applied topically to the hamster cheek pouch and were associated with increased macromolecular extravasation from postcapillary venules due to endothelial cell contraction (23,34). However, extravasation from large veins and petechial hemorrhage were not observed. The mechanism of action of HO· and $O_2(^1\Delta_g)$ on the cheek pouch microvasculature cannot be explained only by induced histamine and bradykinin release or by the production of the prostaglandins mentioned.

We suggest that in the cheek pouch model the extracellular generation of O_2^- and H_2O_2 results in the formation of HO· and possibly $O_2(^1\Delta_g)$ (Fig. 6). This occurs since the extracellular space has only small amounts of superoxide dismutase and catalase (20), and chelated metal complexes are plentiful. Hydroxyl radical and $O_2(^1\Delta_g)$ may then interact with the unsaturated lipids of cellular membranes, releasing hydroperoxides and arachidonic acid either through stimulation of phospholipase A or the disruption of a large area of membrane surface. The arachidonic acid to prostaglandin cascade would then be activated. The vasoconstriction associated with the addition of active xanthine oxidase alone or with extrinsic substrate is maximal about 3–5 min after addition and relaxes 5 min later, suggesting the presence of a short-lived active vasoconstricting agent, which may be thromboxane A_2 or a similar substance. Some of these compounds may also induce a reversible endothelial cell contraction. The increased arteriolar leukocyte adhesion may be a response to an alteration (peroxidation) of the endothelial cell membrane and possibly associated with the production of a serum chemotactic factor described by McCord in an earlier chapter. The timing of the petechial hemorrhages is reminiscent of results reported by Kellogg and Fridovich (13) in which erythrocytes exposed to a xanthine oxidase radical-generating system lysed 2–3 hr after exposure. Intramembrane free-radical chain peroxidation may be initiated by HO· and $O_2(^1\Delta_g)$, which, if uncontrolled by intrinsic scavengers, may eventually lead to endothelial barrier disruption and subsequent hemorrhage.

It seems reasonable to draw a parallel between the results of extracellular enzymatic generation of active oxygen species on the microvasculature and the results of their release and generation from activated inflammatory cells aggregated at sites of inflammation. It is suggested that the permeability changes and resultant edema observed during the inflammatory response may in part be related to the extracellular release of O_2^- from activated polymorphonuclear leukocytes and other cells. This results in further generation of HO· and possibly $O_2(^1\Delta_g)$, which may mediate the cellular and biopolymer damage resulting in altered microvascular permeability.

ACKNOWLEDGMENTS

We are grateful to Rickard Djursäter for valuable technical assistance and to Asa Lindquist for careful typing and preparation of the manuscript. This work was supported by the Canadian Medical Research Council.

REFERENCES

1. Babior, B. M. (1978). Oxygen-dependent microbial killing by phagocytes. Part I. *N. Engl. J. Med.* **298:**659.
2. Sbarra, A. J., and Karnovsky, M. L. (1959). The biochemical basis of phagocytosis. I. Metabolic changes during the ingestion of particles by polymorphonuclear leukocytes. *J. Biol. Chem.* **234:**1355.
3. Segal, A. W., and Coade, S. B. (1978). Kinetics of oxygen consumption by phagocytosing human neutrophils. *Biochem. Biophys. Res. Commun.* **84:**611.
4. Babior, B. M., Kipnes, R. S., and Curnutte, J. T. (1973). Biological defense mechanisms. The production by leukocytes of superoxide, a potential bactericidal agent. *J. Clin. Invest.* **52:**741.
5. Johnston, R. B., Keele, B. B., Misra, H. P., Lehmeyer, J. E., Webb, L. S., Baehner, R. L., and Rajagopalan, K. V. (1975). The role of superoxide anion generation in phagocy-

tic bactericidal activity. Studies with normal and chronic granulomatous disease leukocytes. *J. Clin. Invest.* **55**:1357.

6. Root, R. K., and Metcalf, J. A. (1977). H_2O_2 release from human granulocytes during phagocytosis. Relationship to superoxide anion formation and cellular catabolism of H_2O_2: Studies with normal and cytochalasin B-treated cells. *J. Clin. Invest.* **60**:1266.

7. Khan, A. U. (1970). Singlet molecular oxygen from superoxide anion and sensitized fluorescence of organic molecules. *Science* **168**:476.

8. Beauchamp, C., and Fridovich, I. (1970). A mechanism for the production of ethylene from methional. The generation of the hydroxyl radical by xanthine oxidase. *J. Biol. Chem.* **245**:4641.

9. Haber, F., and Weiss, J. (1934). The catalytic decomposition of hydrogen peroxide by iron salts. *Proc. R. Soc. London, Ser. A* **147**:332.

10. McCord, J. M., and Day, E. D. (1978). Superoxide-dependent production of hydroxyl radical catalyzed by iron-EDTA complex. *FEBS Lett.* **86**:139.

11. Tauber, A. I., and Babior, B. M. (1977). Evidence for hydroxyl radical production by human neutrophils. *J. Clin. Invest.* **60**:374.

12. Weiss, S. J., Rustagi, P. K., and LoBuglio, A. F. (1978). Human granulocyte generation of hydroxyl radical. *J. Exp. Med.* **147**:316.

13. Kellogg, E. W., and Fridovich, I. (1977). Liposome oxidation and erythrocyte lysis by enzymatically generated superoxide and hydrogen peroxide. *J. Biol. Chem.* **252**:6721.

14. Rosen, H., and Klebanoff, S. J. (1977). Formation of singlet oxygen by the myeloperoxidase mediated anti-microbial system. *J. Biol. Chem.* **252**:4803.

15. Allen, R. C., Stjernhölm, R. L., and Steele, R. W. (1972). Evidence for the generation of an electronic excitation state(s) in human polymorphonuclear leukocytes and its participation in bactericidal activity. *Biochem. Biophys. Res. Commun.* **47**:679.

16. Babior, B. M., Curnutte, J. T., and Kipnes, R. S. (1975). Biological defense mechanisms. Evidence for the participation of superoxide in bacterial killing by xanthing oxidase. *J. Lab. Clin. Med.* **85**:235.

17. Krinsky, N. I. (1974). Singlet excited oxygen as a mediator of the antibacterial action of leukocytes. *Science* **186**:363.

18. Salin, M. I., and McCord, J. M. (1975). Free radicals and inflammation. Protection of phagocytosing leukocytes by superoxide dismutase. *J. Clin. Invest.* **56**:1319.

19. Del Maestro, R. F., Arfors, K.-E., and Lindblom, R. (1979). Free radical depolymerization of hyaluronic acid. Influence of scavenger substances. *Bibl. Anat.* **18**:217.

20. McCord, J. M. (1974). Free radicals and inflammation: Protection of synovial fluid by superoxide dismutase. *Science* **185**:529.

21. Morgan, A. R., Cone, R. L., and Elgert, T. M. (1976). The mechanism of DNA strand breakage by Vitamin C and superoxide and the protective roles of catalase and superoxide dismutase. *Nucleic Acids Res.* **3**:1139.

22. Duling, B. R. (1973). The preparation and use of the hamster cheek pouch for studies of the microcirculation. *Microvasc. Res.* **5**:423.

23. Svensjö, E. (1978). "Characterization of Leakage of Macromolecules in Postcapillary Venules" Doctoral thesis, University of Upsala. Almquist & Wiksell, Stockholm.

24. Svensjö, E., Sharpe, D. E., and Arfors, K.-E. (1973). Leakage induced by histamine in the postcapillary venules of the hamster cheek pouch. *Microvasc. Res.* **6**:261.

25. Svensjö, E., Arfors, K.-E., Arturson, G., and Rutili, G. (1978). The hamster cheek pouch preparation as a model for studies of macromolecular permeability of the microvasculature. *Upsala J. Med. Sci.* **83**:71.

26. Fridovich, I. (1970). Quantitative aspects of the production of superoxide anion radical by milk xanthine oxidase. *J. Biol. Chem.* **215**:4053.

27. Crapo, J. D., McCord, J. M., and Fridovich, I. (1978). Preparation and assay of superoxide dismutase *In* "Methods in Enzymology" (S. Fleischer and L. Parker, eds.), Vol. 53, p. 382. Academic Press, New York.
28. Massey, V. (1959). The microestimation of succinate and the extinction coefficient of cytochrome C. *Biochim. Biophys. Acta* **34**:355.
29. Dixon, W. J.,and Massey, F. J. (1957). "Introduction to Statistical Analysis," p. 289. McGraw-Hill, New York.
30. Bray, R. C. (1963). Xanthine oxidase. *In* "The Enzymes" (P. H. Boyer, H. Lardy, and K. Myrbäck, eds.), Vol. 7, p. 533. Academic Press, New York.
31. McCord, J. M., and Fridovich, I. (1969). Superoxide dismutase. An enzymatic function for erythrocuprein (hemocuprein). *J. Biol. Chem.* **244**:6049.
32. Dorfman, L. M., and Adams, G. E. (1973). "Reactivity of Hydroxyl Radical in Aqueous Solutions," NSRDS-NBS No. 46. U. S. Dep. of Commerce, National Bureau of Standards, Washington, D.C.
33. Bellůs, D. (1978). Quenchers of singlet oxygen—A critical review. *In* "Singlet Oxygen" (B. Ranby and J. F. Rabek, eds.), p. 86. Wiley, New York.
34. Majno, G., and Palade, G. E. (1961). Studies on inflammation. I. Effect of histamine and serotonin on vascular permeability: An electron microscopic study. *J. Biophys. Biochem. Cytol.* **11**:571.

DISCUSSION

PROCTOR: My colleague at the Shriners' Burns Institute, Jim Hilton, has found that under experimental conditions superoxide dismutase inhibits burn-induced loss of plasma volume when it is administered before the burn but catalase is effective when administered both before and after the burn. This process does not appear to be inhibited by cyclo-oxygenase inhibitors such as indomethacin, so it may be mediated through the lipoxygenase system. Have you tried indomethacin in this system?

DEL MAESTRO: We are presently testing the influence of indomethacin in the *in vivo* test system. A specific arteriolar vasoconstriction occurs about 5 min after the addition of active xanthine oxidase or hypoxanthine and xanthine oxidase which may be related to prostaglandin (perhaps thromboxane A_2) and which may result from free-radical-induced release of arachidonic acid from cellular membranes.

CUTLER: The superoxide dismutase you added was on the surface of the hamster skin. What would be the effect of superoxide dismutase if it were injected directly into the blood? Do you think that superoxide dismutase applied to the surface of the skin can penetrate the skin and enter the cells? Is this the mode of protection?

DEL MAESTRO: We have not used intravenous superoxide dismutase, so we do not know what the effect of this would be. Since the half-life of intravenously administered superoxide dismutase is very short (see the chapter by McCord, this volume), we thought that direct application would provide more adequate levels of superoxide dismutase in the extracellular space where we had generated the O_2^-. Dr. Petkau (Chapter 14) will address the question of the entry of exogenous superoxide dismutase into cells, which does appear to occur. However, since the radicals are generated extracellularly in the model system we have used and the superoxide dismutase is administered topically, it is most likely scavenged at the extracellular level.

KUEHL: You have introduced prostaglandins with no effect. Have you applied arachidonic acid itself, which should yield both oxygen-centered radicals and other components of the arachidonic acid cascade? Our colleagues in France (Dr. Chibret *et al.*) have found that the administration of arachidonic acid subcutaneously causes protein leakage, an effect reversed by systemic administration of the scavenger compound MK-447.

DEL MAESTRO: I did not mean to give the impression that prostaglandins applied topically had no effect. In fact, PGE_1, PGE_2, and PGF_2 cause extravasation of cellular macromolecules but only from *postcapillary venules*. Extravasation from larger veins, was not seen and hemorrhage did not occur. The influence of the prostaglandins at the level of the microcirculation does not appear to be at the same site as the effect of the free radicals or free-radical-generated products. We are presently testing the influence of arachidonic acid on the extravasation of tissue macromolecules in our model system and hope to use MK-447.

Chapter 11

Studies on a Destructive Oxidant Released in the Enzymatic Reduction of Prostaglandin G$_2$ and Other Hydroperoxy Acids

FREDERICK A. KUEHL, JR., EDWARD A.
HAM, ROBERT W. EGAN, HARRY W.
DOUGHERTY, ROBERT J. BONNEY, AND
JOHN L. HUMES

INTRODUCTION

Prostaglandins are formed by the oxygenation of certain unsaturated fatty acids by a microsomal enzyme complex present in virtually every cell type. Most of the earlier studies were done on the E- and F-type prostaglandins. Later the intermediates, endoperoxides PGG$_2$ and PGH$_2$, the structures of which were proposed by Samuelsson in 1965 (23), were isolated and found to possess significant biological activity. More recently, thromboxane A$_2$ (TXA$_2$), which strictly speaking is not a prostaglandin because it does not have a prostanoic acid structure, and prostacyclin (PGI$_2$) have been isolated. Interest is now focused on these two new products because of their extreme biological potency and the fact that their actions appear to be in direct opposition to each other. Thromboxane A$_2$ contracts aortic strips and triggers platelet aggregation whereas, at very low levels, prostacyclin prevents these actions.

PATHOLOGY OF OXYGEN

The subscript following the abbreviation for a prostaglandin denotes the number of double bonds present in the prostanoic acid skeleton. Thus, in the scheme shown in Fig. 1, that derived from arachidonic acid, we are dealing with PGE_2 and related products. When the substrate fatty acid is eicosatrienoic acid, in which the 5,6 double bond is absent, PGE_1 and related products result. Eicosatrienoic acid cannot be converted to prostacyclin, nor does it yield a thromboxane possessing biological activity. These facts, along with the low levels of eicosatrienoic acid in tissues, emphasize the unique importance of arachidonic acid among the unsaturated fatty acids as the truly relevant precursor of the prostaglandin biosynthetic pathway *in vivo*. The acceptance of this view is indicated by the general use of the term "arachidonic acid cascade" to describe the series of enzymatic reactions shown in Fig. 1.

In this chapter, we describe some of our work on a heretofore ignored by-product released during the synthesis of prostaglandins and thromboxanes. We provide evidence that this substance, an oxidizing species released during the peroxidatic reduction of the endoperoxide PGG_2, hydroperoxy acids, and hydrogen peroxide, may itself play an important role in inflammation, atherosclerosis, hypertension, and other diseases in which lipoperoxidation is an important factor.

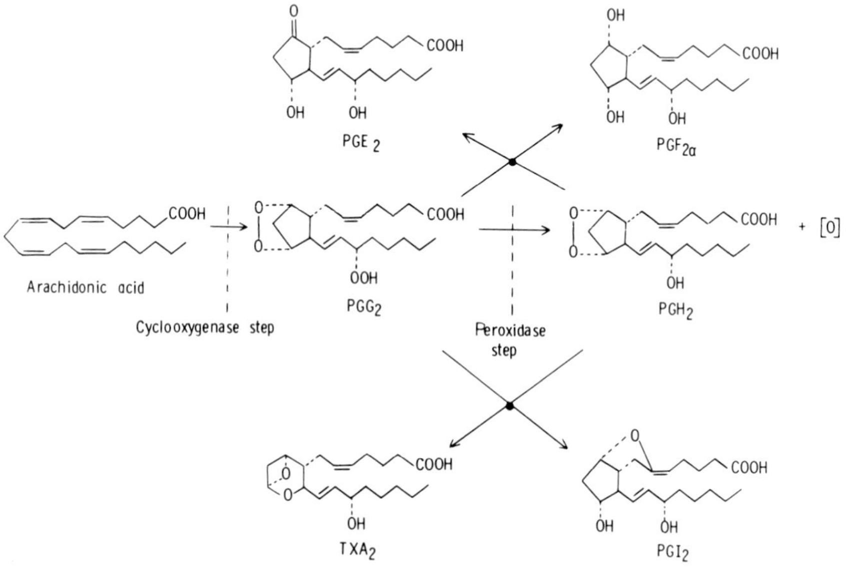

Fig. 1. Prostaglandin biosynthetic pathway.

DETECTION OF OXIDIZING SPECIES

The first data on an oxidizing species of the prostaglandin biosynthetic pathway were derived from studies with an experimental drug, an active antiinflammatory agent in animal models of inflammation. This compound, MK-447 (2-aminomethyl-4-*tert*-butyl-6-iodophenol), was found to be incapable of inhibiting the synthesis of prostaglandins *in vitro* as do indomethacin, aspirin, and other nonsteroidal antiinflammatory agents (18). On the contrary, it stimulated the synthesis of prostaglandins in the *in vitro* prostaglandin synthase assay. When a comparison was made of the separated products following the enzymatic oxygenation of arachidonic acid, the effect of MK-447 was to increase the utilization of substrate arachidonic acid, a reflection of enhanced cyclooxygenase activity, and to facilitate even more markedly the conversion of PGG_2 to PGH_2, a reflection of increased peroxidase activity. A number of radical scavengers, including phenol, methional, and aminopyrine, had an effect similar to that of MK-447, suggesting that they prevent the deactivation of the cyclooxygenase and peroxidase components of prostaglandin synthase by an oxidizing moiety generated during the enzymatic sequence (4,5). The site of oxidant release at the peroxidase was pinpointed by measuring the direct conversion of PGG_2 to PGH_2. In this peroxidatic step significant deactivation of the enzyme occurred, an action prevented by MK-447. Evidence

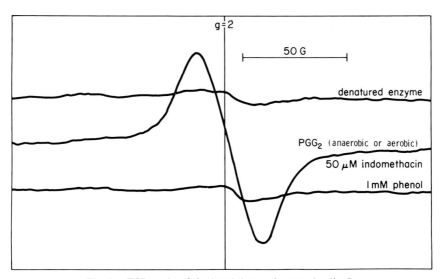

Fig. 2.   ESR study of the breakdown of prostaglandin G_2.

that the peroxidatic reduction is a free-radical-related event is presented in Fig. 2. In this experiment the reaction was quenched by freezing to − 176°C to give the EPR signal shown, an effect observed only in the presence of PGG$_2$ and active enzyme. At present, we have no knowledge of the nature of the radical observed in the EPR spectrum but consider that its formation is secondary to that of the oxidizing species, which itself is a radical.

The correlation between the actions of a number of compounds scavenging the oxidizing moiety [O$_x$] and antiedema activity in the mouse ear is depicted in Table I. In this model, inflammation is induced by topical administration of phorbol myristate acetate, and the edema measured by the weight of ear punches compared to that of the untreated control (18,26). Evidence of a scavenging action was established by the capacity of topically administered compounds to stimulate the conversion of PGG$_2$ to PGH$_2$ and blunt the ESR signal associated with [O$_x$] formation. A wide variety of compounds, including sodium iodide, are active in both parameters.

SUBSTRATES FOR THE PEROXIDATIC REACTION

Having established that PGG$_2$ releases an oxidizing species [O$_x$] on reaction with the peroxidase component of prostaglandin synthase, we

TABLE I

Comparison of Actions of Oxidant Scavengers

Compound	Concentration (mM)	% change in PGG$_2$ → PGH$_2$	Depression of EPR signal	Antiinflammatory action in mouse ear assay
Phenol	0.5	610	+	+
Aminopyrine	1.0	570	+	NT[b]
Promethazine	0.1	525	+	+
Lipoic acid[a]	0.1	465	+	+
Methional	0.2	345	+	NT
Sodium iodide[a]	0.25	393	+	+
Sulindac sulfide	0.1	525	+	+

[a] Egan *et al.* (5a).
[b] Not tested.

examined the enzyme for substrate specificity (19). The parameters studied were conversion of hydroperoxy to hydroxy acid, release of $[O_x]$ as measured by the ESR signal, and deactivation of enzymes. The compounds shown in Fig. 3 are all substrates for the peroxidase and are shown in order of decreasing reactivity with the enzyme. Prostaglandin G_1, the precursor of the PGE_1 series, like PGG_2, is an excellent substrate. 15-Hydroperoxyarachidonic acid (15-HPETE), the principal product of the reaction of arachidonic acid with soybean lipoxygenase, is also an excellent substrate. 12-Hydroperoxyarachidonic acid is a product of the reaction of arachidonic acid with a lipoxygenase present in platelets. As expected, 15-hydroperoxy-PGE_1 (15-$HPGE_1$) is a relatively poor substrate, an observation consistent with the belief that PGH_1 and not PGG_1 is the preferred substrate for PGE isomerase (Fig. 1). The finding that hydrogen peroxide is also a substrate demonstrates that the peroxidase associated with prostaglandin synthase is nonspecific and thus capable of generating $[O_x]$ from a number of hydroperoxy compounds. The reaction of H_2O_2 with this peroxidase raises the possibility that the same destructive species could obtain following dismutation of superoxide to H_2O_2 independent of the arachidonic acid cascade.

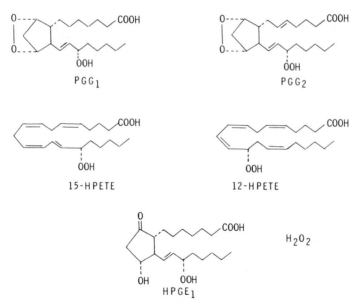

Fig. 3.   Substrates for prostaglandin peroxidase.

NATURE OF [O$_x$]

As a step in the direction of establishing the nature of the [O$_x$], we were interested in determining what substances are sensitive to its action. Since cyclooxygenase and peroxidase enzymes are susceptible to destruction by [O$_x$], amino acid constituents sensitive to such oxidation appeared to be logical targets (5). Tryptophan was shown to be by far the most susceptible to oxidation of the amino acids studied. It was surprising that methionine and cysteine were relatively resistant. There have been several published reports on the fatty acid-dependent oxygenation of a wide variety of organic compounds by the prostaglandin synthase reaction (5,20,24). Such oxygenation can most likely be attributed to [O$_x$] released in the peroxidatic conversion of PGG$_2$ to PGH$_2$. These data are consistent with the character of [O$_x$] as a short-lived, extremely potent, but very nonspecific oxidizing agent. Both methional and aminopyrine are free-radical scavengers and have been suggested to have a specificity for hydroxyl radical (HO$^{.}$) (1,8). Although [O$_x$] does oxidize these substrates and releases ethylene from the former, there is little evidence to support this alleged specificity. In fact, the use of methional for the purpose of identifying HO$^{.}$ has been the subject of critical studies in a recent report (22). We turned, therefore, to other targets of this oxidant. The sulfide of sulindac [5-flouro-2-methyl-1-(4-methylthiobenzylidene)-3-indenylacetic acid], a nonsteroidal antiinflammatory agent, was converted exclusively to its sulfoxide by [O$_x$] (5). Thus, with [^{14}C]sulindac sulfide as a scavenger, it was possible to measure quantitatively the reduction of the hydroperoxide and simultaneous oxidation of the sulfide. As shown in Table II,

TABLE II

Quantitative Comparison of 15-HPE$_1$ Reduction and Sulindac Sulfide Oxidation

15-HPE$_1$ (nmol)	Sulindac sulfide (nmol)	Protein (mg)	15-HPE$_1$ reduced (nmol)	Sulindac sulfide oxidized (nmol)	Ratio[a]
150	100	0	0	0	—
150	—	0.56	25	—	—
150	50	0.56	56	29	0.52
150	100	0.56	97	77	0.79
150	150	0.56	132	125	0.95

[a] The molar ratio of 15-HPE$_1$ reduced to sulindac sulfide oxidized.

the reduction of 15-HPE$_1$ and simultaneous oxidation of sulindac sulfide varies depending on the enzyme and sulfide levels. However, it is apparent that, when 132 nmol of 15-HPE$_1$ are reduced, 125 nmol of sulindac sulfide are oxidized. Since the peroxidase reaction appears to take place in the absence of oxygen (i.e., under nitrogen purging conditions such that the oxygenation of arachidonic acid does not occur), these data obtained with sulindac sulfide imply that both oxygens of the hydroperoxide are accounted for in the reaction products, one in the remaining hydroxyl and the other in the sulfoxide. The stoichiometry of this peroxidase reaction and the apparent lack of a requirement for external oxygen imply a scission between the two oxygen atoms of the hydroperoxy acid. Such a homolytic cleavage, in which external oxygen is not involved and neither oxygen atom from ROOH is converted to by-products, may be interpreted to favor [O$_x$] as equivalent to a hydroxyl radical or capable of generating such an oxidant. This interpretation was supported by the finding that treatment of reduced sulindac with potassium superoxide oxidizes it to the sulfoxide. This reagent is capable of generating HO˙ by a transition-metal-catalyzed equivalent of the Haber–Weiss reaction. Other products of this reaction, H$_2$O$_2$ and superoxide, have no oxidizing action on reduced sulindac.

PATHOLOGICAL ASPECTS OF [O$_x$]

Circulatory Diseases

The destruction by [O$_x$] of the cyclooxygenase and peroxidase components would be expected to have little pathological significance, since the effect would essentially mimic the action of nonsteroidal antiinflammatory agents, i.e., would block to a limited extent the total prostaglandin biosynthetic pathway (see Fig. 1). On the other hand, recent reports that the balance between TXA$_2$ and PGI$_2$ may be important in atherosclerosis and hypertension made it clear that selective sensitivity of PGI$_2$ synthase but not TXA$_2$ synthase to [O$_x$] could be an important pathological aspect of these diseases (21). We have established that prostacyclin synthase is, in fact, uniquely sensitive to deactivation by [O$_x$], whereas thromboxane A$_2$ synthase is completely resistant to its action (9). On these grounds it is reasonable to suggest that circulatory diseases that appear to be related to lipid peroxidation may result from the preferential deactivation of prostacyclin synthase secondary to release of HO˙ from PGG$_2$ or other hydroperoxy acids by the peroxidatic reaction.

Inflammation

In considering the possible targets of $[O_x]$ in inflammatory processes, it is obvious, as noted earlier, that an inhibitory effect at the cyclooxygenase or peroxidase step is not relevant. The unique sensitivity of prostacyclin synthase to such deactivation cannot be important either, since there is an increasing body of evidence suggesting that PGI_2 is itself an inflammatory mediator (3). A target of $[O_x]$ that might be of relevance to the prostaglandin biosynthetic pathway could be that associated with the release of substrate arachidonic acid. It is well established that prostaglandins are not formed directly from phospholipids; arachidonic acid must first be made available to the cyclooxygenase in free form. The action of glucocorticoids in blocking prostaglandin synthesis in intact cells occurs at this locus; it blocks the release of free arachidonic acid. Studies in our laboratory have shown that the cultured macrophage, a relevant cell in inflammatory processes, when challenged with the inflammatory stimulus zymosan or phorbol myristate acetate, releases large amounts of PGE_2 and PGI_2 (12,13). This release is depressed by incorporation of glucocorticoids in the medium.

It is obvious that the initial reaction of the above-mentioned inflammatory stimuli is to stimulate the release of free arachidonic acid. The possibility that $[O_x]$ is involved in this phenomenon was suggested by the finding that a number of scavengers of $[O_x]$, including MK-447, inhibit the synthesis of prostaglandins, an action not consistent with their stimulatory effect on prostaglandin biosynthesis *in vitro*. To explore the phenomenon in a more direct manner, the lecithin pool of mouse peritoneal macrophages was prelabeled with $[^3H]$arachidonic acid. These cells were challenged with zymosan in the presence of indomethacin to prevent prostaglandin formation. As shown in Table III, under these conditions free $[^3H]$arachidonic acid was released into the medium, a phenomenon reversed by inclusion of the scavengers promethazine and iodide in the medium. These data imply that zymosan-induced release of arachidonic acid is mediated by $[O_x]$, which we now believe to be HO·. Since the release of arachidonic acid from these intact cells occurred in the presence of indomethacin, an inhibitor of the cyclooxygenase, it is clear that $[O_x]$, if involved, is not derived from PGG_2. A reaction of another hydroperoxy acid or H_2O_2 with the peroxidase component of prostaglandin synthase or an undefined peroxidase, a step not subject to blockade by indomethacin, would appear to be the source of $[O_x]$ in this instance. Since there is a large body of evidence that zymosan stimulates the release of superoxide (O_2^-) from macrophages (17), it is attractive to suggest that the HO· $([O_x])$ purported to trigger arachidonic acid release from membrane phospho-

TABLE III

Inhibition of Zymosan-Induced Deacylation by Radical Scavengers and Glucocorticoids[a]

Additions to reaction mixture	Drug concentration (μM)	[³H]Arachidonic acid release (cpm)	Inhibition (%)
No additions	—	375 ± 10	—
Zymosan	—	1612 ± 137	—
Zymosan + dexamethazone	1	1019 ± 146	48
Zymosan + promethazine	70	942 ± 127	55
Zymosan + KI	50,000	974 ± 112	52

[a] Indomethacin, 3 μM, in all cultures. Zymosan concentration, 100 μg/ml.

lipid originates from O_2^- via a Haber–Weiss type reaction or by the reaction of H_2O_2 with a peroxidase, perhaps that associated with prostaglandin synthase.

To explore this alternative source of HO˙ from O_2^-, human polymorphonuclear leukocytes (PMN's) were studied for $[O_x]$ release. As with macrophages, when challenged with zymosan, PMN's release copious quantities of O_2^- and H_2O_2 (25); however, their capacity to synthesize prostaglandins is three orders of magnitude lower than that of macrophages (2,27). Zymosan-treated PMN's were shown to release an oxidizing moiety in the presence of indomethacin, an observation precluding the derivation of HO˙ via the prostaglandin cyclooxygenase–peroxidase pathway (i.e., via PGG_2). As seen in Table IV, this oxygen species is capable

TABLE IV

Oxidation of Sulindac Sulfide by Activated PMN's

Reaction mixture[a]	Sulfoxide produced (nmol)		
	Expt. I	Expt. II	Expt. III
PMN's (5 × 10⁶ cells)	0.7 ± 0.1	0.7 ± 0.1	0.3 ± 0.2
PMN's + Z	4.5 ± 0.0	8.4 ± 0.3	14.2 ± 1.2
PMN's + Z + SOD (50 μg/ml)	4.6 ± 0.02	7.7 ± 0.7	—
PMN's + Z + catalase (3000 U/ml)	0.7 ± 0.4	0.8 ± 0.2	—
PMN's + Z + catalase + SOD	0.5 ± 0.3	0.7 ± 0.1	—
PMN's + Z + indomethacin (1 × 10⁻⁵ M)	—	—	10.0 ± 0.4

[a] Abbreviations: Z, zymosan; SOD, superoxide dismutase.

of oxidizing sulindac sulfide. The failure of superoxide dismutase to block oxidation of sulindac sulfide is consistent with *in vitro* studies with this scavenger and implies that HO⋅ is not being formed by the reaction between H_2O_2 and O_2^- (Haber–Weiss type of reaction). In sharp contrast, the marked depression of oxidation in the presence of catalase emphasizes the role of H_2O_2 in facilitating this reaction. However, since sulindac sulfide is insensitive to direct oxidation by H_2O_2, the data are most consistent with a reaction between H_2O_2 and an undelineated peroxidase to yield HO⋅, which in some way alters membrane phospholipids to trigger the release of arachidonic acid.

BIOLOGICAL STUDIES

In exploring alternate targets of HO⋅ generated from the peroxidatic reaction, it is of interest to consider the early concepts of Ferreira and Vane (7). Their studies showing that combinations of PGE_1 with bradykinin are required to elicit full edematous and pain responses led to the suggestion that PGE's play a modulating role in inflammatory processes. In view of the fact that bradykinin can lead to the release of arachidonic acid from membranes (11), we have modified this concept (Fig. 4) by replacing bradykinin with what we consider to be the appropriate components of the arachidonic acid cascade (19). By itself, PGE_2 can induce vasodilation and therefore cause the redness and heat associated with inflammation. However, since PGI_2 is more potent than PGE_2 in raising cyclic AMP levels, a role of PGI_2 in the vasodilation associated with inflammatory processes seems likely. Clearly, edema is dependent on vasodilation for its fullest expression. Nevertheless, it is evident that the edematous response may be elicited in the absence of a significant increase in vasodilation, since edema can occur in the absence of redness.

An alternate approach to the use of scavengers to relate $[O_x]$ to inflammation would be to determine whether administered $[O_x]$ itself could cause symptoms of inflammation. Linoleic acid was shown many years

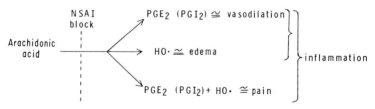

Fig. 4. Proposed role of prostaglandins and related products in inflammation.

ago to react with the prostaglandin synthase complex to yield hydroperoxy acids (10). Although its ω-6-associated double bonds enable it to
yield hydroperoxy acids, the double bond necessary for cyclization to
prostaglandins is absent. Thus, this acid is not converted directly to prostaglandins and yet can yield $[O_x]$, an action blocked by indomethacin.

From the mouse ear edema model of inflammation, it can be seen
Fig. 5a) that a relatively high level of arachidonic acid alone causes a substantial increase in weight (19). Of course, arachidonic acid has the potential for producing both PGE_2 and $[O_x]$ among other products. In Fig. 5b,
the same level of linoleic acid alone is shown to be essentially without effect. However, in combination with a level of PGE_2 that has little effect,
linoleic acid can cause a significant edematous response. These results
imply that combinations of PGE_2 and HO' are required to elicit a full response. The data in Fig. 5a show that the response to arachidonic acid is
blocked by either indomethacin or MK-447, either of which is capable of
blocking the accumulation of HO', indomethacin by its action at the cyclooxygenase, and MK-447 by its scavenging of $[O_x]$ formed. In Fig. 5b,
we see similar results when PGE_2 is added and linoleic acid is used as the
source of HO'. These findings are consistent with the concept that HO' is
a component of the edematous response, although its precise target is not
readily apparent.

The hypothesis that PGE's sensitize peripheral pain receptors to the ac-

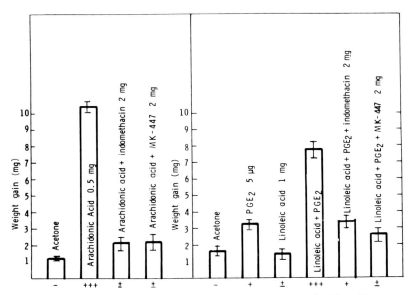

Fig. 5. Edema induced by (a) arachidonic acid and (b) linoleic acid.

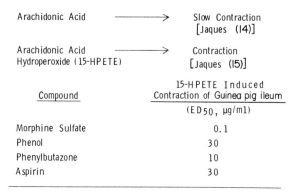

| Arachidonic Acid | ⟶ | Slow Contraction
[Jaques (14)] |
| Arachidonic Acid
Hydroperoxide (15-HPETE) | ⟶ | Contraction
[Jaques (15)] |

Compound	15-HPETE Induced Contraction of Guinea pig ileum
	(ED50, µg/ml)
Morphine Sulfate	0.1
Phenol	30
Phenylbutazone	10
Aspirin	30

Fig. 6. Effect of compounds on contraction of guinea pig ileum.

tion of other mediators such as bradykinin appears to be quite well accepted (7). In addition, the 1972 report by Ferreira that 15-HPETE causes an instantaneous but short-lived painful response when injected subdermally into human beings (6) suggested a possible interrelationship between PGE's and HO·. The potential of 15-HPETE for producing HO· was discussed earlier.

The relationship between pain and the contractile response of the guinea pig ileum, described by Jaques (14), was chosen as an *in vitro* model of pain in these studies. As indicated in Fig. 6 arachidonic acid induces a slow contraction of this tissue, which could be a reflection of the time required to generate PGE_2 and/or HO·. The more rapid response to 15-HPETE implies that HO· may trigger this response (15). The finding that morphine inhibits this contractile response implies that this action involves an opiate receptor in the guinea pig ileum. Inhibition by phenol is consistent with its role as a scavenger of $[O_x]$ (16). Finally, the effects of phenylbutazone and aspirin implicate a role for prostaglandins.

Thus, if one accepts the role of $[O_x]$ in causing pain as suggested by these *in vitro* studies, one of its sites of action must relate to the production of PGE_2 (or PGI_2) to explain the effect of NSAI on contraction induced by 15-HPETE. These data are consistent with studies on the macrophage implicating HO· as a mediator of arachidonic acid release in the guinea pig ileum.

CONCLUSION

Contrary to current dogma that peroxidases convert hydroperoxides to a lower oxidative state, the enzyme associated with prostaglandin synthase converts substrate hydroperoxides to a more lethal oxidizing moiety $[O_x]$. There is evidence that $[O_x]$ is the hydroxyl radical $HO^.$, a designation consistent with its highly potent oxidative capacity and the indiscriminant nature of its action. The $[O_x]$ is released by the reaction of a number of hydroperoxides, including H_2O_2, with the peroxidatic enzyme of prostaglandin synthase, an action that may be common to other mammalian peroxidases. The data indicate that $HO^.$ released from macrophages in response to an inflammatory stimulus triggers the release of arachidonic acid from membrane phospholipids, an action reversed by scavengers of $HO^.$.

The uniquely sensitive nature of prostacyclin synthase to deactivation by $HO^.$ in contrast to the resistance of thromboxane A_2 synthase to this oxidant suggests that its elaboration from the peroxidase component of prostaglandin synthesis may have pathological significance in such diseases as atherosclerosis and hypertension, in which lipoperoxidation occurs. However, the destructive action of $HO^.$ on the enzymes of the prostaglandin biosynthetic pathway does not readily explain its inflammatory effect. Studies with the macrophage suggest that the truly relevant action of $HO^.$ is that of stimulating the release of arachidonic acid from membrane phospholipids and thus triggering the arachidonic acid cascade. The reaction of H_2O_2 with a peroxidase to yield $HO^.$ offers an enzymatic alternative to the Haber–Weiss reaction as a source of $HO^.$ from O_2^-.

Clearly, further knowledge of other targets of $HO^.$ action is required before the origin and precise role of $HO^.$ in inflammation and other diseases can be explained.

REFERENCES

1. Beauchamp, C., and Fridovich, I. (1970). A mechanism for the production of ethylene from methional. *J. Biol. Chem.* **245:**4641–4646.
2. Bonney, R. J., Wightman, P., Davies, P., Sadowski, S. J., Kuehl, F. A., Jr., and Humes, J. L. (1976). The release of prostaglandins and lysosomal enzymes by cultured mouse peritoneal macrophages exposed to zymosan. *Biochem. J.* **176:**433–442.
3. Davidson, E. M., Ford-Hutchinson, A. W., Smith, M. J. H., and Walker, J. R. (1978). Prostacyclin (PGI₂) a potential mediator of inflammation. *BPS Proc.* p. 437.
4. Egan, R. W., Paxton, J., and Kuehl, F. A., Jr. (1976). Mechanism for irreversible self-deactivation of prostaglandin synthetase. *J. Biol. Chem.* **251:**7329–7335.
5. Egan, R. W., Gale, P. H., and Kuehl, F. A., Jr. (1979). Reduction of hydroperoxide in the prostaglandin biosynthetic pathway by a microsomal peroxidase. *J. Biol. Chem.* **254:**3295–3302.
5a. Egan, R. W., Gale, P. H., Beveridge, G. C., Phillips, and Marnett, L. J. (1982). *Prostaglandins* (in press).

6. Ferreira, S. H. (1972). Prostaglandins, aspirin-like drugs and analgesia. *Nature (London) New Biol.* **240:**200–203.

7. Ferreira, S. H., and Vane, J. R. (1974). New aspects of the mode of action of nonsteroid anti-inflammatory drugs. *Annu. Rev. Pharmacol.* **14:**57–73.

8. Griffin, B. W. (1977). Free radical intermediate in the N-demethylation of aminopyrine by horseradish peroxidase-hydrogen peroxide. *FEBS Lett.* **74:**139–143.

9. Ham, E. A., Egan, R. W., Soderman, D. D., Gale, P. H., and Kuehl, F. A., Jr. (1979). Peroxidase-dependent deactivation of prostacyclin synthetase. *J. Biol. Chem.* **254:** 2191–2194.

10. Hamberg, M., and Samuelsson, B. (1967). Oxygenation of unsaturated fatty acids by the vesicular gland of sheep. *J. Biol. Chem.* **242:**5344–5354.

11. Hong, S. L., and Levine, L. (1976). Stimulation of prostaglandin synthesis by bradykinin and thrombin and their mechanism of action on MC5-5 fibroblasts. *J. Biol. Chem.* **251:**5814–5816.

12. Humes, J. L., Bonney, R. J., Pelus, L., Dahlgren, M. E., Sadowski, S. J., Kuehl, F. A., Jr., and Davies, P. (1977). Macrophages synthesize and release prostaglandins in response to inflammatory stimuli. *Nature (London)* **269:**141–151.

13. Humes, J. L., Davies, P., Bonney, R. J., and Kuehl, F. A., Jr. (1978). Phorbol myristate acetate (PMA) stimulates the release of arachidonic acid and its cyclooxygenation products by macrophages. *Fed. Proc., Fed. Am. Soc. Exp. Biol.* **37:**1318 (abstr.).

14. Jaques, R. (1959). Arachidonic acid in unsaturated fatty acid which produces slow contraction of smooth muscle and causes pain. *Helv. Physiol. Acta* **17:**255–267.

15. Jaques, R. (1965). Suppression by morphine and other analgesic compounds of the smooth muscle contraction produced by arachidonic acid release. *Helv. Physiol. Acta* **23:**156–162.

16. Jaques, R. (1977). Inhibitory effect of enkephalins on contractions of the guinea pig ileum elicited by PGE_1. *Agents Actions* **7:**317–319.

17. Johnson, P. B., Jr. (1978). Oxygen metabolism and microbicidal activity of macrophages. *Fed. Proc., Fed. Am. Soc. Exp. Biol.* **37:**2759–2764.

18. Kuehl, F. A. Jr., Humes, J. L., Egan, R. W., Ham, E. A., Beveridge, G. C., and Van Arman, C. G. (1977). Role of prostaglandin endoperoxide PGG_2 in inflammatory processes. *Nature (London)* **265:**170–173.

19. Kuehl, F. A. Jr., Humes, J. L., Torchiana, M. L., Ham, E. A., and Egan, R. W. (1979). Oxygen-centered radicals in inflammatory processes. *In* "Inflammation" (G. Weissman, R. Paoletti, and B. Samuelsson, eds.), pp. 419–430. Raven, New York.

20. Marnett, L. J., Wlodawer, P., and Samuelsson, B. (1975). Co-oxygenation of organic substrates by the prostaglandin synthetase of sheep seminal vesicles. *J. Biol. Chem.* **250:**8510–8517.

21. Moncada, S., Korbat, R., Bunting, S., and Vane, J. R. (1978). Prostacyclin is a circulating hormone. *Nature (London)* **273:**767–768.

22. Pryor, W. A., and Tang, R. H. (1978). Ethylene formation from methional. *Biochem. Biophys. Res. Commun.* **81:**498–503.

23. Samuelsson, B. (1965). On the incorporation of oxygen in the conversion of 8,11,14-eicosatrienoic acid to prostaglandin E_1. *J. Am. Chem. Soc.* **87:**3011–3013.

24. Takeguchi, C., and Sih, C. J. (1972). A rapid spectrophotometric assay for prostaglandin synthetase: Application to the study of non-steroidal antiinflammatory agents. *Prostaglandins* **2:**169–184.

25. Tauber, A. I., and Babior, B. M. (1977). Evidence for hydroxyl radical production by human neutrophils. *J. Clin. Invest.* **60:**374–379.

26. Van Arman, C. G. (1974). Anti-inflammatory drugs. *Clin. Pharmacol. Ther.* **16:**900–904.

27. Zurier, R. B., and Sayadoff, D. M. (1975). Release of prostaglandins from human poly-morphonuclear leukocytes. *Inflammation* **1**:93–101.

DISCUSSION

FOOTE: The nature of your inhibitors suggests that the active species resembles a reactive species such as a peracid; thus, it would be an OH^+ donor rather than $HO\cdot$, so that the enzyme could act as a Lewis acid:

$$R\ddot{O}OH \rightleftharpoons R\ddot{O}\text{-}OH \quad \varnothing\text{:}X \longrightarrow HO\text{-}\overset{+}{X} \longrightarrow product$$

radicals $\longleftarrow$ E / E$^-$

To test this possibility, I suggest that you assess whether the activity of the inhibitor parallels the rate of reduction of peracetic acid by the inhibitor. This is a common type of peroxidase activity.

KUEHL: As long as we can obtain the same oxidizing species from hydrogen peroxides and, on the basis of our present data, exclude the requirement for an external source of oxygen, this possibility is compatible with our thinking.

PROCTOR: In connection with preliminary evidence obtained from Dr. James Hilton (University of Texas, Galveston) that burn-induced loss of plasma volume associated with the release of free fatty acids is inhibited by catalase but not by indomethacin, have you looked at the effect of any straight-chain fatty acid hydroperoxides in relation to this system?

KUEHL: I'm not quite sure what you mean by straight-chain hydroperoxy fatty acids. However, in addition to arachidonic acid, linolenic and linoleic acids form hydroperoxy fatty acids on reaction with prostaglandin synthase. These products in turn react with the peroxidase to generate the same oxidizing species as arachidonic acid.

BABIOR: Could the oxidation by polymorphonuclear leukocytes be due to myeloperoxidase?

KUEHL: We are currently exploring this possibility.

PIETTE: Were you able to observe your ESR spectra at room temperature? It would appear from its g value that the radical is not an oxygen-containing species. It is probably an alkyl-type of radical similar to those observed with all one-electron peroxidase oxidations of a variety of substrates. Does ascorbic acid inhibit the radical?

KUEHL: It is not possible to obtain an observable spectrum at room temperature because the reaction is too rapid. Ascorbic acid does inhibit the signal.

ŌYANAGUI: The Haber–Weiss reaction is active in alkaline reactions. Areas of tissue inflammation are said to be acidic. How is it possible, then, that the Haber–Weiss reaction contributes significantly to the generation of HO in inflammed areas *in vivo?*

KUEHL: I don't feel qualified to assess the role of the Haber–Weiss reaction. Our data suggest the possibility of an enzymatic alternative to the Haber–Weiss reaction as a source of HO in inflammation.

DEMOPOULOS: We have found that corticosteroids are antioxidants and prevent the oxidation of polyunsaturated fatty acids while they are still attached to phospholipids. Do you think this may be relevant to the effects of steroids on phospholipid synthesis? Can radicals breach the ester bond, and can we do without phospholipase?

KUEHL: I do not know if radicals can breach the ester bond.

MICHELSON: Ultraviolet light can breach phosphate–ester covalent bonds.

ŌYANAGUI: The activation of arachidonic acid by active oxygen radicals is apparently required to obtain maximum prostaglandin synthesis. Have you some comments on this point?

KUEHL: Dr. William Lands (University of Michigan) has provided evidence that a hydroperoxide is necessary to initiate the cyclooxygenase reaction. Consistant with this concept, we have found that high levels of phenol compounds (which act as scavengers of oxygen radicals) inhibit cyclooxygenase at low substrate levels. To rule out the possibility that scavengers are inhibiting cyclooxygenase rather than arachidonic acid release from macrophages, we employed fully inhibitory doses of indomethacin, which permitted a direct readout of arachidonic acid release.

Chapter 12

An *in Vivo* Enzymatic Probe for Superoxide and Peroxide Production by Chemotherapeutic Agents

JOHN E. MCGINNESS, PETER H. PROCTOR,
HARRY B. DEMOPOULOS, JAMES A.
HOKANSON, AND NGUYEN T. VAN

INTRODUCTION

Oxygen is no longer considered to be without risk to aerobic living systems which require oxygen to sustain life. The biochemical nature of toxic active oxygen species and its medical implications have opened a new area of medical investigation. The topic of this chapter, however, is restricted to superoxide (O_2^-) and hydrogen peroxide (H_2O_2), two important species of active oxygen, and the enzymes superoxide dismutase and catalase, which have evolved to protect aerobic cells from these two toxic species.

A number of chemotherapeutic agents have been shown to stimulate the production of O_2^- [1,2]. The data presented here relate only to the anticancer drugs *cis*-platinum and adriamycin. In addition to having antitumor activity, *cis*-platinum and adriamycin are toxic to the host. At present there is only limited information as to the precise relationship between toxicity directed toward the tumor and toxicity toward the host. The possibility that the cardiac toxicity of adriamycin might be suppressed with-

PATHOLOGY OF OXYGEN

out interfering with the antitumor activity was explored using a pretreatment with reduced vitamin E (3). The use of vitamin E, however, has not completely solved the clinical problem, and more basic information is required.

The enzymes superoxide dismutase and catalase can provide answers to a number of important questions. Injections of superoxide dismutase and catalase can be expected to increase the extracellular levels of these enzymes. The specificity of the enzymes makes it possible to carry out an independent evaluation of the role of O_2^- and H_2O_2 in the toxicity of anticancer drugs. Our final goal is to develop a set of extracellular and intracellular antioxidants that can be used to evaluate the specific role of each type of active oxygen species. One important step in this direction is understanding the extracellular contribution of O_2^- and H_2O_2 to the toxicity of adriamycin and *cis*-platinum (3,5). In this chapter, we present results obtained by increasing the extracellular levels of either superoxide dismutase or catalase (or both) and then challenging the animals with *cis*-platinum and adriamycin. The response was found to depend on both dose and time.

CHEMOTHERAPEUTIC AGENTS

cis-Diaminodichloroplatinum(II)

The molecular events that occur in *cis*-platinum-induced nephrotoxicity are not known. Both superoxide and hydrogen peroxide appear to be generated. The nephrotoxicity associated with acute doses of *cis*-platinum (up to 10 mg/kg) is ameliorated by superoxide dismutase. Previously reported results are briefly summarized as follows (6,7). Increased survival was correlated more closely with the capacity of superoxide dismutase to minimize *cis*-platinum-induced diarrhea than with the measured kidney toxicity. Examination of the pathological kidney tissue, however, did show that less damage was present in the rats receiving *cis*-platinum and superoxide dismutase than in the rats receiving *cis*-platinum alone.

Although O_2^- production appears to be stimulated by *cis*-platinum, it alone cannot account for the nephrotoxicity. Studies of the effects of chronic administration of *cis*-platinum (5 mg/kg) revealed a synergistic toxicity when the *cis*-platinum was combined with superoxide dismutase. Since superoxide dismutase can convert O_2^- to H_2O_2 and O_2, a study of the combined effects of *cis*-platinum, superoxide dismutase, and catalase was undertaken (Fig. 1). The synergistic toxicity observed with chronic

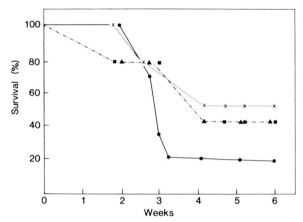

Fig. 1. Percent survival of Sprague–Dawley rats receiving three-weekly ip injections of 5 mg/kg *cis*-diaminodichloroplatinum(II) (CDDP). The mortality was greatest for rats receiving superoxide dismutase (SOD) and *cis*-platinum. Key: ▲, CDDP only; ●, CDDP + 1.0 mg/kg SOD; X, CDDP + 1.0 mg/kg catalase; ■, CDDP + 1.0 mg/kg SOD + 1.0 mg/kg catalase.

application of *cis*-platinum and superoxide dismutase was reversed by catalase. Catalase appeared to offer some protection at these doses but was far less effective than might be expected if H_2O_2 alone were responsible for the chronic toxicity.

Since the greatest toxic effects observed were obtained with superoxide dismutase and *cis*-platinum, a tumor experiment was undertaken with these two drugs. A transplantable leiomyosarcoma (accession no. 14072, experimental no. LX 7330-M09-TB-MU) from Syrian hamster ductus deferens tissues (8,9) was injected into the hamsters subcutaneously in the hind area. Superoxide dismutase did not interfere with the antitumor action of *cis*-platinum at these doses (Fig. 2).

Adriamycin

During our initial work with *cis*-platinum, the observation that O_2^- is produced *in vitro* by adriamycin appeared in print (5). We began experiments with adriamycin *in vivo* in combination with superoxide dismutase and *cis*-platinum. Our first observation was that the cardiac toxicity induced by three pulse doses of 5 mg/kg adriamycin was ameliorated by daily im injections of 1 mg/kg superoxide dismutase and 1 mg/kg catalase (Table I). Representative photomicrographs were prepared from sections cut across the entire heart, which was fixed in formalin while still beating.

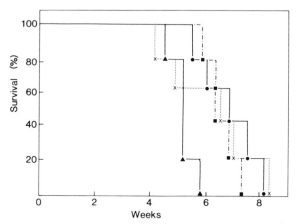

Fig. 2.   Percent survival of tumor-bearing Syrian hamsters receiving 5 mg/kg *cis*-diamino-dichloroplatinum(II) in three-weekly injections. Rate of survival increased with both *cis*-platinum and the enzyme superoxide dismutase. The antitumor activity of the *cis*-platinum was not affected by these agents. Key: ■, CDDP + 10^6 tumor cells; X, 1 mg/kg SOD + 10^6 tumor cells; ●, CDDP + 1 mg/kg SOD + 10^6 tumor cells; ▲, 10^6 tumor cells.

All hearts were fixed and stained at the same time. Micrographs of the tissue, stained with hematoxylin and eosin, were taken from the muscle tissue of the wall of the left ventricle to show longitudinal muscle bundles and cross-sectional muscle bundles (Fig. 3). The damaged hearts show decreased eosinophilic staining and no infiltration by leukocytes (Fig. 3A, C).

Chronic administration of adriamycin consisted of three doses of 4 mg/kg given at 1-week intervals. The survival data indicate that superoxide dismutase alone increased the toxicity of adriamycin on a chronic schedule at this dose (Fig. 4). Catalase enhanced survival. Treatment with superoxide dismutase and catalase appeared to support a slightly higher

TABLE I

Effects of Superoxide Dismutase plus Catalase on Adriamycin Cardiotoxicity[a]

Number of rats	Treatment	% affected	Extent[b]
6	Adriamycin alone	83 (5/6)	20 ± 10
6	Adriamycin with superoxide dismutase plus catalase	16 (1/6)	15

[a] Masked pathology analysis of heart sections of rats receiving 1 mg/kg superoxide dismutase and 1 mg/kg catalase in addition to 5 mg/kg adriamycin in three-weekly doses.

[b] Extent refers to the approximate percentage of myocardial fibers affected.

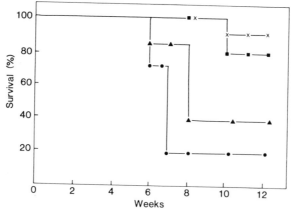

Fig. 4. Percent survival of 12 rats per group receiving 4 mg/kg adriamycin in three-weekly doses. Mortality was greatest for rats receiving 1 mg/kg superoxide dismutase in addition to adriamycin. The combination of 1 mg/kg catalase and adriamycin significantly reduced the mortality ($p < .01$). The greatest protection was seen with superoxide dismutase and catalase together. Experiment was terminated at 12 weeks for necropsy. Key: ▲, adriamycin only; ●, adriamycin + 1 mg/kg SOD; ■, adriamycin + 1 mg/kg catalase; X, adriamycin + 1 mg/kg SOD + 1 mg/kg catalase.

survival than treatment with catalase alone. One rat from each group was necropsied. The rat receiving adriamycin alone was found to have extreme congestion of all myocardial and subequicardial vessels. At this lower level of adriamycin (12 mg/kg total) the hearts did not show the muscle damage seen in the experiment with three-weekly injections of 5 mg/kg. The rats receiving catalase and superoxide dismutase plus catalase were free of heart congestion. Peritonitis was observed with adriamycin and superoxide dismutase or adriamycin and catalase. The combination of superoxide dismutase and catalase seemed to prevent the adriamycin-associated peritonitis under these experimental conditions. A single pulse dose of adriamycin (10 mg/kg) produced significant mortality within 6 weeks and was chosen as the test dose to study the effects of superoxide dismutase and catalase treatment. The dose–response data with adriamycin and superoxide dismutase are presented in Fig. 5. Animals treated with superoxide dismutase were spared during the first few weeks. These animals showed no diarrhea or other signs of illness until the fourth week. Superoxide dismutase was administered every day. Since these data were obtained, we have found that posttreatment should be discontinued after 2 weeks. The dose–response data with catalase and adriamycin are presented in Fig. 6. Even with large doses of catalase little protection was evident. The activity of catalase was 64,000 units/mg, and that of superox-

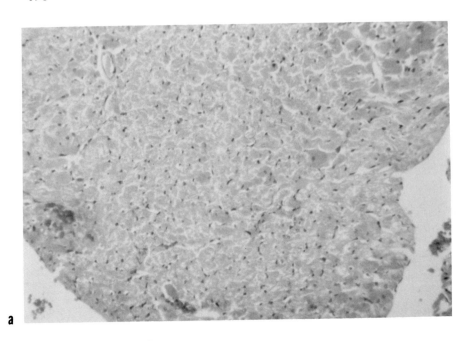

a

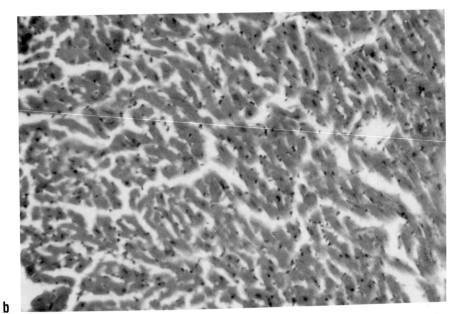

b

Fig. 3. Micrographs of representative muscle tissue (hematoxylin and eosin stained) taken from the wall of the left ventricle of the rats described in Table I. The adriamycin produces decreased eosinophilic staining and no polymorphonuclear leukocytic infiltration.

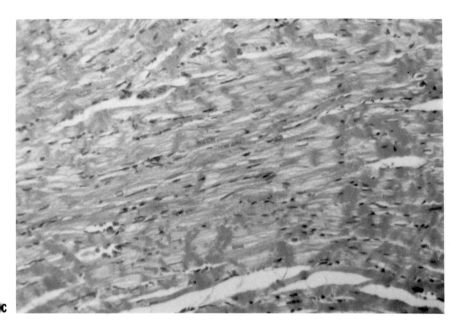

c

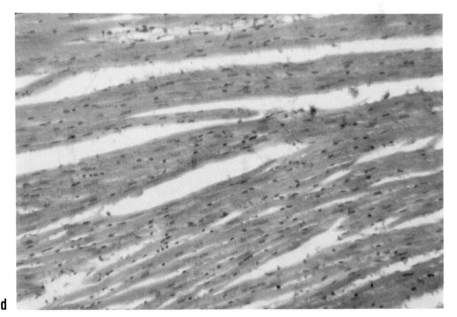

d

(a) Adriamycin treated (cross section). (b) Treated with adriamycin, superoxide, and catalase (cross section). (c) Adriamycin treated (longitudinal section). (d) Treated with adriamycin, superoxide, and catalase (longitudinal section).

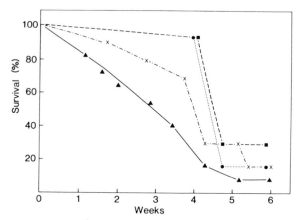

Fig. 5. Percent survival of 36 Lewis inbred rats (300 g weight) receiving a single ip dose of 10 mg/kg adriamycin and daily im injections of superoxide dismutase as indicated. Key: ▲, adriamycin only; X, adriamycin + 0.04 mg/kg SOD; ●, adriamycin + 0.4 mg/kg SOD; ■, adriamycin + 4.0 mg/kg SOD.

ide dismutase was 3300 units/mg. The catalase experiment extended to a higher enzymatic activity.

A survival and necropsy experiment was conducted with superoxide dismutase, catalase, and adriamycin (Fig. 7). Superoxide dismutase and catalase were administered for 2 weeks; then catalase alone was administered. Necropsy was performed on two rats from each group at 18 days,

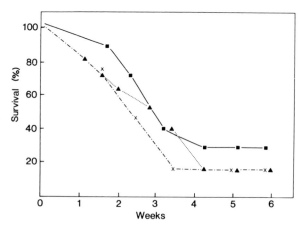

Fig. 6. Percent survival of 36 Lewis inbred rats (300 g weight) receiving a single ip dose of 10 mg/kg adriamycin. Catalase was administered im daily at the doses indicated. Key: ▲, adriamycin only; X, adriamycin + 0.1 mg/kg catalase; ■, adriamycin + 1.0 mg/kg catalase.

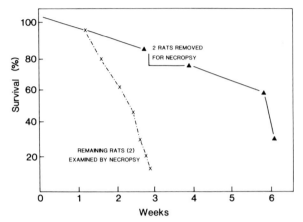

Fig. 7. Percent survival of rats treated with 10 mg/kg adriamycin (high dose) in a single ip injection. The enzymes superoxide dismutase (1 mg/kg) and catalase (1 mg/kg) significantly enhanced survival. Key: X—·—X, adriamycin only; ▲—△, adriamycin plus enzymes.

the point of maximum survival difference. The remaining rats receiving superoxide dismutase, catalase, and adriamycin survived for 6 weeks, which is 2 weeks longer than those given superoxide dismutase alone. Experiments are now in progress to determine whether the increased life span was due to the action of catalase or to the limited exposure to superoxide dismutase or both. The necropsy showed no cardiac damage with the ip injection of 10 mg/kg adriamycin. Death appeared to be due to peritonitis and diarrhea. The animals receiving superoxide dismutase and catalase as described were free of both peritonitis and diarrhea for 5 weeks following injection of 10 mg/kg adriamycin.

Bleomycin

Experimental evidence indicates that superoxide dismutase and catalase can inhibit double-strand DNA breaks by bleomycin (10). In an experiment with 28 mice we administered bleomycin each week for 6 weeks. The mice were split into two groups of 14, each having seven males and seven females. At the end of the 6 weeks all of the females were pregnant in the group receiving bleomycin combined with 1 mg/kg superoxide dismutase and 1 mg/kg catalase. None of the females became pregnant in the group receiving bleomycin alone. These observations support the suggested role of H_2O_2 and O_2^- in the action of bleomycin (11).

SUMMARY

The data obtained with superoxide dismutase and catalase reveal a complicated time- and dose-dependent relation to *cis*-platinum and adriamycin toxicity. The first reaction to these drugs appears to involve O_2^-. Toxicity that is expressed at later times with high doses appears to involve hydrogen peroxide. There are at least three stages of toxicity. At the first stage, when superoxide dismutase is most protective, catalase does not show much effect. There is a second or intermediate stage in which catalase and superoxide dismutase together produce the best results. This is observed when superoxide dismutase alone increases the toxicity. The third stage involved interrupted administration of superoxide dismutase. Superoxide dismutase can even prevent catalase from being effective if it is continued after the animals begin to die. Since our discovery that superoxide dismutase and catalase can affect the toxicity of *cis*-platinum (6), the capacity of *cis*-platinum to deplete sulfhydryl groups has been reported. The effect of superoxide dismutase and catalase on lipid peroxidation following glutathione (GSH) depletion was measured by the resulting malondialdehyde (MDA) levels (13). Superoxide dismutase and catalase did not inhibit MDA production even when combined. These results show the clear difference between acute *cis*-platinum toxicity, in which superoxide dismutase and catalase are effective, and chronic *cis*-platinum toxicity, in which they have a limited effect.

The schedule of administration as well as the dose of the administered drug is important. Vitamin E is more effective if given in more than one pretreatment (14). The effect of a single vitamin E injection was reported only to delay toxicity (15). A role for GSH in adriamycin toxicity has been reported (16), and an elevation of serum lipid peroxide levels associated with adriamycin treatment can apparently be ameliorated by vitamin E (17). However, when vitamin E application was chronic, this attempt to protect against cardiac toxicity in the rabbit failed (18). Our observation that superoxide dismutase and catalase ameliorated or at least delayed cardiac toxicity suggests that O_2^- and H_2O_2 are more important in chronic adriamycin toxicity than in the toxicity of *cis*-platinum.

The pathology studies after adriamycin administration showed mitochondria in the area where tissue has been damaged (19). We have reported an age-dependent retinal degeneration induced by adriamycin with a similar pathological pattern. Vessels are unaltered, phagocytes are not found, and intact mitochondria are present among remnant photoreceptor discs and remnant photoreceptor nuclei (20). The retinal degeneration does appear to be ameliorated by HR (Z12004), which also enhances survival and maintains a more normal differential white blood cell count. HR (Z12004) was tested further when it was discovered that the administration of this agent after adriamycin administration provided protection. We now know that vitamin E is most effective when given before adriamycin (21), whereas superoxide dismutase and catalase are most effective when given before and after adriamycin. We therefore conclude that the demonstrated dependence on schedule does not allow a complete assessment of a potential ameliorative agent to be made until it has been tested both before and after administration of the anticancer agent. Any compound that cannot be used after adriamycin administration may not be effective in chronic administration. Finally, we have found that such agents as superoxide dismutase, catalase, and HR (Z12004) can be used after adriamycin administration.

REFERENCES

1. Bachur, N. R., Gordon, S. L., and Gee, M. V. (1977). Anthracycline antibiotic augmentation of microsomal electron transport and free radical formation. *Mol. Pharmacol.* **13**:901.
2. Bachur, N. R., Gordon, S. L., and Gee, M. V. (1978). A general mechanism for microsomal activation of quinone anticancer agents to free radicals. *Cancer Res.* **38**:1745.
3. Myers, C. E., McGuire, W. P., Liss, R. H., Ifrim, I., Grotzinger, K., and Young, R. C. (1977). Adriamycin: The role of lipid peroxidation in cardiac toxicity and tumor response. *Science* **197**:165.
5. Lenas, L., and Page, J. A. (1976). Cardiotoxicity of adriamycin and related anthracyclines. *Cancer Treat. Rev.* **3**:111.
6. McGinness, J. E., Proctor, P. H., Demopoulos, H. B., Hokanson, J. A., and Kirkpatrick, D. S. (1978). Amelioration of *cis*-platinum nephrotoxicity by orgotein superoxide dismutase. *Physiol. Chem. Phys.* **10**:No. 3.
7. McGinness, J. E., Proctor, P. H., Demopoulos, H. B., Hokanson, J. A., and Kirkpatrick, D. S. (1979). Enzymatic evidence for free radical production by *cis*-platinum *in vivo. Adv. Med. Oncol., Res. Educ., Proc. Int. Cancer Cong. 12th, 1978* p. 155.
8. Norris, J. H., Gorski, J., and Kohler, P. O. (1974). Androgen receptors in a Syrian hamster ductus deferens tumour cell line. *Nature (London)* **248**:422.
9. Norris, J. H., and Kohler, P. O. (1977). The coexistence of androgen and glucocorticoid receptors in the DDT cloned cell line. *Endocrinology* **100**:613.
10. Lown, J. W., and Sim, S. K. (1979). The mechanism of cleavage on DNA by the antitumor agents bleomycin and neocarcinostatin. *Adv. Med. Oncol., Res. Educ., Proc. Int. Cancer Congr. 12th, 1978* Abstract, p. 151.
11. Yamanaka, N., Kato, T., Nishida, K., and Ota, K. (1978). Enhancement of DNA chain breakage by bleomycin A$_2$ in the presence of microsomes and reduced nicotinamide adenine dinucleotide phosphate. *Cancer Res.* **38**:3900.
12. Levi, J. Jacobs, C., Kalman, S. M., McTigue, M., and Weiner, M. W. (1980). Mecha-

nism of cis-platinum nephrotoxicity. I. Effects of sulfhydryl groups in rat kidneys. *J. Pharmacol. Exp. Ther.* **213**(3):545–550.

13. Younes, M., and Siegers, C. P. (1981). Mechanistic aspects of enhanced lipid peroxidation following glutathione depletion in vivo. *Chem.-Biol. Interact.* **34**:257.

14. Wang, Y. M., Madanat, F. F., Kimball, J. C., Gleiser, C. A., Ali, M. K., Kaufman, M. W., and van Eys, J. (1980). Effects of vitamin E against adriamycin-induced toxicity in rabbits. *Cancer Res.* **49**:1022.

15. Mimnaugh, E. G., Siddik, Z. H., Drew, R., Sikic, B. I., and Gram, T. E. (1979). The effects of α-tocopherol on the toxicity, disposition, and metabolism of adriamycin in mice. *Toxicol. Appl. Pharmacol.* **49**:119.

16. Wells, P. G., Boerth, R. C., Oates, J. A., and Harbison, R. D. (1980). Toxicologic enhancement by a combination of drugs which deplete hepatic glutathione: Acetaminophen and doxorubicin (adriamycin). *Toxicol. Appl. Pharmacol.* **54**:197.

17. Yamanaka, N., Kato, T., Nishida, K., Funjikawa, T., Fukushima, M., and Ota, K. (1979). Elevation of serum lipid peroxide level associated with doxorubicin toxicity and its amelioration by (*dl*)-α-tocopheryl acetate or coenzyme Q10 in mouse (doxorubicin, toxicity, lipid peroxide tocopherol, coenzyme Q10). *Cancer Chemother. Pharmacol.* **3**:223.

18. Breed, J. G. S., Zimmerman, A. N. E., Dormans, J. A. M. A., and Pinedo, H. M. (1980). Failure of the antioxidant vitamin E to protect against adriamycin-induced cardiotoxicity in the rabbit. *Cancer Res.* **40**:2033.

19. Billingham, M. E. (1979). Endomyocardial changes in anthracycline-treated patients with and without irradiation. *Front. Radiat. Ther. Oncol.* **13**:67.

20. McGinness, J., Kretzer, F., and Mehta, R. (1981). An adriamycin induced retinal degeneration. *Proc. AACR Meet.* AACR Abstract, No. 1210.

21. McGinness, J., Benjamin, R., Wang, Y. T., and Grossie, B. (1980). The dose schedule dependence of adriamycin toxicity with superoxide dismutase and vitamin E. *Proc. AACR Meet.*

DISCUSSION

BABIOR: Did you measure pharmacokinetics in these studies? Did you look for a nonspecific effect of protein? These types of controls are *crucial* to any interpretation of your data.

McGINNESS: As I pointed out, these experiments were intended to be exploratory. I am presenting the preliminary experimental results. Before we can offer a reasonable interpretation we need more information. We do see opposite effects with superoxide dismutase and catalase, which argues against nonspecific protein effects. Also, I would like to point out that the observable pharmacokinetics of superoxide dismutase are not simply related to its course of action, so perhaps this is not such a "crucial" question, although it is definitely an important one and one that we wish to answer.

PROCTOR: I would like to point out that there is an internal control in this experiment, namely, the experiment with superoxide dismutase and adriamycin. In any case, the total concentration of added protein is so low that it is very unlikely that it would perceptibly increase plasma total protein.

ŌYANAGUI: You said that the animals died of cancer, but what was the real cause of death in your experimental model? Was it thrombosis?

McGINNESS: This study involved the induction of toxicity by anti-cancer drugs. Rats receiving *cis*-platinum died of kidney toxicity. Rats receiving adriamycin died of cardiac toxicity with chronic doses and extravasation toxicity at high doses given intraperitoneally.

FRIDOVICH: Have you considered using acatalasic mice or animals whose catalase has been depleted with 3-aminotriazole to see whether they are more susceptible than normal animals to the toxicity of adriamycin? This would lend even more validity to the very impressive results you have already achieved.

McGINNESS: I appreciate the suggestion. Yes, we have thought of using acatalasic animals and will try such experiments. If we are looking at extracellular effects, we may not see effects due to differences inside the cells. For example, acatalasic mice do not seem to be more sensitive to high-pressure oxygen.

SCHMIDT: Your dose schedules for adriamycin with respect to both the dose and frequency are quite different (greater) from those used clinically. Can you explain your choice of dose schedules?

McGINNESS: I used values reported in the literature for Sprague–Dawley rats.

McLENNAN: What is known about the tissue distribution of catalase after intramuscular injection? Because it is a large molecule, it does not cross the normal endothelial membrane.

McGINNESS: Very little work has been done *in vivo* with catalase. I do not know the serum clearance time. In the case of toxicity resulting in membrane damage, however, the tissue distribution can be markedly altered.

DEMOPOULOS: Catalase, like any other protein, can be picked up by the lymphatics. It then enters the bloodstream. At sites of damage, such as the heart in adriamycin toxicity, the vessels leak, and there may be a "beneficial" leakage of plasma that contains free catalase into the injured site.

MICHELSON: You mentioned that injection of superoxide dismutase into solid tumors increased survival but did not decrease tumor size. Some time ago we injected superoxide dismutase into melanomas (in hamsters) and benzopyrene-induced tumors (in mice). Very marked tumor regression accompanied increased survival, *but* very similar results were obtained with denatured superoxide dismutase. Second, we have begun a program using adriamycin and superoxide dismutase packaged together in a liposome so that both agents are conveyed together to the same site. You have convinced me that I should add catalase to these liposomes.

McGINNESS: I would like to see how this works out. It sounds very promising.

PIETTE: What is the evidence that O_2^- is produced by *cis*-platinum, bleomycin, and adriamycin?

McGINNESS: The species produced by adriamycin has an electron spin resonance spectrum identical to the known spectrum for O_2^-. Bleomycin-induced DNA degradation is inhibited by superoxide dismutase and catalase. Finally, protection from *cis*-platinum toxicity is provided by superoxide dismutase. In all these cases the final toxic species is not known.

COHEN: In our limited experience with adriamycin, using Swiss–Webster mice and doses similar to yours (experiments of M. Bail), we observed the disappearance of the epididymal fat pad and decreased body weight. It seemed that many of our animals were starving to death. Do you monitor food intake in your experiments? Is starvation a factor in your survival curves?

McGINNESS: No, we monitor food intake and weights of the rats. Sprague–Dawley rats tolerate these doses. Animals that show the highest blood urea nitrogen levels die first. Furthermore, the time scale for toxicity correlates with the final pathology reports. We find dramatic differences among species for tolerance to these drugs.

PROCTOR: I would like to clarify the rationale for using superoxide dismutase and catalase for *cis*-platinum nephrotoxicity. First of all, *cis*-platinum does *not* produce O_2^-. However, Ōyanagui has shown that platinum compounds can stimulate O_2^- production by phagocytes. Likewise, *cis*-platinum is ototoxic as well as nephrotoxic; there is some evidence that deafness may be related to a free-radical mechanism.

FRIDOVICH: What is the chemical structure of *cis*-platinum?

McGINNESS:

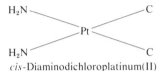

cis-Diaminodichloroplatinum(II)

RILEY: With regard to Gerald Cohen's question concerning the nutritional status of the experimental animals, we have been seriously concerned with these experimental parameters. In routine monitoring of food as well as water consumption, we have observed that certain tumors produce a conspicuous anorexia that is reflected in a significant voluntary reduction in food and thus caloric intake. This is known to have effects on tumor behavior. Interestingly, each tumor type has an individual capacity to affect the appetite centers. For example, some tumors have minimal or no capacity to alter food and water consumption, whereas other tumor strains may even stimulate the appetite centers to produce an increase in food consumption as a fraction of increasing tumor mass. Associated stress factors may be stimulated by alterations in food consumption, resulting in an increase in plasma corticosterone levels, destruction of T cells, thymus involution, and an impairment in immunocompetence that may have significant influences on tumor–drug responses.

McGINNESS: This topic is being actively investigated at the University of Texas Cancer Center in connection with patient care. With respect to our rats, we had to use hematological analysis to determine when to sacrifice rats for pathological examination since no behavioral differences were apparent.

JONES: It has been shown that cadmium salts injected into Sprague–Dawley rats affect the immune response in various ways relative to the time of antigen injection. For example, Ca^{2+} injected subcutaneously in very small doses daily for 2 weeks before injection of human γ-globulin (HGG) significantly enhanced both the primary and secondary anti-HGG responses, whereas HGG injected 1 week after or at the same time of Cd^{2+} treatment significantly suppressed the primary response but not the secondary response. Knowing this, one wonders what effect the *cis*-platinum used in your model had on the immune system? Did you measure this effect? Also, do you know if catalase is immunogenic? If it is, there is a relation between the immune system and the effect of *cis*-platinum; the latter may be associated with the catalase effects that you observed in your model.

McGINNESS: This is an exciting suggestion. The striking difference in the effects of acute and chronic treatment made us think about the immune response. We were unaware of the work you have described. It suggests a number of interesting experiments.

Chapter 13

The Use of Superoxide Dismutase
in the Treatment of Cancer

LARRY W. OBERLEY, SUSAN W. H. C.
LEUTHAUSER, GARRY R. BUETTNER, JOHN
R. J. SORENSON, TERRY D. OBERLEY, AND
ISABEL B. BIZE

INTRODUCTION

The enzyme superoxide dismutase (superoxide oxidoreductase, EC 1.15.1.1) is believed to be present in all oxygen-metabolizing cells but lacking in most obligate anaerobes, presumably because its physiological function is to provide a defense against the potentially damaging reactivity of the superoxide radical (O_2^-) generated by aerobic metabolic reactions (1). Superoxide dismutase (SOD) catalyzes the following reaction (2):

$$O_2^- + O_2^- + 2H^+ \rightarrow H_2O_2 + O_2$$

Four different forms of superoxide dismutase have been found to date (4). One of these, which is found in the cytosol and intermembrane space of mitochondria of eukaryotic cells, contains copper and zinc (CuZnSOD) and is entirely unrelated, except in its activity, to the other three. An example of this superoxide dismutase is the erythrocuprein found in bovine and human red blood cells. There are two kinds of superoxide dismutase that contain manganese (MnSOD). One of these is found largely in the matrix of mitochondria (5), and the other in the matrix of bacteria such as

207

PATHOLOGY OF OXYGEN
Copyright © 1982 by Academic Press, Inc.
All rights of reproduction in any form reserved.
ISBN 0-12-068620-1

Escherichia coli (6) and *Streptococcus mutans* (7). The fourth type of superoxide dismutase contains iron (FeSOD) and has been found in the periplasmic space of *E. coli* (8,9). The purpose of this chapter is to review the role of superoxide dismutase in the treatment of cancer and to discuss how knowledge of the levels of this enzyme in tumor cells may lead to potentially better treatment.

LEVELS OF SUPEROXIDE DISMUTASE AND SUPEROXIDE RADICAL IN CANCER CELLS

Many comparisons have been made between superoxide dismutase activities in normal and in malignant cells. A typical pattern has emerged from these studies. Cancer cells have in general smaller amounts of both CuZnSOD and MnSOD than do their normal cell counterparts. Exceptions to this pattern have been found in the case of CuZnSOD but not in the case of MnSOD. The activity of MnSOD is greatly reduced in *in vivo, in vitro,* spontaneous, transplanted, virally induced, and chemically induced tumors (unpublished observations). This work has been the subject of a recent review (10). A typical example is the mouse liver system (11). Normal mouse liver was found to contain 122 ± 12 units of CuZnSOD activity per milligram protein and 35 ± 5 units of MnSOD activity per milligram protein. Regenerating liver, a rapidly dividing normal cell system, also contained both CuZnSOD and MnSOD. However, the superoxide dismutase activity varied with time after partial hepatectomy. The amount of CuZnSOD was greatly diminished 4 days after surgery, a time at which a nearly synchronous wave of cell division occurs, whereas MnSOD was present at all times after surgery and did not decrease. In contrast, H6 hepatoma tumor cells contain a greatly diminished amount of CuZnSOD and no detectable MnSOD. Isolated mitochondria from normal liver cells contained a large amount of superoxide dismutase activity, but isolated mitochondria from H6 hepatoma mitochondria contained no measureable superoxide dismutase activity. Thus, in this system, a loss of MnSOD was representative of tumor tissue and not of any form of normal tissue.

We have questioned the significance of these enzyme changes because the cancer cell exhibits numerous enzyme alterations. Why is superoxide dismutase any more important than any other enzyme? The answer may be that superoxide dismutase is fundamentally different from most other enzymes in that it is a *protective* enzyme. Indeed, Fridovich has provided substantial evidence that this enzyme is necessary for life in all oxygen-metabolizing cells (3). We believe that the loss of the enzymatic activity of superoxide dismutase in cancer cells leads to changes in key subcellular structures because of the presence of oxygen-derived radicals.

However, superoxide dismutase is a protective enzyme only if its substrate, O_2^-, is present in the cancer cell. If O_2^- is not produced in the cancer cell, then a loss of MnSOD should not have any harmful effects. In this case, research should focus on the loss of superoxide-producing capacity and not on the loss of MnSOD. From these considerations, it can be seen that, in order to establish that the loss of MnSOD is important in malignancy, it is also necessary to show the production of superoxide in tumor cell mitochondria. Dionisi *et al.* (12) have shown that two tumor types have the capacity to produce superoxide. Using adrenochrome formation as an indicator of O_2^- production, we have been able to show that mouse H6 hepatoma tumor mitochondria also produce superoxide. The data are shown in Table I, which indicates the amount of adrenochrome formed each minute per milligram of submitochondrial particles isolated from H6 hepatoma. In all cases studied, superoxide dismutase inhibited adrenochrome formation, showing that O_2^- was responsible for the reaction. Antimycin A (an inhibitor of electron transport) alone caused superoxide production in a reaction system that contained tissue, epinephrine, and diethylenetriaminepentaacetic acid. Succinate enhanced the amount of O_2^- produced by a factor of 3. Antimycin A caused more O_2^- production

TABLE I

Adrenochrome Formation in Submitochondrial Particles[a]

Reactants	$-$SOD	$+$SOD
Succinate	1.44	Not done
Antimycin A	0.96	0.00
Succinate + antimycin A	2.88	0.19
Succinate + rotenone	1.44	Not done
NADH + antimycin A	1.44	0.34
NADH + rotenone	1.15	Not done

[a] Membrane fragments (0.5 mg protein per milliliter) from mouse H6 hepatoma tissue were in all cases suspended in 0.25 M sucrose, 50 mM HEPES, pH 7.5, 0.5 mM diethylenetriamine pentaacetic acid, and 1 mM epinephrine. In some of the tubes, 3 mM succinate, 2.5 μg/ml antimycin A, 13 μM NADH, or 2 μM rotenone was also added. Measurements were performed in a Cary 15 spectrophotometer at both 480 and 575 nm. Values are given in nanomoles adrenochrome formed per minute per milligram of submitochondrial particles.

than rotenone, and succinate was a more effective substrate than NADH. These results, as well as those of Dionisi, show that cancer cells have the capacity to produce O_2^-.

A diminished amount of MnSOD coupled with superoxide production appears to be a general characteristic of the tumor cells studied. This undoubtedly leads to changes in subcellular structures because of the presence of oxygen-derived chemical species (such as hydroxyl radical, singlet oxygen, and hydroperoxides). These changes are in turn probably responsible for at least part of the phenotypic properties of the cancer cell.

TREATMENT OF CANCER

We have described a general characteristic of the tumor cell: a diminished amount of MnSOD coupled with superoxide production. What use can we make of this in the treatment of cancer? Three different techniques are being used at present: (a) production of an excess flux of O_2^- or other superoxide-derived radicals in tumor cells, (b) inhibition of CuZnSOD, and (c) addition of superoxide dismutase activity to tumor cells.

The first technique is the oldest and was actually developed long before the association of cytotoxicity with O_2^- was known. Many antitumor agents produce or cause the production of O_2^- or superoxide-derived radicals such as HO·. If an equal amount of O_2^- or superoxide-derived radicals can be delivered to both cancer cells and normal cells, the cancer cells should be preferentially killed because they have lower MnSOD activity. An example of this type of mechanism is the action of the anticancer agent bleomycin, a glycopeptide antibiotic thought to be cytotoxic to tumor cells because of DNA chain breakage. *In vitro* DNA chain breakage by bleomycin was shown to be enhanced by the addition of xanthine–xanthine oxidase (13). The effect of the xanthine oxidase system disappeared completely when superoxide dismutase was added. From these results, it was concluded that superoxide radical is one of the mediators for the enhancement of the DNA chain breakage action of bleomycin. Sausville *et al.* have shown that DNA degradation by bleomycin requires oxygen and Fe(II) (14). Reducing agents such as ascorbate and H_2O_2, as well as O_2^-, greatly increase the DNA degradation. These observations have led Sausville *et al.* to propose the following model for the action of bleomycin (14). Bleomycin can bind to DNA in the absence of metal ion or reducing agent. Iron(II) can then attach to the bleomycin and thus form a ternary complex. The ternary complex can produce a species that degrades DNA.

Reducing agents, including O_2^-, enhance the breakage by regenerating Fe(II) from Fe(III) and thus continuing the reaction. The nature of the toxic species is not identified in this model. Since the mechanism is similar to that observed by us (15) and others (16–18) for the production of hydroxyl radical from xanthine–xanthine oxidase, the authors thought that this radical might also be responsible for the degradation of DNA by bleomycin. Using the technique of spin trapping, we have observed that bleomycin and Fe(II) produce HO· (19). Because of the high reactivity of HO·, it is likely that this radical is responsible for the toxicity caused by bleomycin. Since bleomycin binds preferentially to DNA, the net result is a site-specific free radical. As mentioned earlier, reducing agents such as H_2O_2 and O_2^- are necessary for bleomycin to degrade DNA effectively. What is the source of reducing agent in the tumor cell? Since tumor cells apparently have a lower level of MnSOD and many have a diminished amount of CuZnSOD, tumor cells should have a greatly increased level of O_2^-. Moreover, O_2^- has been shown to be produced in tumor cell nuclei (20). The increased level of O_2^- in tumor cells as compared to normal cells may explain the differential toxicity exhibited between normal and malignant cells upon treatment with bleomycin.

There are many other examples of antitumor agents that produce superoxide or superoxide-derived radicals. The antitumor antibiotic streptonigrin causes DNA strand breaks *in vivo* (21). This antibiotic has been shown to generate the superoxide anion upon reduction and autoxidation *in vitro* (22,23), and the superoxide anion has been shown to cause strand breaks in closed circular double-stranded DNA (24,25). These observations have led to the formulation of a mechanism in which antibiotic generates superoxide during a reduction–oxidation cycle, and this radical brings about single-strand breaks (22,25). It was also shown that superoxide radicals are formed by the redox cycling of the antitumor anthracycline antibiotics daunomycin and adriamycin (26). It was found that NADPH and purified cytochrome *P*-450 reductase caused oxygen consumption from these drugs in excess of the amount of drug present. A reduction–autoxidation of sulfite may be initiated. The latter reaction was inhibited by superoxide dismutase, suggesting that O_2^- was formed. Hydrogen peroxide was also generated, presumably by nonenzymatic dismutation of superoxide. Rat liver microsomes also catalyzed this redox cycling, which was accompanied by the peroxidation of lipids. These experiments suggested that the formation of oxygen radicals followed by lipid peroxidation may be the basis for the cardiotoxic effects of these drugs.

Thayer has shown that adriamycin stimulates superoxide formation in submitochondrial particles (27). At a concentration of 400 μM, adriamycin stimulated the rate of O_2^- formation sixfold to 25 nmol/min mg. Measurements of the relative catalase activity of blood-free tissues of rabbits and rats indicated that heart contained 2–4% of the catalase activity of liver or kidney. The author concluded that an enhanced production of O_2^- and H_2O_2 and the relatively low catalase content of heart tissue may be factors in the cardiotoxicity induced by adriamycin chemotherapy.

Bachur *et al.* (28) extended these measurements and proposed a unifying theory for their mechanisms of action. They found that the highly active quinone-containing anticancer drugs, adriamycin, daunorubicin, carminomycin, rubidazone, nogalamycin, aclacinomycin A, and steffimycin (benzathraquinones), mitomycin C and streptonigrin (*N*-heterocyclic quinones), and lapachol (naphthaquinone) interacted with mammalian microsomes and functioned as free-radical carriers. These quinone drugs augmented the flow of electrons from reduced nicotinamide adenine dinucleotide phosphate to molecular oxygen. This reaction was catalyzed by microsomal protein and produced a free-radical intermediate form of the drugs as determined by ESR spectroscopy. Several nonquinone anticancer agents were tested and found to be inactive in this system. Since quinone anticancer drugs are associated with chromosomal damage that appears to be dependent on the metabolic activation of these drugs, the authors proposed that intracellular activation of these drugs to a free-radical state is primary to their cytotoxic activity. Because of their high affinity and selective binding to nucleic acids, these drugs, as free radicals, have the potential to be "site-specific free radicals" that bind to DNA or RNA and either react directly or generate oxygen-dependent free radicals such as O_2^- or $HO^{\cdot}$ to cause the damage associated with their cytotoxic actions.

Thus, a large number of anticancer drugs seem to involve O_2^- or O_2^--derived radicals in their mode of action. The differential toxicity of O_2^- to tumor cells as compared to normal cells may be brought about by the lack of MnSOD in tumor cells. This, perhaps coupled with increased O_2^- production in tumor cells, can easily explain their mechanism of action.

All of these anticancer drugs that involve superoxide are also toxic to normal cells and are associated with later induction of cancer. Thus, the capacity to kill tumor cells is less than optimal because the concentrations of drugs that can be used are limited by the damage to normal cells. Since damage to normal cells is also caused by superoxide or superoxide-derived radicals, it is conceivable that normal tissue could be protected by the administration of superoxide dismutase. Of course, in this type of therapy, one must be concerned with whether superoxide dismutase will also affect the antitumor action of the drug. There has been one report that superoxide dismutaste can prevent damage to normal cells. McGinness *et al.* have reported that a subcutaneous dose of CuZnSOD lowers the nephrotoxicity induced by a 5.0 mg/kg dose of the antitumor agent *cis*-platinum (29). The toxicity of *cis*-platinum was studied by comparative measurements of blood urea nitrogen, change in body weight, and renal histology. The results support a role for oxygen radicals in the nephrotoxicity of *cis*-platinum.

A second method that makes use of the inherent differences between normal and tumor cells in superoxide dismutase activity was proposed by Lin and associates (30). They inhibited CuZnSOD with diethyl dithiocarbamate (DDC). Since normal cells still have MnSOD, they were expected to survive this treatment, whereas tumor cells, having only CuZnSOD, were not. The authors carried out preliminary experiments with normal Chinese hamster cells (DON). The cytotoxic effect of DDC on DON cells was dependent on the DDC concentration and exposure time. After 8–10 days of incubation with 10^{-9} M DDC, no change in DON cell survival was noted; however, incubation with 10^{-4} M DDC showed marked toxicity. When DDC-treated cells were irradiated, they showed a lower percentage survival than cells that were treated with radiation or DDC alone. The combined effects of hyperthermia and DDC were dramatic. Cells treated 8 min at 43°C with 10^{-4} M DDC or 10 min at 47°C with 10^{-5} M DDC showed a significant decrease in survival. These results suggested that DDC may be a powerful sensitization agent in tumor therapy. However, it still has not been shown whether DDC alone or in combination with other anticancer agents will kill more tumor cells than normal cells. Without such differential toxicity, it is difficult to believe that this therapy will be successful because the damage to normal tissue will be too severe.

The third potential method of treatment involves the addition of superoxide dismutase to tumor cells. The proposed mechanism of action is radically different from those of the two techniques already discussed. The latter two involved using differences in superoxide dismutase activities to kill tumor cells preferentially. The third method does not involve cytotoxicity, but rather addition of superoxide dismutase to tumor cells to try to halt cell division. The rationale of this approach is simply that the level of MnSOD is diminished in tumor cells. This enzyme could be responsible for part of the cancer cell phenotype, and it is possible that the addition of superoxide dismutase to these tumor cells would cause cessation of cell division.

In order to test this method, it is necessary to use a compound that has superoxide dismutase activity and penetrates the cell. The most likely candidate, natural CuZnSOD, would not be expected to be effective because of low penetrability into cells (31). Nonetheless, the enzyme was tested and, surprisingly, was found to have some effect on tumor growth.

Treatment with a single intratumor injection of CuZnSOD 1 hr after intramuscular injection of 4×10^6 sarcoma 180 tumor cells had a small effect
on tumor growth (Fig. 1). It also increased animal survival by approximately 20% (Fig. 2). The group treated with superoxide dismutase had
19% long-term survivors (more than 90 days); the saline-treated group had
0% long-term survivors.

Similar experiments with Ehrlich ascites carcinoma cells produced little
effects on tumor growth, but the animals treated with superoxide dismutase survived longer. Preliminary evidence indicates that this is because
of better encapsulation of the tumor in the group treated with superoxide
dismutase, with less metastasis resulting. Thus, it appears that natural
CuZnSOD does have an effect, although it is small.

If we could find a compound with superoxide dismutase activity that
could penetrate the cell, our results might be more dramatic. For this reason, we investigated the copper coordination compounds that have been
studied by Dr. John Sorenson for many years because of their antiarthritic
and antiulcer activities (32); these compounds have high superoxide dismutase activity (33,34). Recently we synthesized copper coordination
compounds with high penetrability. Our preliminary evidence indicates
that these compounds have a dramatic effect on tumor growth. Figure 3
shows the results of the first experiments. Tumors were induced in CBA
mice by intramuscular injection of 5×10^6 Ehrlich ascites tumor cells.
These tumors were then treated by an injection of 1 mg of copper coordination compound at 1 hr, 1 day, 2 days, 3 days, and 4 days. Three compounds were tested: $copper(II)_2(aspirinate)_4(DMSO)_4$, $copper(II)_2(aspi-$

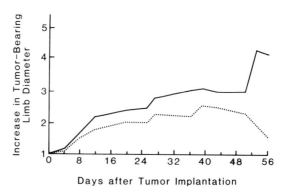

Days after Tumor Implantation

Fig. 1.   Effect of superoxide dismutase treatment on tumor growth. Average tumor size
was measured as a function of time after tumor implantation. Sarcoma 180 cells (4×10^6)
were injected intramuscularly into male CF1 mice; CuZnSOD (---) or saline (—) was given
intramuscularly 1 hr after implantation of the tumor. Each experimental group contained 16
animals.

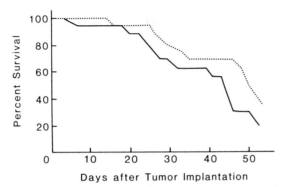

Fig. 2. Effect of superoxide dismutase treatment on cumulative mortality of tumor-bearing mice. Animal survival was monitored as a function of time after tumor implantation. Sarcoma 180 cells (4×10^6) were injected intramuscularly into male CF1 mice; SOD (---) or saline (—) was given intramuscularly 1 hr after implantation of the tumor. Each experimental group contained 16 animals. Survival time of the animals treated with superoxide dismutase was significantly greater than that of the saline-treated animals, as evaluated by the Smirorov test ($p = 0.05$).

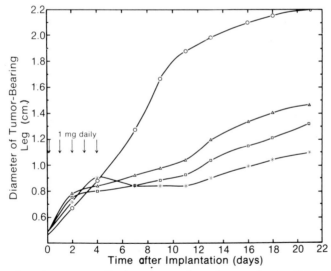

Fig. 3. Effect of copper coordination compounds on the growth of Ehrlich ascites tumor cells in CBA mice. Average tumor size in centimeters was determined as a function of time after tumor implantation. Ehrlich ascites tumor cells (5×10^6) were injected intramuscularly into male CBA mice. A 10% solution of Tween 80 in saline or 1 mg of copper coordination compound in Tween 80 was given intramuscularly at 1 hr, 1 day, 2 days, 3 days, and 4 days after tumor implantation; 0.2 ml was injected in each case. Each experimental group contained four animals. Key: $\bigcirc$, 10% Tween 80–saline; $\triangle$, Cu(II)$_2$(aspirinate)$_4$(DMSO)$_4$; $\square$, Cu(II)$_2$(aspirinate)$_4$(pyridine)$_4$; *, Cu(II)(3,5-diisopropyl salicylate)$_2$.

rinate)$_4$(pyridine)$_4$, copper(II)(3,5-diisopropyl salicylate)$_2$. The three compounds have quite different degrees of lipid solubility, the copper(II)$_2$(aspirinate)$_4$(DMSO)$_4$ being the least soluble and copper(II) (3,5-diisopropyl salicylate)$_2$ being the most soluble. The degree of inhibition of tumor growth follows the same order as the degree of lipid solubility, the aspirinate–DMSO compound being the least effective and diisopropyl salicylate the most effective. Histological studies indicate that these compounds function not by killing cells but by inhibiting cell division. Furthermore, there was no evidence of an inflammatory infiltrate in treated or control tumors. We have not established the mechanism of action of these compounds, but we can say that compounds with superoxide dismutase activity that penetrate the cell appear to inhibit tumor cell growth.

The idea that copper coordination compounds can be used as antitumor agents is not new; many other copper compounds have been shown to have antitumor activity (35–37). However, all of these studies have centered on compounds that are cytotoxic; copper coordination compounds that are not cytotoxic but only inhibit cell division have not been studied in detail (38). Compounds that are not cytotoxic must be administered continuously, whereas cytotoxic compounds can be given only intermittently. This represents a fundamentally new approach to cancer therapy.

It appears that this type of therapy has distinct possibilities for cancer treatment. However, all of these compounds exhibit toxicity at high doses (32), so chronic long-term administration may also have deleterious side effects. For this reason, it is still very desirable to use naturally occurring superoxide dismutase, which is metabolized by natural processes. Thus, encapsulating superoxide dismutase in liposomes may ultimately lead to the best treatment of cancer.

ACKNOWLEDGMENTS

Studies from our laboratory described in this chapter were supported by grants from the Alexander Medical Foundation, the National Institutes of Health, DHEW (no. 2 T 32 CA 09125), and the International Copper Research Association (J.R.J.).

REFERENCES

1. McCord, J. M., Keele, B. B., and Fridovich, I. (1971). An enzyme based theory of obligate anaerobiosis: The physiological function of superoxide dismutase. *Proc. Natl. Acad. Sci. U.S.A.* **68**:1024.

2. McCord, J. M., and Fridovich, I. (1969). Superoxide dismutase. An enzymatic function for erythrocuprein (hemocuprein). *J. Biol. Chem.* **244**:6049.

3. Fridovich, I. (1975). Superoxide dismutase. *Annu. Rev. Biochem.* **44**:147.

4. Fridovich, I. (1974). Superoxide dismutase. *Adv. Enzymol.* **41**:35–97.

5. Weisiger, R. A., and Fridovich, I. (1973). Superoxide dismutase: Organelle specificity. *J. Biol. Chem.* **248**:3582.

6. Keele, B. B., Jr., McCord, J. M., and Fridovich, I. (1972). Superoxide dismutase from *Escherichia coli* B. A new manganese-containing enzyme. *J. Biol. Chem.* **245**:6176.

7. Vance, P. G., Keele, B. B., Jr., and Rajayopalan, K. V. (1972). Superoxide dismutase from *Streptococcus mutans*. *J. Biol. Chem.* **247**:4782.

8. Yost, F. J., Jr., and Fridovich, I. (1973). An iron-containing superoxide dismutase from *Escherichia coli*. *J. Biol. Chem.* **248**:4905.

9. Gregory, E. M., Yost, F. J., and Fridovich, I. (1973). The superoxide dismutase of *Escherichia coli*. Intracellular localizations and functions. *J. Bacteriol.* **115**:987.

10. Oberley, L. W., and Buettner, G. R. (1979). The role of superoxide dismutase in cancer: A review. *Cancer Res.* **39**:1141.

11. Oberley, L. W., Bize, I. B., and Sahu, S. K. (1978). Superoxide dismutase activity of normal murine liver, regenerating liver, and H6 hepatoma. *J. Natl. Cancer Inst.* **61**:375.

12. Dionisi, D., Galeotti, T., Terranove, T., and Azzi, A. (1975). Superoxide radicals and hydrogen peroxide formation in mitochondria from normal and neoplastic tissues. *Biochim. Biophys. Acta* **403**:292.

13. Ishida, R., and Takahashi, T. (1975). Increased DNA chain breakage by combined action of bleomycin and superoxide radical. *Biochem. Biophys. Res. Commun.* **66**:1432.

14. Sausville, E. A., Peisach, J., and Horwitz, S. B. (1978). Effect of chelating agents and metal ions on the degradation of DNA by bleomycin. *Biochemistry* **17**:2740.

15. Buettner, G. R., Oberley, L. W., and Leuthauser, S. W. H. C. (1978). The effect of iron on the distribution of superoxide and hydroxyl radicals as seen by spin trapping and on the superoxide dismutase assay. *Photochem. Photobiol.* **28**:693.

16. Fong, K. L., McCay, P. B., and Poyer, J. L. (1973). Evidence that peroxidation of lysosomal membranes is initiated by hydroxyl free radicals produced during flavin enzyme activity. *J. Biol. Chem.* **248**:7792.

17. Halliwell, B. (1978). Superoxide-dependent formation of hydroxyl radicals in the presence of iron chelates: Is it a mechanism for hydroxyl radical production in biochemical systems? *FEBS Lett.* **92**:321.

18. McCord, J. M., and Day, E. D. (1978). Superoxide-dependent production of hydroxyl radical catalyzed by iron–EDTA complex. *FEBS Lett.* **86**:139.

19. Oberley, L. W., and Buettner, G. R. (1979). The production of hydroxyl radical by bleomycin and iron(II). *FEBS Lett.* **97**:47.

20. Bartoli, G. M., Galeotti, T., and Azzi, A. (1977). Production of superoxide anions and hydrogen peroxide in Ehrlich ascites tumor cell nuclei. *Biochim. Biophys. Acta* **497**:622.

21. Cohen, M. M., Shaw, M. W., and Craig, A. P. (1963). The effects of streptonigrin on cultured human leukocytes. *Proc. Natl. Acad. Sci. U.S.A.* **50**:16.

22. White, J. R., Vaughan, T. O., and Yeh, W. S. (1971). Superoxide radical in the mechanism of action of streptonigrin. *Fed. Proc., Fed. Am. Soc. Exp. Biol.* **30**:1145.

23. Gregory, E. M., and Fridovich, I. (1973). Oxygen toxicity and the superoxide dismutase. *J. Bacteriol.* **114**:1193.

24. Yeh, S. W. (1971). The *in vitro* effect of streptonigrin on DNA. Ph.D. Thesis, University of North Carolina at Chapel Hill.

25. Cone, R., Hasan, S. K., Lown, J. W., and Morgan, A. R. (1976). The mechanism of the degradation of DNA by streptonigrin. *Can. J. Biochem.* **54**:219.

26. Goodman, J., and Hochstein, P. (1977). Generation of free radicals and lipid peroxidation by redox cycling of adriamycin and daunomycin. *Biochem. Biophys. Res. Commun.* **77**:797.

27. Thayer, W. S. (1977). Adriamycin stimulated superoxide formation in submitochondrial particles. *Chem.-Biol. Interact.* **19**:265.

28. Bachur, N. R., Gordon, S. L., and Gee, M. W. (1978). A general mechanism for microsomal activation of quinone anticancer agents to free radicals. *Cancer Res.* **38**:1745.

29. McGinness, J. E., Proctor, P. H., Demopoulos, H. B., Hokanson, J. A., and Kirkpatrick, D. S. (1978). Amelioration of *cis*-platinum nephrotoxicity by orgotein (superoxide dismutase). *Physiol. Chem. Phy.* **10**:267.

30. Lin, P. S., Kwock, L., Ciborowski, L., and Butterfield, C. (1978). Sensitization effects of diethyldithiocarbamate. *Radiat. Res.* **74**:515.

31. Petkau, A., Chelack, W. S., Kelly, K., Barefoot, C., and Monasterski, L. (1977). Tissue distribution of bovine ^{125}I-superoxide dismutase in mice. *Res. Commun. Chem. Pathol. Pharmacol.* **17**:125.

32. Sorenson, J. R. J. (1975). Some copper coordination compounds and their anti-inflammatory and antiulcer activities. *Inflammation (N.Y.)* **1**:317.

33. DeAlvare, L. R., Goda, L., and Kimura, T. (1976). Mechanism of superoxide anion scavenging reaction by bis-(salicylato)-copper-(II)complex. *Biochem. Biophys. Res. Commun.* **69**:687.

34. Weser, U., Richter, C., Wendel, A., and Younes, M. (1978). Reactivity of anti-inflammatory and superoxide dismutase active Cu(II)-salicylates. *Bioinorg. Chem.* **8**:201.

35. French, F. A., and Blanz, E. J. J. (1974). α-(*N*)-Formylheterogromatic thiosemicarbazones. Inhibition of tumor-derived ribonucleoside diphosphate reductase and correlation with in vivo antitumor activity. *J. Med. Chem.* **17**:172.

36. Antholine, W. E., Knight, J. M., and Petering, D. H. (1976). Inhibition of tumor cell transplantability by iron and copper complexes of 5-substituted 2-formylpyridine thiosemicarbazone. *J. Med. Chem.* **19**:335.

37. Coats, E. A., Milstein, S. R., Holbein, B., McDonald, J., Reed, R., and Petering, H. G. (1976). Comparative analysis of the cytotoxicity of substituted [phenylglyoxalbis(4-methyl-3-thiosemicarbazone)] copper(II) chelates. *J. Med. Chem.* **19**:131.

38. Minkel, D. T., Saryan, L. A., and Petering, D. H. (1978). Structure-function correlations in the reaction of bis(thiosemicarbazonate) copper(II) complexes with Ehrlich ascites tumor cells. *Cancer Res.* **38**:124.

DISCUSSION

FRIDOVICH: Congratulations on your exciting work. Have you considered that the Warburg phenomenon, that is, lactate production by tumor cells (even under aerobic conditions), might be explained by the lack of MnSOD from tumor mitochondria? Thus, tumor mitochondria would suffer self-inflicted damage due to unscavenged O_2^- generated within the mitochondria. The tumor cell would then have to rely on the cytoplasmic fermentation (Embden–Meyerhof pathway) for its energy supply.

OBERLEY: We have considered this possibility and believe that it is very likely that the high glycolytic rate of tumors is caused by mitochondrial damage. We are at present examining tumors with varyious rates of glycolysis, and our results show that the degree of mitochondrial damage and the level of MnSOD correlate well with the rate of glycolysis. Thus, tumors with a high glycolytic rate show a low level of MnSOD and significant mitochondrial damage.

ŌYANAGUI: I have observed the existence of electron release to an unknown compound in the mitochondria of a variety of liver tumor cells at the cytochrome oxidase site. Is there a possibility of O_2^- involvement at this site? Also, what is the superoxide dismutase content in the cultured cells of normal origin?

OBERLEY: Normally, electrons are not donated singly to oxygen at the cytochrome oxidase site. However, tumor cell mitochondrial membranes may be damaged, so that leakage from the cytochrome chain may occur; thus, your observation could be consistent with my observations on the lack of MnSOD in tumor cells. In answer to your second question, the one study that was done indicated that tissue culture cells of normal origin had both CuZnSOD and MnSOD. The content of each was about the same as in the *in vivo* cells.

PIETRONIGRO: If your hypothesis concerning bleomycin antitumor effectiveness is correct, one would expect to see an oxygen effect with respect to tumor cell killing. Has this been observed?

OBERLEY: I believe that an oxygen effect has been seen in connection with *in vitro* DNA breakage, but I don't know if one has been seen in association with cell killing.

PIETRONIGRO: Since the formation of the "active" bleomycin–Fe^{2+}–O_2 complex seems independent of DNA binding, one may expect to see bleomycin damage at other cellular sites, especially those producing reducing species, including O_2^-. In this regard, do you know whether bleomycin damaged either tumor or lung mitochondria?

OBERLEY: I don't know of any data on this. Perhaps some DNA might be damaged, including both the nuclear or mitochondrial DNA.

DEL MAESTRO: Could the level of superoxide dismutase in tumor cells be a reflection of the O_2^- content in which the tumor cells are living *in vivo* rather than a genetic DNA effect?

OBERLEY: This possibility has been considered by us and others. Dr. Petkau has shown that total superoxide dismutase activity increases as it goes from the poorly oxygenated center of mammary tumor to the well-oxygenated periphery of the tumor. However, we have observed in preliminary studies that, in H6 hepatoma tumors, the levels of MnSOD do not seem to vary much in the tumor; so the answer to your question is that it is possible, but the evidence so far does not point in that direction.

PROCTOR: This is very exciting work. Bleomycin is of particular interest in cancer chemotherapy because it is uniquely active against cells in the G_0 (nonreplicating) tumor population. Under ordinary circumstances, these are very difficult to kill chemotherapeutically. There is a tendency for anoxic tumor cells to be in the G_0 phase. Perhaps this is related to their sensitivity to bleomycin-induced radicals since the content of intracellular protective systems may be diminished. I wonder what the content of superoxide dismutase and associated enzymes is as a function of the cell cycle, since both bleomycin and adriamycin seem to be cycle-dependent cytotoxic agents.

SHEREMATA: Dr. Oberley's observations prompt me to make a comment on a recent study made in collaboration with Dr. Stanley Skoryna and Dr. K. Tanaka at McGill University. Manganese deficiency is a well-recognized cause of seizures in foraging animals. It has also been induced in a variety of laboratory animals, including rats. These observations led us to study levels of manganese and magnesium in the serum of humans with epileptic seizures. Newborn infants in status epilepticus had barely detectable levels (< 5 ng/ml) of these elements. In children or adults with idiopathic epilepsy, intermediate levels (10–20 ng/ml) were observed. Others who had isolated seizures after trauma or surgery had only slightly decreased levels (20–35 ng/ml). Effective anticonvulsant therapy did not alter these levels. In children, however, there was a definite rise in manganese, possibly reflecting unrelated factors. In view of the abrupt rise in blood and tissue oxygen levels following delivery, these observations suggest that an absence of manganese-containing superoxide dismutase may result in the abrupt appearance of O_2^- and neuronal membrane damage, leading to depolarization and seizure activity. It should be mentioned that manganese serum levels bore no relationship to the presence or absence of seizures.

Our observations also relate to the fact that brain tumors frequently produce seizures. However, malignant, infiltrating tumors of brain may not. This fact does cloud the issue somewhat. We must study MnSOD in these tumors including the edematous and normal surrounding brain tissue, as well as in normal brain. The evidence nevertheless points to the importance of MnSOD deficiency in the genesis of seizures.

CUTLER: You have put forth a very interesting model suggesting that low superoxide dismutase levels may be responsible for some of the characteristics of tumors (transformed) cells. I wonder if the reverse might be true, that is, that an initial low value of superoxide dismutase could lead to transformation. According to such a model, a low superoxide dismutase level would lead to tumor formation but would not be responsible for its maintenance.

OBERLEY: The model you suggest is as plausible as the one we have suggested. Experimentally, all we know is that superoxide dismutase levels are altered. It is possible that changes in DNA lead to a loss of MnSOD or that a loss of MnSOD leads to DNA damage from oxygen-derived radicals. We have no real evidence for either model at the present time.

Chapter 14

Superoxide Dismutase and Radiosensitivity: Implications for Human Mammary Carcinomas

ABRAM PETKAU, WILLIAM S. CHELACK,
KENNETH KELLY, AND HENRY G.
FRIESEN

INTRODUCTION

Developing strategies for the radiotherapeutic management of tumors requires a continuing interest in factors that determine tissue sensitivity to ionizing radiation. Some of this interest has focused on superoxide dismutase (1–5) in view of this enzyme's antioxidant activity (6) and its utilization in the radioprotection of subcellular components (7,8), cells (9–14), and animals (13,15,16). To develop this interest further, we show that cellular radiosensitivity is related to the amount of endogenous superoxide dismutase(s) present and use the enzyme as a probe to identify critical subcellular regions using mouse bone marrow stem cells as a model. If the foregoing relationship is generalized and one also assumes that cellular and tissue radiosensitivities are related, then assays of superoxide dismutase activity in tumors and host tissues are desirable for assessing the role of the enzyme in any differential radiosensitivity that may exist between a tumor and its host tissue. In this chapter, we present data on superoxide dismutase assays of human fibroids, mammary carcinomas, and their host tissues to show that significantly different levels of activity exist between

PATHOLOGY OF OXYGEN

human mammary carcinomas and their host tissue but not between fibroids and normal myometrium.

UPTAKE OF EXOGENOUS
SUPEROXIDE DISMUTASE

Cell Isolation

Bone marrow cells from a sufficient number of femurs of Swiss white female mice were eluted with McCoy's 5A medium (Flow Laboratories, Rockville, Maryland) containing 15% fetal calf serum (Grand Island Biological Company, Grand Island, New York). The medium and eluted cells were stored on ice. The cells were sedimented by centrifugation at 4000 g for 5 min, and the erythrocytes were differentially lysed by resuspending the pellet for 30 sec in 3 vol of distilled water at 4°C, after which 1 vol of 3.6% NaCl at 4°C was added. The cells were sedimented again and washed twice in normal saline. For incubations with bovine CuZnSOD (supplied by Dr. J. V. Bannister, Malta), the washed cells were suspended in normal saline containing the appropriate concentration of superoxide dismutase and incubated for 1 hr at 37°C. When ^{125}I-labeled superoxide dismutase was used, the cells were also suspended in normal saline containing the appropriate concentration of unlabeled superoxide dismutase plus labeled superoxide dismutase (10) at a final activity of $\sim 8 \times 10^7$ cpm/ml. Incubations were also for 1 hr at 37°C. After the incubations, the cells were washed three times in normal saline. The cell number was determined by counting an aliquot in a hemocytometer. The final pellets were used for subcellular fractionation procedures, except for one aliquot, which was usually retained in appropriate runs to determine the uptake of exogenous superoxide dismutase.

Isolation of Mitochondria and
Cytoplasmic Membranes

Mitochondrial and cytoplasmic membrane fractions were prepared using a modification of the method described by Rest and Spitznagel (17). Pellets of cells, incubated with or without exogenous superoxide dismutase for 1 hr at 37°C and then washed as above, were suspended in 0.34 M sucrose and disrupted with a motor-driven Teflon pestle in a glass homogenizer operated for 45-sec bursts at 1900 rpm until greater than 90% disruption of cells was achieved. The cell homogenate in 1-ml aliquots was layered on a sucrose density gradient of 30–40% in 2% steps of 1 ml each. Centrifugation was for 2 hr in a Beckman L4 centrifuge using a 50.1 rotor operated at 25,000 rpm. The two uppermost bands were collected, the top band comprising the membrane fraction and the next one consisting of mitochondria as revealed by transmission electron microscopy (17,18). The membrane and mitochondrial preparations compared well with the published observations (17,19,20). It was noted, however, that in many of the mitochondria the matrix material was partially or wholly absent. Therefore, the uptake of exogenous superoxide dismutase and the level of endogenous superoxide dismutase in the mitochondria were probably underestimated. The membrane and mitochondrial fractions were separately diluted with 3 vol of normal saline and sedimented by centrifugation at 160,000 g for 2 hr. The pellets were suspended in normal saline and disrupted by sonication, frozen, thawed, and centrifuged at 12,000 g for 2 min. The supernatants were assayed either for endogenous superoxide dismutase by the nitro blue tetrazolium–riboflavin–methionine method (21) or for exogenous superoxide dismutase by a direct competitive radioimmunoassay (22) or, when applicable, by counting and profiling the ^{125}I activity (10,22).

Isolation of Nuclei

Nuclei of bone marrow cells were prepared using a modification of the method described by Monneron and d'Alayer (20). Buffer consisting of 50 mM Tris–HCl, pH 7.4, 25 mM KCl, and 5 mM MgCl$_2$ (TKM buffer) was used in the preparation of the sucrose density gradients as well as in the sucrose solutions (STKM) required for suspending the cells and subcellular fractions. The cell pellets, prepared as described above, were suspended in TKM-buffered 60% sucrose (60% STKM) and homogenized in an ice-cold glass-Teflon homogenizer operated at 4500 rpm. More than 90% of the cells were disrupted after 10 strokes. The cell homogenate was diluted with TKM to 40% STKM. Step gradients of STKM of 1 ml each were prepared and consisted of 60% STKM, 50% STKM, followed by the cell homogenate and overlayered successively by 35 and 22.5% STKM. The gradient was spun for 2 hr in a 50.1 rotor at 30,000 rpm. The gradient was discarded, and the nuclear pellet at the bottom of the tube was resuspended in normal saline, disrupted by sonication, frozen, thawed, and centrifuged for 2 min at 12,000 g. The supernatant was assayed for endogenous or exogenous superoxide dismutase as above. Light microscopy of orcein-stained suspensions of the pellet indicated that it contained mostly nuclei with less than 0.5% of undisrupted cells. In some runs, the supernatant was subjected, to disc gel electrophoresis (23) in Tris–borate EDTA buffer, pH 8.6 (24), in order to display the characteristic staining bands of the exogenous superoxide dismutase in the nuclear fraction.

Variation and Assay of Endogenous Superoxide Dismutase

To vary the level of endogenous superoxide dismutase from the normal level in bone marrow cells of adult Swiss white female mice (25), the donor animals were placed beforehand in one of the following environments: 85% O_2 for 3 days, 4.5% O_2 for 2 days, or 8% O_2 for 2 weeks. Normal weanling mice of the same strain were also used as a source of bone marrow cells. The nucleated cells were isolated and purified as above and assayed for endogenous superoxide dismutase as described (21). *In vitro* survival studies of bone marrow cells, X-irradiated in air at 37°C, were done concurrently as previously described (13) in order to establish a correlation between the endogenous superoxide dismutase and cell radiosensitivity as expressed by loss of colony-forming ability.

Assay of Endogenous Superoxide Dismutase in Human Tumors

Samples of spontaneous mammary carcinoma in human females were obtained either as fresh-frozen $(-20°C)$ specimens through Dr. D. W. Penner, Pathology Department, Health Sciences Centre, Winnipeg, or as frozen remnants of the estrogen receptor assay service directed by Dr. H. G. Friesen. In general, the former specimens were much larger than necessary, whereas the latter were in the range 0.25–2.2 g. Samples of normal human female mammary tissue were made available at mammoplasty operations (courtesy of Dr. M. F. Stranc) and were collected, fresh-frozen at $-20°C$, through the kind cooperation of the Pathology Department, Health Sciences Centre, Winnipeg. This department also provided uterine fibroid material and myometrial tissue as they became available following elective surgery.

Weighed samples of the tissues were minced, homogenized in 5 parts of distilled water to 1 part of tissue (v/w), first in a high-speed Sorval homogenizer and then with an ultrasonic probe. The homogenates were centrifuged at 5000 *g* for 10 min and the supernatants recovered. These were assayed for total protein (26) and superoxide dismutase (21). The latter determinations were done in 0.02 m*M* KCN, final concentration. The estrogen receptor in breast tissue and mammary carcinomas was measured as previously described (27).

Radiosensitive L5178Y leukemia cells were obtained from Dr. W. Hryniuk (Manitoba Cancer Treatment and Research Foundation, Winnipeg) and maintained *in vivo* in DBA male mice. The leukemia cells were harvested from the ascites fluid at a cell count of $> 10^9$ nucleated cells per milliliter, differentially lysed of red cells and washed as above, and assayed for endogenous superoxide dismutase as above.

UPTAKE AND BIOLOGICAL EFFECT OF EXOGENOUS SUPEROXIDE DISMUTASE

We had previously shown that exogenous (bovine) superoxide dismutase increased the D_0* of mouse bone marrow stem cells from 105 ± 6 to 290 ± 34 rads (13). Of this increase in D_0, 143 ± 28 rads were attributable to the enzyme acting outside the cell, and the balance of 42 ± 11 rads was ostensibly due to its intracellular activity (13). Of the two general sites of action, the latter is much more ($172/0.4 = 430$ times) efficient (Table 1).

In view of the cellular uptake of exogenous superoxide dismutase and its higher protection efficiency inside the cell, it was of interest to trace the enzyme into such subcellular fractions as nuclei, mitochondria, and cytoplasmic membranes. This was accomplished by using two independent methods: ^{125}I-labeled superoxide dismutase as tracer and radioimmu-

TABLE I

Extracellular and Intracellular Efficiency of Bovine Superoxide Dismutase Protection of Bone Marrow (Stem) Cells X-irradiated in Air

Bovine Superoxide Dismutase		Increase in D_0^a (mean $\pm \sigma$)	Protection efficiency[b] (ion pairs/molecule of enyzme)
Location	Amount		
Outside cell	6.4×10^{14} molecules/ml	143 ± 38	0.4
Inside cell	520 ± 47 molecules/cell	42 ± 11	172

[a] Control value, 105 ± 6 rads (13).

[b] Protection efficiency, increase in D_0/number of enzyme molecules $\times$ grams.

* The D_0 is the dose required to reduce survival to 37% in the region where the logarithm of survival is a linear function of the radiation dose. In mouse bone marrow stem cells, the logarithmic response starts at low doses since these cells have little or no shoulder (13).

noassay (10,22). The advantages of using the latter technique are that there is no reaction with murine superoxide dismutase and that enzymatically active bovine superoxide dismutase can be detected (22). Figure 1 shows the characteristic curve for the inhibition of the reaction of rabbit antibovine superoxide dismutase with ^{125}I-labeled bovine superoxide dismutase by a standard of pure bovine superoxide dismutase. Figures 2a, b, c, and d show, respectively, typical inhibition curves for exogenous superoxide dismutase in extracts of cells, nuclei, membranes, and mitochondria isolated from mouse bone marrow cells after being incubated with bovine CuZnSOD for 1 hr at 37°C *in vitro*. The parallelism of these curves with the standard (Fig. 1) was established within 95% confidence limits by analysis of covariance of the linear regressions of the inhibition curves in the 20–80% range (22). The 50% inhibition point was used to calculate the amount of bovine superoxide dismutase in the samples.

Table II summarizes the uptake of bovine superoxide dismutase by mouse bone marrow cells and their nuclear, mitochondrial, and mem-

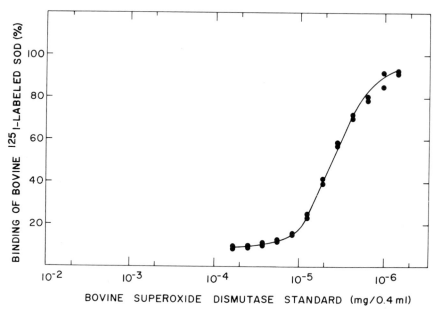

Fig. 1. Characteristic curve for the inhibition of the reaction of rabbit antibovine superoxide dismutase with ^{125}I-labeled bovine superoxide dismutase by a standard of purified bovine superoxide dismutase. Rabbit anti-superoxide dismutase (0.4 ml) was incubated in duplicate with 0.4 ml of serial dilutions of superoxide dismutase standard for 4 hr at 37°C, then with 2 μl of ^{125}I-labeled superoxide dismutase (169,000 cpm) overnight at room temperature, and finally with 0.15 ml of SARb-4B for 4 hr at 37°C before the solid phase was washed three times with 1.0 ml assay buffer and the bound radioactivity measured (22).

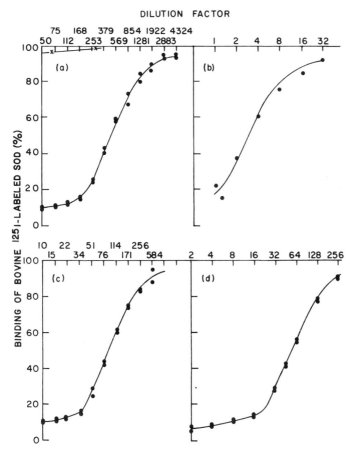

Fig. 2. Inhibition curves for exogenous superoxide dismutase in extracts from bone marrow of (a) 1.2×10^8 cells incubated with bovine superoxide dismutase at 10 mg/ml; (b) nuclei of 1.3×10^9 cells incubated with bovine superoxide dismutase at 0.5 mg/ml; (c) cytoplasmic membranes from 6.1×10^8 cells incubated with bovine superoxide dismutase at 10 mg/ml; and (d) mitochondria from 6.1×10^8 cells incubated with bovine superoxide dismutase at 10 mg/ml. Incubations for 1 hr at 37°C. Curve X—X in panel (a) represents control for cells without exogenous superoxide dismutase. Sample size in (b) insufficient for duplicates.

brane fractions as measured by radioimmunoassay and ^{125}I labeling. The uptakes, normalized to an exogenous superoxide dismutase concentration of 15.3 μM, are expressed in molecules per cell using 32,600 as the molecular weight of the bovine superoxide dismutase and the number of cells actually disrupted during the subcellular fractionation procedures. The uptakes as measured by the two methods are in quantitative agreement within experimental error. Further evidence that intact and enzymatically

TABLE II

Subcellular Uptake of Exogenous Bovine Superoxide Dismutase by Swiss Mice Bone Marrow Cells in 1 hr at 37°C Compared with Endogenous Enzyme Levels[a]

Cell compartment	Endogenous (molecules/cell × 10^5)			Exogenous (molecules/cell × 10^3)					
				By ^{125}I label			By radioimmunoassay		
	N	Mean ± σ	%	N	Mean ± σ	% increase[b]	N	Mean ± σ	% increase[b]
Cell	5	5.4 ± 1.7	100	6	45 ± 35	8.3	7	46 ± 19	8.5
Nucleus	3	2.9 ± 2.3	54	3	2.1 ± 1.1	0.7	3	1.8 ± 0.5	0.6
Membrane	3	0.29 ± 0.3	5	3	1.5 ± 1.2	5.1	4	1.4 ± 0.5	4.5
Mitochondria	3	0.14 ± 0.13	2.5	3	1.2 ± 1.1	8.5	4	0.5 ± 0.2	3.6

[a] Concentration of bovine enzyme in medium, 15.3 μM.
[b] Mean increase relative to the endogenous amount within the compartment.

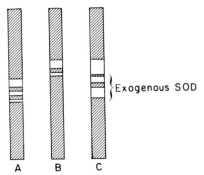

Fig. 3. Superoxide dismutase activity bands on polyacrylamide gel electrophoresis of: (A) 10 μg of purified superoxide dismutase from bovine erythrocytes; (B) superoxide dismutase extracted from the nuclei of 7.4 × 10⁶ bone marrow cells; and (C) superoxide dismutase extracted from the nuclei of 3.7 × 10⁶ bone marrow cells after treatment with bovine superoxide dismutase at 10 mg/ml for 1 hr at 37°C. The bands due to the bovine superoxide dismutase are identifiable by comparison with gel (A) and are not present in (B).

active bovine superoxide dismutase enters the mouse bone marrow cells is given in Fig. 3, in which the electrophoretic separation of the exogenous and endogenous superoxide dismutases in the nuclear fraction is shown.

Table II also gives the extent to which the total superoxide dismutase activity in bone marrow cells is elevated following treatment with bovine superoxide dismutase at 15.3 μM. The amount of endogenous and exogenous superoxide dismutases in the cells and their subcellular fractions are tabulated in absolute and relative terms. The increment in activity (percent increase) is highest in intact cells and lowest in the nuclear fraction, with membranes and mitochondria in between. The uptake of exogenous superoxide dismutase by the three subcellular organelles amounts to ≈ 10% of that which is taken up by the cells; the remaining 90% was presumably in the cytosol. The increment in the nuclear fraction is relatively small. In terms of the law of mass action, these results suggest that radioprotection of the bone marrow stem cells by bovine superoxide dismutase acting intracellularly is at least in part due to its activity in the cytosol, the cytoplasmic membranes, and/or mitochondria. Entry of exogenous superoxide dismutase into mitochondria for radioprotective purposes may be particularly significant in view of the possibility of unquenched superoxide radical formation during oxygen metabolism (28,29).

The possibility of a radioprotective role for exogenous superoxide dismutase outside the cell nucleus would be further strengthened by showing that the protection efficiency of the endogenous enzyme is not as high as that of the exogenous one. To calculate the protection efficiency of the endogenous superoxide dismutase, it was necessary to develop a correlation between the radiation response of the bone marrow cells and their superoxide dismutase content. It was found that the latter could be increased from the normal value of $5.4 \pm 1.7 \times 10^5$ to $11.3 \pm 3.1 \times 10^5$ molecules per cell by subjecting the donor mice beforehand to different concentrations of oxygen for variable periods of time (Table III). This change in superoxide dismutase content was accompanied by an increase in survival after X irradiation *in vitro* (Table III). Figure 4 is a graphical presentation of this relationship, which is best-fitted by the equation $y = 43.5$ $\ln x - 461$, at a correlation coefficient of 0.95. The correlation assumes that the superoxide dismutase level in bone marrow stem cells behaves and is the same as that in nucleated bone marrow cells in general. The ratio of the former to the latter in our experience was $\sim 1.3 \times 10^{-4}$, consistent with the published value (30). The equation passes through the (x, y) coordinates of $(10^6, 140)$ and $(10^5, 40)$, from which the slope of the line is

$$\frac{(140 - 40) \text{ rads}}{(10^6 - 10^5) \text{ molecules/cell}} = 111 \ \mu\text{rads/molecule} \times \text{cell}$$

Since 1 rad $= 6.2418 \times 10^{13}$ eV/g and the weight of the stem cell may be taken as 1150×10^{-2} g (12,13), *the value of* 111 μrads/molecule $\times$ cell is equivalent to

$$\frac{111 \times 10^{-6} \text{ rad} \times 6.2418 \times 13^{13} \text{ eV/g}}{1150 \times 10^{-12} \text{ g} \times \text{a molecule of enzyme}} = 7.9 \text{ eV/molecule}$$

or 0.24 ion pair per molecule of enzyme at 33.7 eV/ion pair.

The value of 0.24 ion pair per molecule of endogenous superoxide dis-

TABLE III

Correlation of *in Vitro* Radioresistance of Swiss Mice Bone Marrow Stem Cells with Endogenous Superoxide Dismutase

History of stem cell donors	Endogenous enzyme (molecules/cell $\times 10^5$)		Radioresistance, D_0 (rads)	
	N	Mean $\pm \sigma$	N	Mean $\pm \sigma$
Normal	5	5.4 ± 1.7	8	105 ± 11
In 85% O_2 for 3 days	6	7.5 ± 0.8	10	133 ± 4
Normal weanling mice	4	8.2 ± 1.6	6	134 ± 9
In 4.5% O_2 for 2 days	6	11.3 ± 3.1	4	143 ± 4
In 8% O_2 for 2 weeks	6	10.6 ± 4	3	149 ± 4

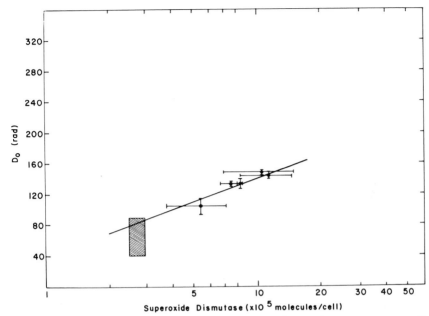

Fig. 4. Correlation of the *in vitro* radioresistance (D_0) of mouse bone marrow stem cells with their endogenous superoxide dismutase content (data from Table III). Equation of best-fitted line through the points is $y = 43.5 \ln x - 461$; correlation coefficient is 0.95. The shaded rectangle represents L5178Y mouse leukemia cells in terms of their superoxide dismutase content (width of area), as measured by us, and the D_0 values (height of area), as reported in the literature (32–35).

mutase is 716 times lower than that for exogenous superoxide dismutase acting intracellularly (Table IV) and suggests that the juxtaposition of the endogenous enzyme near (macro) molecular targets, critical to radiation survival and cellular proliferation, is relatively poor, possibly because of suboptimal compartmentalization. Moreover, the larger increments in activity following enzyme treatment occur in subcellular fractions of mem-

TABLE IV

Comparison of Protection Efficiencies of Bovine Superoxide Dismutase and the Endogenous Enzyme inside Bone Marrow Stem Cells of Swiss Mice

Type of superoxide dismutase	Amount (molecules per cell)	Increase in D_0 (rads)	Protection efficiency (ion pairs/molecule of enzyme)
Bovine	520 ± 47	42	$\left.\begin{array}{c} 172 \\ 0.24 \end{array}\right\} \rightarrow \dfrac{172}{0.24} = 716$
Endogenous	$10^5 \rightarrow 10^6$	100	

branes and mitochondria, suggesting that these structures could benefit the most from entry of the exogenous enzyme. The use of superoxide dismutase as a therapeutic agent to probe subcellular regions for critically important responses to radiation therefore seems promising and may lead to an understanding of the mechanism(s) whereby the enzyme inhibits radiation-induced cell transformation (9) and chromsomal aberrations (31).

The shaded rectangle in Fig. 4 defines the radioresistance of L5178Y mouse leukemia cells (32–35) and their superoxide dismutase content as determined in this study. This area is intercepted by extrapolating the line through the points of Fig. 4 to lower coordinates. Although this agreement may be coincidental because the leukemia cells were grown in mice of another strain (DBA), the fact remains that the lymphoblastic L5178Y cells contain less superoxide dismutase and are also less radioresistant than normal bone marrow stem cells. Since the stem cells in turn contain less superoxide dismutase and are less radioresistant than well-differentiated lymphocytes and granulocytes (12), it follows that, among lymphoblastic (L5178Y) leukemia cells, stem cells, lymphocytes, and granulocytes, the leukemia cells contain the least superoxide dismutase and are the most sensitive to radiation. Qualitatively, therefore, the type of correlation depicted in Fig. 4 extends from leukemia cells through stem cells to mature blood cells.

The foregoing observation raises the issue as to whether superoxide dismutase activity levels determine the relative radiosensitivities of tissues and tumors. Sykes *et al.* (5) have noted that human tissues with low superoxide dismutase content, such as bone marrow and spleen, are generally more sensitive to radiation than those with high enzyme activity and have reported assay data on superoxide dismutase in a variety of human tissues. In general, their data also support the existence of a relationship between the radiation sensitivity of tumors and their superoxide dismutase content. In addition to their results and observations, comparative data on superoxide dismutase content of tumor and host tissue are required as a first step in exploring the enzymatic basis for any difference in radiosensitivity that may exist. We have measured the total protein and superoxide dismutase in human uterine fibroids and spontaneous mammary carcinomas and related the results to the respective host tissues. Table V summarizes the data on normal myometrial tissue and uterine fibroids. It shows that there is no difference in protein and superoxide dismutase levels between the nonneoplastic fibroids and uterine tissues. Table VI summarizes similar data for spontaneous breast carcinomas and normal mammary tissue of women. Increases in both protein and superoxide dismutase were found in the carcinomas. The change in total protein, although not statistically significant, is consistent with previous

TABLE V

Comparison of Protein and Superoxide Dismutase Levels in Normal Human Myometrial Tissue and Uterine Fibroids

	Myometrial tissue		Uterine fibroids		
Assay	N	Mean ± σ	N	Mean ± σ	p
Total tissue protein (mg/ml)	14	7.3 ± 4.2	15	7.1 ± 4.1	<.5
Superoxide dismutase (μg/ml)	14	14.3 ± 6.3	15	13.9 ± 5.6	<.5

measurements (36), but its meaning in relation to the nature of malignancy is not clear. Endogenous superoxide dismutase activity is, on average, higher in the carcinomas, and in more than 50% of the tumors is above the normal range of 4.2 ± 4 μg/ml of extract (Table VI) or 21 ± 20 μg/g of wet tissue (Fig. 5). No carcinoma was without a measurable amount of the enzyme. The increase is statistically significant at 99.5% $>p$ > 99% confidence limits. In four of the 30 cases of carcinoma (Table VI), the tumor was submitted as part of a larger specimen of breast tissue, permitting concurrent analysis for superoxide dismutase and protein of both the mammary tissue and the carcinoma. Of the four cases, the total protein and superoxide dismutase activity in the tumor, relative to the adjacent tissue, were unchanged in one case, decreased in another, and elevated in two. The higher superoxide dismutase activity in individual cases of breast carcinoma as compared to mammary tissue is a reason for the statistically significant increase shown in Table VI and provides an enzymatic basis for any differential increase in radioresistance that may exist in such carcinomas.

The statistically significant increase in superoxide dismutase within neoplastic breast carcinomas, as compared to mammary tissue, contrasts with the absence of any difference between nonneoplastic tumors (fi-

TABLE VI

Comparison of Protein and Superoxide Dismutase Levels in Normal Human Mammary Tissue and Female Breast Carcinomas

	Normal		Carcinomas		
Assay	N	Mean ± σ	N	Mean ± σ	p
Total tissue protein (mg/ml)	11	2.9 ± 1.4	30	4.3 ± 2.3	<.1
Superoxide dismutase (μg/ml)	11	4.2 ± 4	30	10.4 ± 6.6	<.01

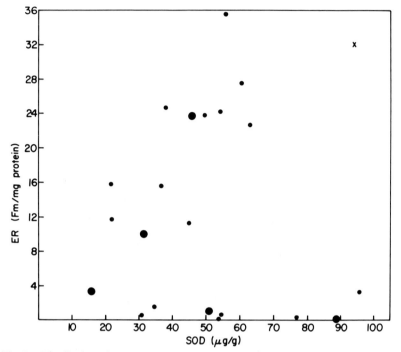

Fig. 5. Distribution of estrogen receptor assay (ER) and endogenous superoxide dismutase activity in specimens of mammary carcinomas in women in which both variables were determined. Enzyme activity in normal mammary tissue is 21 ± 20 $\mu g/g$ (Table VI). Key: X, lobular; ●, infiltrating ducts; ●, intraductal.

broids) and normal myometria. Bearing in mind that different organs are being compared, one might say that the contrast is perhaps also a reflection of the more rapid growth of the carcinomas, accompanied possibly by an increase in ribonucleic acids and a higher rate of protein synthesis (37). It is also noted, however, that in animal hepatomas and adenocarcinomas the superoxide dismutase activity is depressed relative to that present in host tissue (2).

SIGNIFICANCE

It is difficult to compare our data on superoxide dismutase activity in human mammary carcinomas with those reported by Sykes *et al.* (5) because the latter are given in units of activity rather than by weight. In addition, Sykes *et al.*'s unit of activity may be larger since their purified enzyme standard from bovine erythrocytes had a lower specific activity than ours (12), as determined by an alternate method (21). Moreover, their extraction procedure inactivated the mitochondrial superoxide dismutase, whereas it was probably present in our extracts. Disc gel electrophoresis of extracts from six carcinomas exhibited the band attributed to the mitochondrial enzyme (38), albeit perhaps in reduced amount. Earlier reports described a decrease or absence of the mitochondrial enzyme in Ehrlich ascites tumor cells (3), Morris hepatoma (39), and W1-38 cells transformed by Simian virus 40 (1). However, the mitochondrial superoxide dismutase in the hepatomas may have been missed by the negative staining technique (40). Isolated mitochondria from Ehrlich ascites tumor cells have been found to exhibit two activity bands on disc gel electrophoresis that are characteristic of the CuZnSOD and are inhibited by 2 mM NaCN (3). The presence of the cyanide-sensitive enzyme in mitochondria is interesting in that the enzyme is synthesized in the cytosol (38) and presumably entered the mitochondria by diffusion, a possibility supported by the evidence presented above for the uptake of exogenous superoxide dismutase by subcellular organelles, including mitochondria. Clearly, more studies on the presence of mitochondrial superoxide dismutase and on the subcellular distribution of the cyanide-sensitive enzyme in tumors are necessary.

Increased superoxide dismutase activity in human mammary carcinomas is important for reasons other than the fact that it suggests a possible decrease in radiosensitivity. The enzyme contributes to the total antioxidant activity of cells and is therefore part of an anticancer surveillance system (41). Furthermore, in dismutating superoxide radicals, the enzyme is expected to inhibit the role of free radicals in carcinogenesis as well as stimulate the cytotoxic peroxide–peroxidase–halide system for tumor destruction. It has been reported that synthesis of a peroxidase endogenous to mammary carcinoma cells is stimulated by estrogen (42–44). The peroxidase was not found in estrogen-deprived tumors (42). There may therefore be a functional interdependence between the antioxidative activity of superoxide dismutase, the peroxide–peroxidase–halide systems of tumor surveillance (41), and the estrogen dependence of tumors. In the majority of cases, the hormone dependence of mammary carcinomas is determined by the presence of estrogen receptors (ER's) (45–47). This line of reasoning suggested correlating the superoxide dismutase activity in the breast carcinomas with their ER levels. The results are shown in Fig. 5 for 22 of the 30 tumors examined (Table VI), involving 16 infiltrating duct, 5 intraductal, and 1 lobular carcinoma (histology the courtesy of Dr. D. W. Penner, Health Sciences Centre, Winnipeg). The range in enzyme activity is substantial, irrespective of whether the tumors are rich or poor in ER's [< 10 fmol/ml protein (48)]. Thus, it appears that, in general, superoxide dismutase is not a specific marker enzyme for ER-rich mammary carcinomas. However, the superoxide dismutase activity in this group does tend to increase with the hormone receptor level. It would be interesting to determine the peroxidase activity in the ER-rich group of tumors, since it has a direct bearing on the efficacy of the superoxide dismutase-stimulated cytotoxic peroxide–peroxidase–halide systems, assuming that superoxide generation, as a potential source of peroxides, goes on, possibly at an accelerated rate (37). This cytotoxic system is presumably weakened in the ER-poor group of tumors if peroxidase activity is absent or impaired (42,43). The variation in superoxide dismutase activity may then more simply affect the extent to which superoxide radicals are used in carcinogenesis through free-radical reactions.

ACKNOWLEDGMENTS

We thank Dr. I. Worsley and H. Cosby for assistance in tissue collection. We also appreciate the technical assistance of R. Zepp, T. P. Copps, S. D. Pleskach, S. Bell, and H. Boux in various stages of this work.

REFERENCES

1. Yamanaka, N., and Deamer, D. (1974). Superoxide dismutase activity in WI-38 cell cultures: Effects of age, trypsinization and SV-40 transformation. *Physiol. Chem. Phys.* **6**:95.
2. Peskin, A. V., Zbarskii, I. B., and Konstantinov, A. A. (1976). Investigation of superoxide dismutase activity in tumoral tissues. *Dokl. Akad. Nauk SSSR* **229**:751.
3. Sahu, S. K., Oberley, L. W., Stevens, R. H., and Riley, E. F. (1977). Brief communication: Superoxide dismutase activity of Ehrlich ascites tumor cells. *JNCI, J. Natl. Cancer Inst.* **58**:1125.
4. Petkau, A., Monasterski, L. G., Kelly, K., and Friesen, H. G. (1977). Modification of superoxide dismutase in rat mammary carcinoma. *Res. Commun. Chem. Pathol. Pharmacol.* **17**:125.
5. Sykes, J. A., McCormack, F. X., Jr., and O'Brien, T. J. (1978). A preliminary study of the superoxide dismutase content of some human tumors. *Cancer Res.* **38**:2759.
6. McCord, J. M., and Fridovich, I. (1969). Superoxide dismutase: An enzymic function for erythrocuprein (hemocuprein). *J. Biol. Chem.* **244**:6049.
7. Petkau, A., and Chelack, W. S. (1976). Radioprotective effect of superoxide dismutase on model phospholipid membranes. *Biochim. Biophys. Acta* **433**:445.
8. Lavelle, F., Michelson, A. M., and Dimitrijevic, L. (1973). Biological protection by superoxide dismutase. *Biochem. Biophys. Res. Commun.* **5**:350.
9. Michelson, A. M., and Buckingham, M. E. (1974). Effects of superoxide radicals on myoblast growth and differentiation. *Biochem. Biophys. Res. Commun.* **58**:1079.

10. Petkau, A., Kelly, K., Chelack, W. S., Pleskach, S. D., Barefoot, C., and Meeker, B. E. (1975). Radioprotection of bone marrow stem cells by superoxide dismutase. *Biochem. Biophys. Res. Commun.* **67**:1167.

11. Petkau, A., Kelly, K., Chelack, W. S., and Barefoot, C. (1976). Protective effect of superoxide dismutase on erythrocytes of X-irradiated mice. *Biochem. Biophys. Res. Commun.* **70**:452.

12. Petkau, A., Chelack, W. S., and Pleskach, S. D. (1978). Protection by superoxide dismutase of white blood cells in X-irradiated mice. *Life Sci.* **22**:867.

13. Petkau, A. (1978). Radiation protection by superoxide dismutase. *Photochem. Photobiol.* **28**:765.

14. Stone, D., Lin, P. S., and Kwock, L. (1978). Radiosensitization of human erythrocytes by diethyldithiocarbamate. *Int. J. Radiat. Biol.* **33**:393.

15. Petkau, A., Chelack, W. S., Pleskach, S. D., Meeker, B. E., and Brady, C. M. (1975). Radioprotection of mice by superoxide dismutase. *Biochem. Biophys. Res. Commun.* **65**:886.

16. Petkau, A., Chelack, W. S., and Pleskach, S. D. (1976). Protection of post-irradiated mice by superoxide dismutase. *Int. J. Radiat. Biol.* **29**:297.

17. Rest, R. F., and Spitznagel, J. K. (1977). Subcellular distribution of superoxide dismutase in human neutrophils. *Biochem. J.* **166**:145.

18. Hayat, M. A., ed. (1972). "Basic Electron Microscopy Techniques," pp. 63–64. Van Nostrand-Reinhold, Princeton, New Jersey.

19. Spitznagel, J. K., Doldorf, F. G., Leffell, M. S., Folds, J. D., Welsh, I. R. H., Cooney, M. H., and Martin, L. E. (1974). Character of azurophil and specific granules purified from human polymorphonuclear leukocytes. *Lab. Invest.* **30**:774.

20. Monneron, A., and d'Alayer, J. (1978). Isolation of plasma and nuclear membranes of thymocytes. *J. Cell Biol.* **77**:211.

21. Beauchamp, C., and Fridovich, I. (1971): Superoxide dismutase: Improved assays and an assay applicable to acrylamide gels. *Anal. Biochem.* **44**:276.

22. Kelly, K., Barefoot, C., Sehon, A., and Petkau, A. (1978). Bovine superoxide dismutase: A radioimmunoassay. *Arch. Biochem. Biophys.* **190**:531.

23. Davis, B. J. (1964). Disc gel electrophoresis: Method and application to human serum proteins. *Ann. N.Y. Acad. Sci.* **121**:404.

24. Beckman, G., Lundgren, E., and Tärnvik, A. (1973). Superoxide dismutase isozymes in different human tissues, their genetic control and intracellular localization. *Hum. Hered.* **23**:338.

25. Gregory, E. M., and Fridovich, I. (1973). Induction of superoxide dismutase by molecular oxygen. *J. Bacteriol.* **114**:543.

26. Schacterle, G. R., and Pollock, R. L. (1978). A simplified method for the quantitative assay of small amounts of protein in biologic material. *Anal. Biochem.* **51**:654.

27. McGuire, W. L., and De La Garza, M. (1978). Improved sensitivity in the measurement of estrogen receptor in human breast cancer. *Clin. Endocrin. Metab.*, **37**:986.

28. Britton, L., Malinowski, D. P., and Fridovich, I. (1978). Superoxide dismutase and oxygen metabolism in *Streptococcus faecalis* and comparisons with other organisms. *J. Bacteriol.* **134**:229.

29. Nohl, H., and Hegner, D. (1978). Do mitochondria produce oxygen radicals *in vivo?* *Eur. J. Biochem.* **82**:563.

30. Covelli, V., and Metalli, P. (1973). A late effect of radiation on the haemopoietic stem cells of the mouse. *Int. J. Radiat. Biol.* **23**:83.

31. Nordenson, I., Beckman, G., and Beckman, L. (1976). The effect of superoxide dismutase and catalase on radiation-induced chromosome breaks. *Hereditas* **82**:125.

32. Lett, J. T., Caldwell, I., Dean, C. J., and Alexander, P. (1967). Rejoining of X-ray induced breaks in the DNA of leukemia cells. *Nature (London)* **214**:790.
33. Veatch, W., and Okada, S. (1969). Radiation-induced breaks of DNA in cultured mammalian cells. *Biophys. J.* **9**:330.
34. Hesselwood, I. P. (1978). DNA strand breaks in resistant and sensitive murine lymphoma cells, detected by the hydroxyapatite chromatographic technique. *Int. J. Radiat. Biol.* **34**:461.
35. Courtenay, V. D. (1969). Radioresistant mutants of L5178Y cells. *Radiat. Res.* **38**:186.
36. Singer, A. L., Sherwin, R. P., Dunn, A. S., and Appleman, M. M. (1976). Cyclic nucleotide phosphodiesterases in neoplastic and nonneoplastic human mammary tissues. *Cancer Res.* **36**:60.
37. Wickramasinghe, R. H., Reddy, P. R. K., Klein, L., and Villee, C. A. (1976). Superoxide anions and other components of human renal adenocarcinoma. *Clin. Biochem.* **9**:24.
38. Weisiger, R. A., and Fridovich, I. (1973). Superoxide dismutase: Organelle specificity. *J. Biol. Chem.* **248**:3582.
39. Dionisi, O., Galeotti, T., Terranova, T., and Azzi, A. (1975). Superoxide radicals and hydrogen peroxide formation in mitochondria from normal and neoplastic tissues. *Biochim. Biophys. Acta* **403**:292.
40. De Rosa, G., Duncan, D. S., Keen, G. L., and Hurley, L. S. (1979). Evaluation of negative staining technique for determination of CN^--insensitive superoxide dismutase activity. *Biochim. Biophys. Acta* **566**:32.
41. Apffel, C. A. (1976). Nonimmunological host defenses: A review. *Cancer Res.* **36**:1527.
42. DeSombre, E. R., Anderson, W. A., and Kang, Y. H. (1975). Identification, subcellular localization, and estrogen regulation of peroxidase in 7,12-dimethylbenz[*a*]anthracene-induced rat mammary tumors. *Cancer Res.* **35**:172.
43. Anderson, W. A., Kang, Y. H., and DeSombre, E. R. (1975). Endogenous peroxidase: Specific marker enzyme for tissues displaying growth dependency on estrogen. *J. Cell Biol.* **64**:668.
44. Lippman, M. E., and Allegra, J. C. (1978). Current concepts in cancer. Receptors in breast cancer. *N. Engl. J. Med.* **229**:930.
45. Friedberg, F. (1977). Hormone receptors. *Horiz. Biochem. Biophys.* **4**:63.
46. Zava, D. T., Chamness, G. C., Horwitz, K. B., and McGuire, W. L. (1977). Human breast cancer: Biologically active estroten receptor in the absence of estrogen? *Science* **196**:663.
47. Lippman, M., Bolan, G., and Huff, K. (1976). Interactions of antiestrogens with human breast cancer in long-term tissue culture. *Cancer Treat. Rep.* **60**:1421.
48. Lippman, M. E., Allegra, J. C., Thompson, E. R., Simon, R., Barlock, A., Green, L., Huff, K. K., Do, H. M. J., Aiken, S. C., and Warren, R. (1978). The relation between estrogen receptors and response rate to cytotoxic chemotherapy in metastatic breast cancer. *N. Engl. J. Med.* **298**:1223.

DISCUSSION

McLENNAN: Could you describe the "normal breast tissue" you used in your studies? Was it glandular breast tissue and therefore equivalent to the breast carcinoma, or was it principally adipose tissue?

PETKAU: Some of the normal breast specimens consisted of glandular tissues whereas, in the remainder, adipose tissue was the principal component.

MICHELSON: I have a number of observations that confirm Dr. Petkau's studies on human breast cancer in a striking way. These results are described in the chapter entitled "Clinical Use of Superoxide Dismutase and Possible Pharmacological Approaches" (this volume). Both of our groups were completely unaware of each other's work and used quite different techniques, yet we obtained similar results and drew similar conclusions, particularly with respect to MnSOD levels.

MEHDI: For your measurements on the intracellular distribution of exogenous superoxide dismutase in bone marrow stem cells, did you measure marker enzymes for the cross-contamination of these preparations? Small fragments of the plasma membrane can be treacherous contaminants and could account for your finding superoxide dismutase in the nuclear and mitochondrial preparations. The purity of your fractions is vital to your interpretations.

PETKAU: For the subcellular fractionation of nucleated bone marrow cells, we used the methods previously applied to the study of enzyme markers. Our preparations were examined by electron microscopy, and the results compared well with published observations. Nonetheless, we do not claim that the membrane fraction, for example, consisted of plasma membranes only. It most likely included other membrane fragments. We believe the nuclear fraction to be markedly free of cytoplasmic membrane fragments, but marker enzymes were not measured.

OBERLEY: In your work on mammary carcinomas, you must be very careful when comparing human or *in vivo* samples because many cell types are present. For proper comparison, you must compare the cancerous cells with the normal cells from which the cancer cells were derived. For example, in chemically induced intestinal tumors, we have found that the tumor tissue has nearly the same MnSOD levels as normal tissue. However, when tumor cells are compared to intestinal villus cells, the MnSOD is greatly reduced.

PETKAU: I agree with you entirely. The optimal comparison must be at the cell-to-cell level. This implies a histological approach, for example, with immunofluorescent antibodies against both types of superoxide dismutase.

FRIDOVICH: What appears to be a discrepancy between your results and those of Dr. Oberley may in fact not be a discrepancy. In most species the MnSOD is restricted to the mitochondria, but in human beings and baboons there is MnSOD in the cytosol also. In mouse and rat liver, therefore, the MnSOD decreases. In human liver it may also decrease. In mouse and rat tissue this represents the total MnSOD, whereas in human beings it does not.

PETKAU: Our assay procedure was aimed at measuring total superoxide dismutase. The MnSOD may well have been depressed, as Dr. Oberley has stated. However, in the extracts of the half-dozen mammary carcinomas that we subjected to disc gel electrophoresis, the MnSOD band was observed. These specimens, from which the extracts were derived, consisted of solid tumor, each composed of a number of different types of cells. The presence of MnSOD may have been due to the presence of the different types of cells, of which not all may have been cancerous. Therefore, the discrepancy may not be real.

RILEY: I would like to respond to the question that was raised earlier in this session concerning the possible relevance of Otto Warburg's studies to the subject matter of this symposium. The controversy over the interpretation of Warburg's findings is, and should be, restricted to the disputed cancer hypothesis and should not detract in any way from the extensive contributions that have made him the unquestioned father of modern biochemistry and for which he received international recognition through the award of the Nobel Prize. One special phase of his later studies is particularly relevant to various studies reported in this symposium. In beautiful, simple studies on the differential response of cancer cells and normal cells to X irradiation, he demonstrated clearly that a striking difference existed in the peroxidase concentration of normal cells and radiosensitive cancer cells. He then postulated that the differential response was due to the production of H_2O_2 by X irradiation. Since normal cells possessed the necessary enzymes to detoxify the H_2O_2 and the radiosensitive cancer cells did not, the differential destruction of the two cell types seemed clear. These studies were undertaken at a time when little was known about O_2^- and superoxide dismutase. It is regrettable that Professor Warburg did not live to see the provocative and stimulating studies presented at this symposium, since many of them represent a logical extension of his early observations. His basic studies on the aerobic and anaerobic glycolysis of tumors and other tissues may also be relevant to the rational therapy of cancer in which active oxygen and related factors may be involved.

PIETRONIGRO: Since many factors are probably involved in protecting cells from free-radical toxicity, is it possible that the oxygen treatment of your animals may have resulted in the induction of other components?

In this regard, have you looked at the survival curves of these cells in nitrogen?

PETKAU: Other factors within the cells may well have changed, e.g., catalase and glutathione peroxidase. However, the plating efficiency of the unirradiated cells remained the same. As to your second question, we did not look for changes in the nitrogen survival curves.

Chapter **15**

Redox Cycling and the Mechanism of Action of Antibiotics in Neoplastic Diseases

JAMES DOROSHOW AND PAUL HOCHSTEIN

INTRODUCTION

The univalent reduction of oxygen during the course of either normal cellular metabolism (1) or consequent to the autoxidation of cellular constituents such as iron (2) has been suggested to be involved in alterations in DNA that lead to the development of cancer. Presumably, such effects would be mediated by a variety of oxygen metabolites, which include, in addition to superoxide, hydrogen peroxide, hydroxyl radicals, and singlet oxygen. In recent years, there has been intense interest in the role of these chemical species in many other cellular processes (3). For example, they have been implicated in the chemotherapeutic actions of numerous naturally occurring and synthetic substances. Among these substances are the group of antibiotics whose interaction with molecular oxygen depends on either quinoid groups or bound metals. In this brief chapter, it is not our intention to provide an exhaustive review of the literature on these agents. Rather, we present concepts and speculations derived, in some instances, from the perspectives of work in our own laboratories.

PATHOLOGY OF OXYGEN

ISBN 0-12-068620-1

BACKGROUND

For the quinoid antibiotics it is abundantly clear that semiquinone forms play a central role in the generation of oxygen radicals and metabolites with cytotoxic potential. Both the oxidation of the hydroquinone forms and the reduction of the quinone may lead to the formation of semiquinone. This is illustrated in Eq. (1).

$$\text{(1)}$$

In addition, semiquinone free radicals may be formed by spontaneous proportionation of equilibrium mixtures of quinone and hydroquinone [Eq. (2)].

$$\text{(2)}$$

Fully reduced quinols may react predominantly in a divalent reduction of oxygen (4), although they may be restricted from doing so in the phospholipid environment of biological membranes (5). On the other hand, the oxidation of semiquinone free radicals should exclusively generate superoxide, assuming that only a single electron is transferred during bimolecular collisions. Spontaneous or enzymatic disproportionation of superoxide accounts for the ultimate formation of hydrogen peroxide in the latter reactions. In turn, the generation of hydrogen peroxide may result in metal-catalyzed hydroxyl radical formation either through interaction with superoxide [Eq. (3)].

$$H_2O_2 + O_2^- \rightarrow {}^\cdot OH + OH^- + {}^1O_2 \tag{3}$$

or through decomposition [Eq. (4)].

$$H_2O_2 \rightarrow {}^\cdot OH + OH^- \tag{4}$$

Each of the quinone antibiotics discussed below is capable of generating a variety of oxygen metabolites by these mechanisms.

The generation of oxygen radicals from metal-containing agents apparently does not involve oxidation of the antibiotic itself. Rather, these radicals are generated during oxidation of the metal component. Such an effect of iron (or copper) is not surprising and is in keeping with the known reactions of heavy metals of this type with molecular oxygen. These reactions, which also ultimately result in peroxide formation, require the reduced forms of the metals, which may be maintained through the activity of enzymes or molecules, such as ascorbate and glutathione, or oxygen radicals themselves.

Investigations of the role of oxygen radicals in biological systems have received enormous impetus in the past 10 years from the discovery of the superoxide dismutases (6) [Eq. (5)].

$$2O_2^- + 2H^+ \rightarrow H_2O_2 + O_2 \tag{5}$$

It has been known for many years that quinol–quinone agents and certain metals form hydrogen peroxide during their oxidation–reduction. However, the formation of peroxide in biological systems was generally thought not to be an event of major consequence because of the activity of the ubiquitous enzyme catalase [Eq. (6)].

$$2H_2O_2 \rightarrow O_2 + 2H_2O \tag{6}$$

This view was substantially altered with the discovery of the enzyme glutathione peroxidase by Gordon Mills in the late 1950's (7) [Eq. (7)].

$$H_2O_2 + 2GSH \rightarrow GSSG + H_2O \tag{7}$$

In his early experiments, the addition of cyanide to inhibit catalase was found to be essential for the demonstration of enzyme activity in homogenates and lysates. It was not until the subsequent demonstration (8) that glutathione peroxidase effectively competes with catalase in the detoxification of hydrogen peroxide, in the absence of cyanide and in intact cells, that peroxide was established as a key intermediate in the cytotoxicity of many chemicals and in the pathophysiology of certain diseases. The recognition of the role of selenium in glutathione peroxidase activity (9) and its capacity to react with organic hydroperoxides (10) have added to the interest in this enzyme. Studies on its role in peroxide detoxification are still underway (11).

Early experiments with erythrocytes from individuals with a genetic deficiency of glucose-6-phosphate dehydrogenase suggested that the autoxidation–reduction of many drugs, including antibiotics, might be of importance in their mechanism of action (12). These cells cannot maintain

reduced glutathione levels, and hence glutathione peroxidase activity, because of their failure to generate NADPH (13). Their sensitivity to dihy-
dric phenols, phenolic amines, and hydrazo and quinoid compounds is
well documented (14). The demonstration that these compounds might
form hydrogen peroxide within cells resolved the apparent paradox of
these disparate agents, which cause oxidative damage to cells when they
are in fact reducing substances (15). It seems clear now that such chemicals act to reduce oxygen to radical species and peroxides, which in turn
interact with cellular constituents to cause alterations in cellular function.
In recent years, two autoxidizable substances in the fava bean (*Vicia
faba*), divicine (2,6-diamino-4,5-dihydroxypyrimidine) and isouramil
(2,4,5-trihydroxy-6-aminopyrimidine), have been associated with oxidant
cell damage in individuals with glucose-6-phosphate dehydrogenase deficiency (16). At least *in vitro,* the oxygen-dependent antibiotics also may
produce oxidant damage in these erythrocytes similar to that observed
with more classical hemolytic agents.

The generation of oxygen radicals and peroxides through oxidation–reduction cycles observed with quinones and other organic substances may
also be observed with certain metals. For example, iron is well known for
its capacity to participate in reactions that generate free radicals. The formation of radicals through the actions of a metal appears to be of importance in the mechanism of action of at least one of the antibiotics
described below, bleomycin. The addition of Fe(II) ions to DNA has been
reported to result in the formation of hydroxyl free radicals, presumably
by a Fenton-type reaction, when hydrogen peroxide is present (17). In
this instance, the attack on DNA by bound iron results in the formation of
aldehydes, which react with thiobarbituric acid and which appear to be
derived from ribose. Although not frequently associated with antibiotic
activity, copper, like iron, has the capacity to generate oxygen free radicals. These radicals have been implicated in the direct therapeutic effects
of this metal (18) as well as in its cytotoxicity (19).

STREPTONIGRIN

Streptonigrin, derived from *Streptomyces flocculus,* was one of the first
quinoid antibiotics whose action was shown to be dependent on oxygen.
Although it has antitumor effects in man (20), its use has been limited because of its toxicity. It is of interest that among its toxic effects is the
development of anemia in individuals deficient in glucose-6-phosphate dehydrogenase (21).

White and colleagues demonstrated that the lethality of streptonigrin increased in the presence of oxygen (22) and that the antibiotic gave rise to an EPR-detectable semiquinone signal in cultures of *Escherichia coli* (23). It was also demonstrated (24) that streptonigrin reduction by hepatic mitochondrial preparations resulted in a cyanide-insensitive, EDTA-sensitive oxidation of intra- and extramitochondrial NADH. These effects were accompanied by the uptake of oxygen and the accumulation of hydrogen peroxide in excess of the amounts of sterptonigrin added. They are consistent with the idea that sterptonigrin undergoes redox cycling to form, at least, its semiquinone. The semiquinone (or hydroquinone) would then react with oxygen to eventually yield peroxide after dismutation of initially formed superoxide.

The idea that superoxide is involved in radical attack that results in DNA degradation in *E. coli* was reinforced by experiments with induced cells, which contained high levels of superoxide dismutase and were more resistant to the antibiotic than uninduced cultures of the organism (25). Although superoxide formed from streptonigrin may cause DNA strand cleavage (26), it has also been noted that catalase completely inhibits the capacity of the antibiotic to cause breakage of DNA (27). This phenomenon, in addition to the fact that copper stimulates the cleavage reaction (28), suggests that hydroxyl radicals, derived from peroxide decomposition or from the interaction of peroxide with semiquinone, may be the chemical species that causes DNA damage and cell death in bacteria.

In human leukemic leukocytes, streptonigrin also results in strand breakage of extractable DNA (29). The antibiotic also has profound inhibitory effects on both DNA and RNA synthesis, as well as on the incorporation of [^{14}C]phenylalanine into protein of intact cells. The issue of whether the effects in human leukemic cells are the consequence of the action of superoxide or hydroxyl radicals derived from hydrogen peroxide is not resolved. In terms of the ultimate cause of cell death in leukemic leukocytes exposed to streptonigrin, this issue may not be of primary importance. Thus, treated leukocytes undergo a rapid depletion of cellular ATP without marked diminution of oxygen consumption (29). This effect apparently results from the oxidation of cellular NADH and consequent bypass of mitochondrial electron transport systems that form ATP. The continued oxygen uptake of cells under these conditions is a consequence of the autoxidation of the reduced forms of streptonigrin. The oxygen utilization is not sensitive to cyanide as would be expected if it were a consequence of mitochondrial cytochrome oxidase activity. The depletion of ATP in treated cells might be sufficient cause for inhibition of DNA, RNA, and protein synthesis *without* implicating the toxic effects of oxygen metabolites. It would be of interest to determine the extent to which the antineoplastic effects of other quinone antibiotics might also involve their reduction and autoxidation and the diversion of NADH (or NADPH) through futile oxidative cycles with loss of nucleotides essential for energy-dependent cellular functions.

ANTHRACYCLINE ANTIBIOTICS

The anthracycline antibiotics doxorubicin and daunorubicin are among the most useful antineoplastic agents known, principally because of their significant therapeutic utility in the treatment of hematogenous malignancies as well as solid tumors of the breast, lung, bone, and thyroid (30). Although the binding of the anthracyclines to DNA by intercalation between adjacent base pairs has consistently been suggested to underlie the chemotherapeutic action of these drugs (30), it has recently been appreciated that these antibiotics have a wide variety of other biochemical effects, including free-radical formation, which may explain their antineoplastic activity as well as their toxic effect on the heart (31).

Handa and Sato initially demonstrated that the anthracycline antibiotics enhance oxygen consumption from hepatic microsomes in the presence of NADPH (32). Subsequent investigations by this group (33), by Goodman and Hochstein (34), and by Bachur and co-workers (35,36) have established that microsomal NADPH cytochrome P-450 reductase acts as an electron shuttle between NADPH and the quinone moiety of the anthracycline drugs, leading to the formation of an anthracycline semiquinone radical. Electron spin resonance studies by several groups have indicated that the anthracycline semiquinone signal may be quite long-lived, even in the presence of biological preparations; this had led to the speculation that the semiquinone radical may itself be membrane bound (33,35,37). The suitability of the anthracyclines as electron acceptors is not surprising since previous studies have revealed that NADPH cytochrome P-450 reductase transfers single electrons to a remarkable array of both natural and synthetic quinones (38). Recent investigations have shown that the conversion of anthracycline drugs to their respective semiquinones may be supported by microsomal and nuclear preparations from several murine tumor systems (39,40), as well as by cardiac sarcoplasmic reticulum (41). Furthermore, it now appears that cytoplasmic and mitochondrial flavin enzymes distinct from NADPH P-450 reductase are also capable of initiating anthracycline activation (39,42). Thus, free-radical formation could be related to effects that anthracycline drugs have been previously demonstrated to produce in essentially all cellular compartments.

Under aerobic conditions, the unshared electron of the anthracycline semiquinone is donated to molecular oxygen to form superoxide anion (34,37,41). As long as aerobic conditions are maintained, cyclical oxidation and reduction of the anthracycline quinone catalytically promotes the production of superoxide and, by dismutation, H_2O_2 (35,43). In the absence of oxygen, semiquinone formation leads to the reductive cleavage of the anthracycline glycosidic bond and deoxyaglycone formation (36,43). Preliminary evidence suggests that hydroxyl radical is also formed in these microsomal systems by way of the metal-catalyzed Haber–Weiss reaction (37).

Bachur has suggested that nuclear oxidation–reduction cycling of the anthracyclines may damage nucleic acids by a free-radical mechanism that would explain the chemotherapeutic effect of these drugs better than intercalation (36). Support for this suggestion comes from studies showing that oxygen radical metabolites produced by redox cycling of the anthracyclines may be responsible for the strand scission of closed, circular DNA found after its treatment with chemically reduced doxorubicin (44) and for the scission of specifically defined 3′-end-labeled DNA fragments by enzymatically activated drug (45). Membrane peroxidation produced by the doxorubicin redox cycle, as shown by Goodman and Hochstein, could also contribute to antineoplastic cytotoxicity (34). Furthermore, the fragmentation of nuclear DNA by anthracycline analogs that localize and cycle only in the cytoplasmic compartment of experimental tumor cells provides presumptive evidence implicating oxygen radicals in the antitumor activity of anthracycline antibiotics (46). However, it has also been reported that the free-radical scavengers α-tocopherol and N-acetylcysteine to not interfere with the chemotherapeutic activity of doxorubicin against murine tumors (47,48) and that DNA fragmentation may not be the major feature of anthracycline-induced nuclear injury (49). Thus, although enhanced oxygen radical formation clearly occurs in neoplastic cells treated with anthracyclines (39), its contribution to the therapeutic efficacy of these drugs remains incompletely understood.

Whereas the role of oxygen radicals in the antineoplastic activity of the anthracycline antibiotics is as yet uncertain, there is now substantial evidence that anthracycline cardiac toxicity may result from unrestrained, drug-induced, cardiac reactive oxygen metabolism (47,50). In the heart, investigations by Thayer (51) and our own laboratory (41) have shown that electron transfer after treatment with doxorubicin *in vitro* is significantly enhanced and leads to a substantial increase in superoxide anion and hydrogen peroxide formation in cardiac mitochondria and sarcoplasmic reticulum, two major sites of damage from doxorubicin (52). Furthermore, the cytotoxic potential of this cardiac oxygen radical production may be magnified by the limited specific activity of cardiac catalase (51) and the inhibition of cardiac glutathione peroxidase activity produced by treatment with doxorubicin *in vivo* (53). The accumulation of drug-induced reactive oxygen radicals in heart cells may also explain the cardiac lipid membrane peroxidation (47), increased hexose monophosphate shunt activity (54), and depletion of cardiac reduced glutathione pools (55) that have been found after doxorubicin administration. Further support for the theory that anthracycline cardiac toxicity is mediated by reactive oxygen metabolites *in vivo* comes from studies showing that treatment with free-radical scavengers such as α-tocopherol and N-acetylcysteine blocks the acute and chromic pathological changes usually observed after anthracycline treatment in mouse or rabbit heart (47,50,56). Thus, oxygen radical formation appears to play an important, and possibly preventable, role in the etiology of the major dose-limiting side effect of this important class of anticancer chemicals. It should be noted that adriamycin has also been reported to inhibit metmyoglobin reductase activity in the heart. Such an effect might also be related to its cardiotoxicity (57).

MITOMYCIN C

Mitomycin C is an antineoplastic antibiotic isolated from *Streptomyces caespitosus* that is currently used for the palliative treatment of disseminated carcinomas of the breast, stomach, or colon (58). The therapeutic activity of mitomycin C has been related to the presence of three reactive groups in the molecule: an aziridine ring, a carbamate moiety, and a quinone. It has been appreciated for some time that NADPH-mediated reductive activation of mitomycin C is necessary for experimental antitumor activity (58), and until recently the reductive transformation of the drug (via the aziridine and carbamate functions) into a bifunctional molecule capable of DNA alkylation and interstrand cross-linking was considered to explain the antineoplastic action of mitomycin C (58). However, several recent studies have indicated that the cyclical oxidation and reduction of the mitomycin C quinone with subsequent oxygen radical formation may contribute substantially to both the mode of action and the toxicity of the drug (59–61).

It is now clear that mitomycin C, like the anthracyclines, is easily reduced to its semiquinone by microsomal NADPH cytochrome P-450 reductase (62). Under anaerobic conditions the semiquinone radical is relatively stable, producing a characteristic ESR spectrum that has been well characterized by Kalyanaraman and colleagues (63). Aerobically, the mitomycin C semiquinone is very short-lived (63), rapidly donating its unpaired electron to molecular oxygen, forming superoxide anion directly (63,64). The hydrogen peroxide that is also formed under these biological conditions probably results from the dismutation of O_2^- rather than the two-electron reduction of oxygen (64). In the presence of trace metal contamination, this leads to hydroxyl radical formation, which has now been demonstrated by spin trapping in systems utilizing both enzymatically and chemically reduced mitomycin C (63,65).

The biological consequences of mitomycin C-enhanced oxygen radical formation are under active investigation. Lown and co-workers have shown that chemically reduced mitomycin C produces single-strand breaks in closed, circular PM2 phage DNA on exposure to oxygen; this is prevented by superoxide dismutase, catalase, and hydroxyl radical scavengers (65,66). Reduced mitomycin C also inactivates bacteriophage ϕX 174 in the presence of cupric ion by DNA strand scission (67). Furthermore, superoxide dismutase, catalase, and reduced thiols have been found to reduce chromosomal breakage significantly in fibroblasts exposed to mitomycin C (68). Thus, it is possible that drug-induced oxygen radical formation may at least partially explain the therapeutic effect of the drug on tumor cell DNA synthesis as well as the known mutagenic potential of mitomycin C (69). It has also been recognized that treatment with mitomycin C may exacerbate the cardiac toxicity of the anthracycline antitumor agents (70). Enhancement of cardiac oxygen radical metabolism by mitomycin C has been suggested as an explanation for this clinical observation (64).

BLEOMYCIN

The bleomycins comprise a group of water-soluble glycopeptides that are particularly effective in the chemotherapy of certain carcinomas and lymphomas. The investigations of several groups suggest that bleomycin damages cells and inhibits their growth through breakage of DNA. It appears that the antibiotic can bind to DNA without causing major damage but that in the presence of iron, oxygen, and reducing agents strand breakage takes place (71). The nature of the iron-binding ligands in DNA is not yet fully clarified (71). Lown and Sim (73) have suggested that superoxide and hydroxyl radicals may play a role in producing DNA damage. The following scheme has been proposed (74) to account for the radical-dependent degradation of DNA by intercalated bleomycin containing iron:

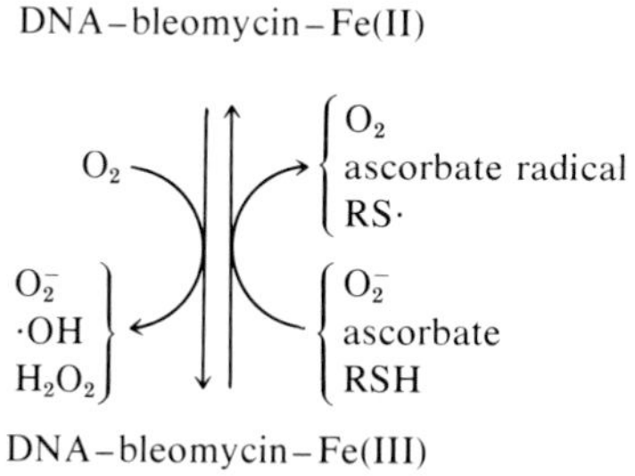

DNA–bleomycin–Fe(II)

DNA–bleomycin–Fe(III)

Implicit in this scheme is the capacity of bleomycin to act as a ferrous oxidase (75) while bound to DNA and cause the reduction of oxygen at the target molecule.

Although the effects of bleomycin that involve iron and oxygen are well documented *in vitro*, there is no good evidence that such reactions take place in cells exposed to the drug. Currently, metal-free bleomycin is used in antineoplastic disease therapy, and the efficacy of bleomycin–Fe as a chemotherapeutic agent has not yet been examined. Thus, the antibiotic must recruit iron from cellular sites. Since the amount of free iron in biological systems is negligible, it remains to be determined whether bleomycin can remove iron from transit pools (transferrin), storage pools (ferritin), or other sequestering molecules (pyrophosphate).

PERSPECTIVES

The effects of quinoid agents, which depend on an interaction with oxygen, are terminated when the quinones are fully reduced and conjugated as esters with sulfate, sugars, and amino acids. In 1963 Hochstein and Ernster observed that dicoumarol inhibited the conjugation of quinones with sulfate (76). Dicoumarol is a potent inhibitor of the enzyme DT diaphorase (77). On the basis of those experiments it was suggested that this unique flavoenzyme might be involved as a quinone reductase in the biological reduction and detoxification of quinones (78). Such a role has been substantiated in experiments with polycyclic hydrocarbons (79) and with the vitamin K derivative menadione (80). Thus, purified preparations of DT diaphorase from liver result, in the presence of NADPH, in the formation of fully reduced menadiol, which is then available for conjugation reactions. On the other hand, preparations of NADPH-cytochrome P-450 reductase, which participate in "one-electron transfer," result in the formation of autoxidizable menadione semiquinone. Apparently only DT diaphorase, because of its unique capacity as a "two-electron transfer" enzyme, can terminate the reaction of quinoid compounds with oxygen by forming more stable hydroquinones. These concepts are diagrammed below. Their general applicability to the actions of quinoid antibiotics in particular tissues and at particular subcellular sites remains to be determined.

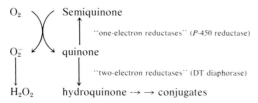

Although our knowledge of autoxidation and detoxification mechanisms is growing rapidly, many large gaps exist in our understanding of drug-induced free-radical toxicity. For example, there is a paucity of information on the stability and the properties of free radicals under physiological conditions. Although DNA is an obvious target in the cytotoxicity of these agents, their effects on other cellular components should not be ignored. It is also not yet clear whether these radicals act directly on sensitive cellular constituents or exert their effects through a secondary event such as lipid peroxidation (81). At least with respect to the mutagenic activity of quinones and diols, the development of new tester strains of *Salmonella typhimurium,* which are sensitive to a variety of radical substances, should prove to be of major import in resolving some of these issues (82).

The past few decades have brought a profound change in our awareness of the role of oxygen in cytotoxic phenomena. It is clear that the years ahead will bring an equal increase in our understanding of the detailed molecular mechanisms involved in the specificity of the chemotherapeutic and cytotoxic actions of radical-generating chemicals.

REFERENCES

1. Totter, J. R. (1980). Spontaneous cancer and its possible relationship to oxygen metabolism. *Proc. Natl. Acad. Sci. U.S.A.* **77**:1763–1767.
2. Hochstein, P. (1981). Nucleotide–iron complexes and lipid peroxidation: mechanisms and biological significance. *Isr. J. Chem.* **21**:52–53.
3. Ciba Foundation Symposium (1979). "Oxygen Free Radicals and Tissue Damage," No. 65. Excerpta Medica, Amsterdam.

4. Misra, H. P., and Fridovich, I. (1972). The univalent reduction of oxygen by reduced flavins and quinones. *J. Biol. Chem.* **247**:188–195.
5. Hochstein, P., Lind, C., and Ernster, L. (1982). In preparation.
6. Fridovich, I. (1974). Superoxide dismutase. *In* "Molecular Mechanisms of Oxygen Activation" (O. Hayaishi, ed.) pp. 453–477. Academic Press, New York.
7. Mills, G. C. (1957). Hemoglobin catabolism. 1. Glutathione peroxidase, an erythrocyte enzyme which protects hemoglobin from oxidative breakdown. *J. Biol. Chem.* **229**:189–197.
8. Cohen, G., and Hochstein, P. (1963). Glutathione peroxidase: The primary agent for the elimination of hydrogen peroxide in erythrocytes. *Biochemistry* **2**:1420–1428.
9. Rotruck, J. T., Pope, A. L., Ganther, H. E., Swanson, A. B., Hateman, D., and Hoekstra, W. G. (1973). Selenium: Biochemical role as a component of glutathione peroxidase. *Science* **179**:588–590.
10. Little, C., and O'Brien, P. J. (1968). An intracellular GSH-peroxidase with a lipid peroxide substrate. *Biochem. Biophys. Res. Commun.* **31**:145–150.
11. Chance, B., Sies, H., and Boveris, A. (1979). Hydroperoxide metabolism in mammalian organs. *Physiol. Rev.* **59**:527–605.
12. Cohen, G., and Hochstein, P. (1963). Glutathone peroxidase: The major pathway of peroxide detoxification of erythrocytes. *Biochemistry* **2**:1420–1428.
13. Cohen, G., and Hochstein, P. (1961). Glucose-6-phosphate dehydrogenase and the detoxification of hydrogen peroxide in human erythrocytes. *Science* **134**:1574–1575.
14. Beutler, E. (1969). Drug-induced hemolytic anemia. *Pharmacol. Rev.* **21**:73–103.
15. Cohen, G., and Hochstein, P. (1964). Generation of hydrogen peroxide in erythrocytes by hemolytic agents. *Biochemistry* **3**:895–900.
16. Mager, J., Chevion, M., and Glaser, G. (1980). Favism. *In* "Toxic Constituents of Plant Foodstuffs" (I. E. Liener, ed.), pp. 265–293. Academic Press, New York.
17. Floyd, R. A. (1981). DNA–Ferrous iron catalyzed hydroxyl free radical formation from hydrogen peroxide. *Biochem. Biophys. Res. Commun.* **99**:1209–1215.
18. Oster, G., and Salgo, M. P. (1977). Copper in mammalian reproduction. *Adv. Pharmacol. Chemother.* **14**:327–409.
19. Hochstein, P., Kumar, K. S., and Forman, S. J. (1980). Lipid peroxidation and the cytotoxicity of copper. *Ann. N.Y. Acad. Sci.* **355**:240–248.
20. Harris, M. N., Medrek, T. J., Golomb, F. M., Gumport, S. L., Postel, A. H., and Wright, J. C. (1965). Chemotherapy with streptonigrin in advanced cancer. *Cancer* **18**:49–57.
21. Laszlo, J., and Hochstein, P., unpublished observations.
22. White, H. L., and White, J. R. (1968). Lethal action and metabolic effects of streptonigrin on *Escherichia coli*. *Mol. Pharmacol.* **4**:549–565.
23. White, J. R., and Dearman, H. (1965). Generation of free radicals from phenazine methosulfate, streptonigrin, and rubiflavin in bacterial suspension. *Proc. Natl. Acad. Sci. U.S.A.* **54**:887–891.
24. Hochstein, P., Laszlo, J., and Miller, M. (1965). A unique, dicoumarol-sensitive, nonphosphorylating oxidation of DPNH and TPNH catalyzed by streptonigrin. *Biochem. Biophys. Res. Commun.* **19**:289–295.
25. Gregory, E. M., and Fridovich, I. (1973). Oxygen toxicity and the superoxide dismutase. *J. Bacteriol.* **114**:1193–1197.
26. White, H. L., and White, J. R. (1966). Interaction of streptonigrin with DNA *in vitro*. *Biochim. Biophys. Acta* **123**:648–651.
27. Cone, R., Hasan, S. K., Lown, J. W., and Morgan, A. R. (1975). The mechanism of the degradation of DNA by streptonigrin. *Can. J. Biochem.* **54**:219–223.

28. Lown, J. W., and Sim, S.-K. (1975). Studies related to antitumor antibiotics. Part VIII. Cleavage of DNA by streptonigrin analogues and the relationship to antineoplastic activity. *Can. J. Biochem.* **54**:446–452.
29. Miller, D. S., Laszlo, J., McCarty, K. S., Guild, W. R., and Hochstein, P. (1967). Mechanism of action of streptonigrin in leukemic cells. *Cancer Res.* **27**:632–638.
30. Carter, S. K. (1975). Adriamycin: A review. *JNCI, J. Natl. Cancer Inst.* **55**:1265–1274.
31. Young, R. C., Ozols, R. F., and Myers, C. E. (1981). The anthracycline antineoplastic drugs. *N. Engl. J. Med.* **305**:139–153.
32. Handa, K., and Sato, S. (1976). Stimulation of microsomal NADPH oxidation by quinone group-containing anticancer chemicals. *Gann* **67**:523–528.
33. Sato, S., Iwaizumi, M., Handa, K., and Tamura, Y. (1977). Electron spin resonance study on the mode of generation of free radicals of daunomycin, adriamycin, and carboquone in NAD(P)H-microsome system. *Gann* **68**:603–608.
34. Goodman, J., and Hochstein, P. (1977). Generation of free radicals and lipid peroxidation by redox cycling of adriamycin and daunomycin. *Biochem. Biophys. Res. Commun.* **77**:797–803.
35. Bachur, N. R., Gordon, S. L., and Gee, M. V. (1977). Anthracycline antibiotic augmentation of microsomal electron transport and free radical formation. *Mol. Pharmacol.* **13**:901–910.
36. Bachur, N. R., Gordon, S. L., Gee, M. V., and Kon, H. (1979). NADPH cytochrome P-450 reductase activation of quinone anticancer agents to free radicals. *Proc. Natl. Acad. Sci. U.S.A.* **76**:954–957.
37. Kalyanaraman, B., Perez-Reyes, E., and Mason, R. P. (1980). Spin-trapping and direct electron spin resonance investigations of the redox metabolism of quinone anticancer drugs. *Biochim. Biophys. Acta* **630**:119–130.
38. Iyanagi, T., and Yamazaki I. (1970). One-electron-transfer reactions in biochemical systems. V. Difference in the mechanism of quinone reduction by the NADH dehydrogenase and the NAD(P)H dehydrogenase (DT-diaphorase). *Biochim. Biophys. Acta* **216**:282–294.
39. Doroshow, J. H. (1981). Effect of doxorubicin on oxygen radical metabolism in Ehrlich ascites tumor cells. *Proc. Am. Assoc. Cancer Res.* **22**:203.
40. Bachur, N. R., Friedman, R. D., and Gee, M. V. (1979). Nuclear catalyzed antibiotic free radical formation. *Proc. Am. Assoc. Cancer Res.* **20**:128.
41. Doroshow, J. H., and Reeves, J. (1981). Daunorubicin-stimulated reactive oxygen metabolism in cardiac sarcosomes. *Biochem. Pharmacol.* **30**:259–262.
42. Pan, S., Pedersen, L., and Bachur, N. R. (1981). Comparative flavoprotein catalysis of anthracycline antibiotic reductive cleavage and oxygen consumption. *Mol. Pharmacol.* **19**:184–186.
43. Komiyama, T., Oki, T., and Inui, T. (1979). A proposed reaction mechanism for the enzymatic reductive cleavage of glycosidic bond in anthracycline antibiotics. *J. Antibiot.* **32**:1219–1222.
44. Lown, J. W., Sim, S., Majumdar, K. C., and Chang, R. (1977). Strand scission of DNA by bound adriamycin and daunorubicin in the presence of reducing agents. *Biochem. Biophys. Res. Commun.* **76**:705–710.
45. Berlin, V., and Haseltine, W. A. (1981). Reduction of adriamycin to a semiquinone-free radical by NADPH cytochrome P-450 reductase produces DNA cleavage in a reaction mediated by molecular oxygen. *J. Biol. Chem.* **256**:4747–4756.
46. Levin, M., Silber, R., Israel, M., Goldfeder, A., Khetarpal, V., and Potmesil, M. (1981). Protein-associated DNA breaks and DNA-protein cross-links caused by DNA nonbinding derivatives of adriamycin in L1210 cells. *Cancer Res.* **41**:1006–1010.

47. Myers, C. E., McGuire, W. P., Liss, R., Ifrim, I., Grotzinger, K., and Young, R. C. (1977). Adriamycin: The role of lipid peroxidation in cardiac toxicity and tumor response. *Science* **197**:165–167.

48. Freeman, R., MacDonald, J. S., Olson, R. D., Boerth, R., Oates, J., and Harbison, R. (1980). Effect of sulfhydryl-containing compounds on the antitumor effects of adriamycin *Toxicol. Appl. Pharmacol.* **54**:168–175.

49. Ross, W., Glaubiger, D., and Kohn, K. (1979). Qualitative and quantitative aspects of intercalator-induced DNA strand breaks. *Biochim. Biophys. Acta* **562**:41–50.

50. Doroshow, J., Locker, G., Ifrim, I., and Myers, C. E. (1981). Prevention of doxorubicin cardiac toxicity in the mouse by *N*-acetylcysteine. *J. Clin. Invest.* **68**:1053–1064.

51. Thayer, W. (1977). Adriamycin stimulated superoxide formation in submitochondrial particles. *Chem.-Biol. Interact.* **19**:265–278.

52. Ferrans, V. (1978). Overview of cardiac pathology in relation to anthracycline cardiotoxicity. *Cancer Treat. Rep.* **62**:955–961.

53. Doroshow, J., Locker, G., and Myers, C. (1980). Enzymatic defenses of the mouse heart against reactive oxygen metabolites: Alterations produced by doxorubicin. *J. Clin. Invest.* **65**:128–135.

54. Burton, G. M., Henderson, C. A., Balcerzak, S. P., and Sagone, A. (1979). Effect of adriamycin on the metabolism of heart slices. *Int. J. Radiat. Oncol. Biol. Phys.* **5**:1287–1289.

55. Wang, Y., Madanat, F., Kimball, J., Gleiser, C., and Ali, M. (1980). Effect of vitamin E against adriamycin-induced toxicity in rabbits. *Cancer Res.* **40**:1022–1027.

56. Van Vleet, J., and Ferrans, V. J. (1980). Evaluation of vitamin E and selenium protection against chronic adriamycin toxicity in rabbits. *Cancer Treat. Rep.* **64**:315–317.

57. Taylor, D., and Hochstein, P. (1978). Inhibition by adriamycin of a metmyoglobin reductase from beef heart. *Biochem. Pharmacol.* **27**:2079–2082.

58. Crooke, S. T., and Bradner, W. T. (1976). Mitomycin C: A review. *Cancer Treat. Rev.* **3**:121–139.

59. Handa, K., and Sato, S. (1976). Stimulation of microsomal NADPH oxidation by quinone group-containing anticancer chemicals. *Gann* **67**:523–528.

60. Tomasz, M. (1976). H_2O_2 generation during the redox cycle of mitomycin C and DNA-bound mitomycin C. *Chem.-Biol. Interact.* **13**:89–97.

61. Bachur, N. R., Gordon, S. L., and Gee, M. V. (1978). A general mechanism for microsomal activation of quinone anticancer agents to free radicals. *Cancer Res.* **38**:1745–1750.

62. Komiyama, T., Oki, T., and Inui, T. (1979). Activation of mitomycin C and quinone drug metabolism by NADPH-cytochrome P-450 reductase. *J. Pharmacobio- Dyn.* **2**:407–410.

63. Kalyanaraman, B., Perez-Reyes, E., and Mason, R. P. (1980). Spin-trapping and direct electron spin resonance investigations of the redox metabolism of quinone anticancer drugs. *Biochim. Biophys. Acta* **630**:119–130.

64. Doroshow, J. (1981). Mitomycin C-enhanced superoxide and hydrogen peroxide formation in rat heart. *J. Pharmacol. Exp. Ther.* **218**:206–211.

65. Lown, J., Sim, S., and Chan, H. (1978). Hydroxyl radical production by free and DNA-bound aminoquinone antibiotics and its role in DNA degradation. Electron spin resonance detection of hydroxyl radicals by spin-trapping. *Can. J. Biochem.* **56**:1042–1047.

66. Lown, J., Begleiter, A., Johnson, D., and Morgan, A. R. (1976). Studies related to antitumor antibiotics. Part V. Reactions of mitomycin C with DNA examined by ethidium fluorescence assay. *Can. J. Biochem.* **54**:110–119.

67. Ueda, K., Morita, J., Yamashita, K., and Komano, T. (1980). Inactivation of bacterio-

phage ϕX 174 by mitomycin C in the presence of sodium hydrosulfite and cupric ions. *Chem.-Biol. Interact.* **29:**145–158.

68. Raj, A., and Heddle, J. (1980). The effect of superoxide dismutase, catalase, and L-cysteine on spontaneous and on mitomycin C induced chromosomal breakage in Fanconi's anemia and normal fibroblasts as measured by the micronucleus method. *Mutat. Res.* **78:**59–66.

69. Seino, Y., Nagao, M., Yahagi, T., Hoshi, A., Kawachi, T., and Sugimura, T. (1978). Mutagenicity of several classes of antitumor agents to *Salmonella typhimurium* TA 98, TA 100, and TA 92. *Cancer Res.* **38:**2148–2156.

70. Buzdar, A., Legha, S., Toshima, C. K., Hortobagyi, G., Yap, H., Krutchik, A., Luna, M., and Blumenschein, G. (1978). Adriamycin and mitomycin C: Possible synergistic cardiotoxicity. *Cancer Treat. Rep.* **62:**1005–1008.

71. Sausville, E. A., Peisach, J., and Horwitz, S. B. (1978). Effect of chelating agents and metal ions on the degradation of DNA by bleomycin. *Biochemistry* **17:**2740–2245.

72. Takita, T., Muraoka, Y., Nakatani, T., Fujii, A., Iitaka, Y., and Umezewa, H. (1978). Chemistry of bleomycin. XIX. Revised structures of bleomycin and phlemoycin. *J. Antibiot.* **31:**801–884.

73. Lown, J. W., and Sim, S.-K. (1977). The mechanism of the bleomycin-induced cleavage of DNA. *Biochem. Biophys. Res. Commun.* **77:**1150–1157.

74. Sausville, E. A., and Horwitz, S. B. (1979). A mechanism for the degradation of DNA by bleomycin. *In* "Effects of Drugs on the Cell Nucleus" (H. Busch, S. T. Crooke, and Y. Daskal, eds.), pp. 181–205. Academic Press, New York.

75. Caspary, W. J., Niziak, C., Lanzo, D. A., Friedman, R., and Bachur, N. R. (1979). Bleomycin A$_2$: A ferrous oxidase. *Mol. Pharmacol.* **16:**256–260.

76. Hochstein, P., and Ernster, L., unpublished observations.

77. Ernster, L., Danielson, L., and Ljunggren, M. (1962). DT diaphorase. 1. Purification from the soluble fraction of rat liver cytoplasm and properties. *Biochim. Biophys. Acta* **58:**171–188.

78. Ernster, L. (1967). DT diaphorase. *In* "Methods in Enzymology" (R. W. Estabrook and M. E. Pullman, eds.), Vol. 10, pp. 309–317. Academic Press, New York.

79. Lind, C., Vadi, H., and Ernster, L. (1978). Metabolism of benzo[*a*]pyrene-3,6-quinone and 3-hydroxybenzo[*a*]pyrene in liver microsomes from 3-methylcholanthrene-treated rats. A possible role of DT diaphorase in the formation of glucuromyl conjugates. *Arch. Biochem. Biophys.* **190:**97–108.

80. Lind, C., Hochstein, P., and Ernster, L. (1982). DT diaphorase: Properties, reaction mechanism, metabolic function. *In* "Oxidases and Related Redox Systems" (T. E. King, H. S. Hason, and M. Morrison, eds.), p. 313–323. Pergamon, Oxford.

81. Hochstein, P., and Jain, S. K. (1981). Association of lipid peroxidation and polymerization of membrane proteins with red cell aging. *Fed. Proc., Fed. Am. Soc. Exp. Biol.* **40:**183–188.

82. Ames, B. N., Hollstein, M. C. and Cathcart, R. (1982). Lipid peroxidation and oxidative damage to DNA. *In* "Lipid Peroxides in Biology and Medicine" (S. Yagi, ed.). Academic Press, New York (in press).

Chapter **16**

Oxygen Free Radicals and the Diabetogenic Action of Alloxan

LAWRENCE J. FISCHER AND ANDREW
W. HARMAN

INTRODUCTION

Alloxan is a cyclic urea analog that produces irreversible damage to the insulin-producing β-cells of the pancreas. A single dose of alloxan administered to most laboratory animal species produces a permanent hyperglycemia. This diabetic state is due to the necrosis of insulin-producing cells, which occurs within 4–6 hr of the alloxan administration. The initial cytotoxic event, however, occurs within 5 min of the injection. At doses that produce necrosis of β-cells and permanent hyperglycemia, there appears to be little damage to other cell types in the pancreas or to cells in other tissues. Alloxan, therefore, is an example of a chemical with a cell-selective toxic action, and this property has been exploited by diabetes researchers for nearly 40 years. A number of reviews of the diabetic action of alloxan are available (1,2).

In spite of intense study, the mechanism of alloxan-induced necrosis in pancreatic β-cells has remained obscure. Recently, however, through work in this and other laboratories an understanding of the mechanism by which alloxan damages cells is beginning to emerge. The purpose of this chapter is to review the pertinent data that imply a role for reactive, free-radical forms of oxygen in the cytotoxic action of alloxan.

261

PATHOLOGY OF OXYGEN
Copyright © 1982 by Academic Press, Inc.
All rights of reproduction in any form reserved.
ISBN 0-12-068620-1

ORIGIN OF THE OXYGEN FREE-RADICAL
HYPOTHESIS FOR ALLOXAN

Cohen and Heikkila reported that dialuric acid, a reduced form of alloxan, upon autoxidation produced superoxide anion (O_2^-), hydrogen peroxide (H_2O_2), and hydroxyl free radical ($\cdot OH$) (3). These potentially toxic species of oxygen, generated *in vitro,* were detected by the usual indirect methods employing superoxide dismutase, catalase, and hydroxyl radical scavengers. It was later shown by the same authors that short-chain alcohols such as ethanol and *n*-butanol, when given to mice before a dose of alloxan, could protect the animals from alloxan-induced diabetes (4). Because these alcohols were known to be scavengers of hydroxyl free radicals, it was suggested that alloxan diabetes may involve the production of $\cdot OH$. It was proposed that alloxan was reduced to dialuric acid *in vivo* and that autoxidation of the latter substance resulted in the generation of O_2^- and ultimately a cytotoxic amount of $\cdot OH$. A variety of chemical substances purported to be hydroxyl radical scavengers, when given before alloxan, have been found to eliminate the appearance of permanent hyperglycemia. Examples of these substances are thiourea (4), N,N'-dimethylurea (5), and dimethylsulfoxide (6). These results were used as additional support for a cytotoxic mechanism based on the generation of $\cdot OH$.

STUDIES USING ISOLATED
PANCREATIC ISLETS

Experiments in which pretreatment with hydroxyl radical scavengers *in vivo* is used in an attempt to protect animals from alloxan can yield results that are difficult to interpret. A variety of substances protect animals from alloxan diabetes (1,2), and many of these are not known to be hydroxyl radical scavengers. In addition, some radical scavengers (e.g., *n*-butanol) protect mice from alloxan diabetes by producing hyperglycemia in the test animal at the time of alloxan injection (7). The production of hyperglycemia has long been recognized as a method of protecting animals from alloxan diabetes (8). In an effort to reduce the variables inherent in *in vivo* systems, we and others have utilized isolated pancreatic islets to investigate whether oxygen free radicals are involved in the action of alloxan.

Exposure of isolated pancreatic islets to alloxan for a short period (e.g., 5 min) produces functional defects that can be assessed relatively easily. Pancreatic islets, obtained from rats or mice by collagenase digestion techniques and exposed to alloxan, show a deficiency in glucose-stimulated insulin secretion (9), glucose oxidation (10), insulin biosynthesis (11), rubidium uptake, and dye exclusion (12). These effects produced by alloxan *in vitro* are thought to be produced by a mechanism similar to that producing the cytotoxic effects of alloxan *in vivo*. Evidence for this similarity in mechanisms includes data showing that a series of hexoses exhibit the same relative capacity to protect from the effects of alloxan when used *in vivo* or *in vitro* (9,11).

Primarily on the basis of the work of Cohen and Heikkila (3,4), a scheme was proposed for the generation of ·OH from alloxan (Fig. 1). This scheme included the facile reduction of alloxan to dialuric acid in the biological milieu and the autoxidation of dialuric acid with the commensurate production of O_2^-. The "iron-catalyzed Haber–Weiss reaction" or "modified Fenton reaction" (13,14) was presumed to be responsible for the production of ·OH. It was postulated that the generation of ·OH would be interrupted by the use of superoxide dismutase, catalase, or the iron chelator diethylenetriaminepentaacetic acid (DETAPAC). Each of these substances would presumably reduce the amount of a different component necessary for the production of ·OH, as shown in Fig. 1. The presence of superoxide dismutase, catalase, or DETAPAC in the pancreatic islet system to which alloxan was to be added should reduce the deleterious effects in insulin-secreting cells caused by the generation of ·OH. In addition, scavengers of ·OH such as N,N'-dimethylurea would be expected to protect pancreatic islets from alloxan.

The capacity of various substances to protect pancreatic β-cells from the effects of alloxan was investigated using islets obtained from rats by the collagenase digestion technique (15). Isolated islets were preincubated for 10 min at 37°C with or without potential protective substances, and

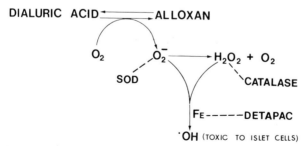

Fig. 1. A simplified scheme for the production of toxic ·OH from alloxan. Sites of probable action for inhibitors of ·OH formation are shown by the dashed lines. In addition to superoxide dismutase, catalase, and DETAPAC, scavengers of ·OH would be expected to reduce the toxicity of alloxan. From Fischer and Hamburger (12), reproduced with permission from the American Diabetes Association, Inc.

this was followed by a 5-min exposure to alloxan. The alloxan-containing solution was removed and the islets placed in a medium with a high concentration of glucose (3 mg/ml) to stimulate insulin release. The amount of insulin released into the medium over a 45-min period was measured by radioimmunoassay.

A summary of the results of these experiments is shown in Fig. 2. A 5-min exposure of pancreatic islets to 0.15 mg/ml of alloxan caused a 70% decrease in subsequent glucose-stimulated insulin release. The presence of superoxide dismutase, catalase, DETAPAC, and the hydroxyl radical scavenger dimethylurea protected the islets from this effect of alloxan. None of the protective treatments, when used without alloxan, had an effect on glucose-stimulated insulin release. In addition, heat inactivation of superoxide dismutase and catalase and prior chelation of iron by DETAPAC eliminated their protective effects [data presented elsewhere (12)]. It was apparent from these results that the protective capacity of superoxide dismutase and catalase involved enzymatic action and, in the case of DETAPAC, chelating capacity.

Not all scavengers of ·OH were found to be effective in protecting islets

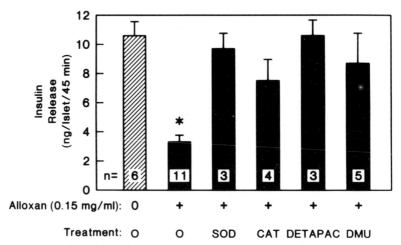

Fig. 2. Protection of isolated islets from alloxan provided by treatment with 1000 U/ml superoxide dismutase (SOD), 50 μg/ml catalase (CAT), 1 mM DETAPAC, and 40 mM dimethylurea (DMU). A plus sign indicates that the alloxan was present during a 5-min exposure period, whereas a zero indicates the absence of alloxan. The protective agents were absent (0) or present for 10 min before and during the alloxan exposure period. After alloxan exposure, the function of pancreatic islets was assessed by measuring glucose-stimulated insulin release over a 45-min period. Results were compiled from Fischer and Hamburger (12,16), with permission from the American Diabetes Association, Inc.

from the effects of alloxan. In our hands, thiourea, mannitol, and n-butanol were not effective, but dimethylurea did protect islets, as shown by the data in Fig. 2. Grankvist *et al.* (17) found that dimethyl sulfoxide, benzoate, and mannitol, all scavengers of ·OH, exhibited some protection from the effects of alloxan on isolated pancreatic islets. The difficulty we had in demonstrating the effectiveness of hydroxyl radical scavengers in the biological system was not unexpected. The extremely reactive ·OH can be expected to interact immediately after its formation with endogenous substances. Exogenously administered scavengers of ·OH apparently must be present in high concentration to scavenge the reactive radicals, and this high concentration is often incompatible with the normal function of living systems. To be effective, the scavenger must not alter the living system and it must be extremely susceptible to radical attack. This combination of characteristics makes it difficult to find biologically effective radical scavengers.

Independent from our work, Grankvist *et al.* have demonstrated that superoxide dismutase, catalase, DETAPAC, and some hydroxyl radical scavengers can protect isolated mouse pancreatic islets from the effects of alloxan exposure (17). The measures of islet cell function used in their experiments were the capacity of islets to accumulate Rb^+ and to exclude trypan blue. Their results led these authors to conclude, as we did, that ·OH produced by an iron-catalyzed reaction involving H_2O_2 and O_2^- is the toxic agent in the isolated islet preparation exposed to alloxan.

It seemed reasonable to suggest that, if alloxan damaged isolated islets through a hydroxyl free-radical mechanism, any agent that generated these toxic radicals should cause alloxan-like effects *in vitro*. The autoxidation of dihydroxyfumarate is known to generate O_2^- and ultimately ·OH (18). We employed dihydroxyfumarate in a series of experiments identical to those we had conducted with alloxan (19). Exposure of isolated pancreatic islets to various concentrations of dihydroxyfumarate for 5 min produced a concentration-dependent reduction in subsequent glucose-stimulated insulin release. The presence of superoxide dismutase, catalase, DETAPAC, and dimethylurea during the exposure period protected the islets from the deleterious effects caused by the production of ·OH (Fig. 3). The controls used in these experiments (not shown here) indicated that the autoxidation process was necessary to inhibit the deleterious effects of dihydroxyfumarate and that the protective effects of superoxide dismutase, catalase, and DETAPAC were dependent on their enzymatic or chelating capacity. The results of these experiments were identical to those observed with alloxan and lend support to the concept that alloxan produces damage to the insulin-secreting cells of the pancreas through the production of ·OH.

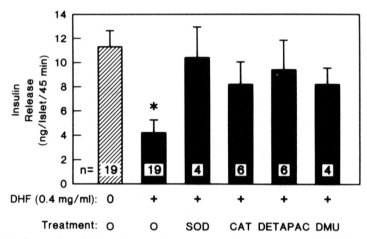

Fig. 3. Protection of isolated pancreatic islets from dihydroxyfumarate (DHF) by treatment with 1000 U/ml superoxide dismutase (SOD), 50 μg/ml catalase (CAT), 1 mM DETAPAC, and 40 mM dimethylurea (DMU). A plus sign indicates that dihydroxyfumarate was present during a 5-min exposure period, whereas a zero indicates its absence. The protective agents were absent (0) or present for 10 min before and during the dihydroxyfumarate exposure period. After dihydroxyfumarate exposure, the function of pancreatic islets was assessed by measuring glucose-stimulated insulin release over a 45-min period. Results were compiled from Fischer and Hamburger (16,19).

SPECIFICITY IN THE ACTION OF ALLOXAN

The action of alloxan *in vivo* exhibits a high degree of cellular specificity. Doses of alloxan that produce a diabetic state in animals through the destruction of insulin-producing pancreatic β-cells cause little or no damage in other tissues (20). Exposure of isolated pancreatic islets to alloxan produces functional impairment of β-cells, but higher concentrations of alloxan *in vitro* are needed to produce a reduction in glucagon release from α-cells (21). The reason for the greater sensitivity of the pancreatic β-cell to the effects of alloxan is not known.

Cell-Specific Accumulation

A mechanism of action for alloxan based on the generation of ·OH in the extracellular space would not be expected to produce toxicity that is highly specific for a single type of cell, i.e., the pancreatic β-cell. Specificity would result, however, if alloxan and/or its toxic products were concentrated at the plasma membrane of, or within, β-cells. Whether alloxan and its degradation products are concentrated in β-cells is unknown because high-resolution autoradiographic or immunohistological studies to localize alloxan *within* the pancreatic islet have not been performed. However, some studies have been performed in an attempt to determine the localization of alloxan in various tissues. There is some evidence that [^{14}C]alloxan is concentrated in the tissue of the endocrine pancreas relative to other tissues (22). Other studies have shown that alloxan concentrations in relatively nonsusceptible tissues such as kidney and liver were higher than in the whole pancreas (23,24). A study of uptake of [^{14}C]alloxan into pancreatic islets isolated from rats showed that alloxan freely entered the endocrine cells (25). Evidence available at this time indicates that alloxan can enter pancreatic islet cells, and this raises the possibility that toxic oxygen free radicals are generated within the insulin-secreting cell.

Endogenous Protective Substances

Another possible reason for the high susceptibility of pancreatic β-cells to the effects of alloxan is that these cells may not have adequate amounts of endogenous protective substances. A relative lack of superoxide dismutase, catalase, glutathione peroxidase, or hydroxyl radical scavengers in β-cells could result in a higher amount of toxic $\cdot$OH being present in those cells as a consequence of the autoxidation of dialuric acid. We have conducted a limited number of experiments to compare the superoxide dismutase and catalase activities in whole pancreas and in isolated pancreatic islets. Enzyme activity in whole pancreas should primarily reflect activity in nonsusceptible acinar (exocrine) cells, whereas isolated islets represent cells of the endocrine pancreas, the majority of which are β-cells. The results in Table I show that catalase activity is not significantly different in whole pancreas and in isolated islets. In contrast, superoxide dismutase activity is significantly higher in endocrine tissue than in whole pancreas. This difference in superoxide dismutase activity between endocrine and exocrine tissue has also been observed by Crouch *et al.* (26). Exposure of isolated pancreatic islets to 0.15 mg/ml alloxan, under conditions that damage islet cell function (12), causes no change in the activity of the enzymes (Table I). This indicates that alloxan exposure does not reduce the activity of superoxide dismutase and catalase within islets even though the insulin secretory and other functions of the tissue have been altered.

Crouch *et al.* (26) have reported that alloxan is capable of inhibiting superoxide dismutase activity after the enzyme has been extracted from

TABLE I

Activity of Superoxide Dismutase and Catalase in Whole Pancreas and Isolated Pancreatic Islets[a]

Preparation	Catalase (units/mg protein)	Superoxide dismutase (units/mg protein)
Whole pancreas[b]	40.7 ± 0.4	10.6 ± 1.7
	($n = 6$)	($n = 3$)
Isolated pancreatic islets[c]	27.9 ± 11.4	67.8 ± 16.5
	($n = 7$)	($n = 3$)
Isolated pancreatic islets treated with alloxan[d]	26.9 ± 3.2	76.4 ± 8.2
	($n = 4$)	($n = 3$)

[a] Activity of superoxide dismutase was measured using the method of McCord and Fridovich (27), and catalase activity by the assay of del Rio *et al.* (28). Protein was measured by the Bradford assay (BioRad, Richmond, California) using bovine serum albumin as a standard.

[b] Pancreas tissue was homogenized in 0.1 M phosphate buffer, pH 7.4, containing a protease inhibitor (phenylmethylsulfonyl fluoride, 0.1 mM). The homogenate was sonicated at 5°C (Sonifer Cell Disrupter-Ultrasonics) and centrifuged (2800 g, 10 min, 4°C) to pellet tissue. The supernatant was assayed for enzyme activity.

[c] Rat pancreatic islets were isolated by collagenase digestion (15). About 400 islets were isolated, the cells disrupted by sonication, the tissue pelleted by centrifugation, and the supernatant assayed for enzyme activity.

[d] Isolated pancreatic islets (400) were exposed to 0.15 mg/ml of alloxan for 5 min as described previously (12). The islets were then treated as described above for measurement of catalase and superoxide dismutase activity.

pancreatic islets. In the same study, it was shown that SOD activity in erythrocytes was reduced at 24 hr, but not at 3 hr after a dose of alloxan was given to rats. It is not clear that these results, which suggest that alloxan can inhibit superoxide dismutase activity, relate to the action of alloxan in pancreatic islets. A reduction of enzyme activity due to high concentrations (0.04 M) of alloxan in a broken cell preparation could be expected, but whether alloxan or its products can reach SOD in similar concentrations in intact cells remains to be demonstrated. The 24-hr delay in the action of alloxan in erythrocytes suggests that the observed reduction in superoxide dismutase activity may be a consequence of alloxan-induced toxicity and not part of the initial toxic event. This seems likely because the cytotoxic action of alloxan occurs within minutes, not hours, after the exposure of cells to the agent.

To summarize the results of the limited number of experiments on the role of superoxide dismutase or catalase in the cell specific action of alloxan, it appears that these protective enzymes are not particularly low in isolated pancreatic islets compared to the whole pancreas or other organs. It is possible, however, that the β-cells of the pancreatic islets contain a very low amount of protective enzymes relative to other pancreatic endocrine cells. Immunocytochemical studies must be conducted to localize the enzymes within the pancreatic islet. An ability of alloxan to markedly inhibit the activity of protective enzymes only within the susceptible β-cells of the endocrine pancreas has not been demonstrated to date. Until that is accomplished, an explanation for the cell-specific action based on enzyme inhibition cannot be accepted.

Finally, a consideration of endogenous protective substances in cells must include reduced glutathione (GSH). This substance is present in pancreatic islets (29), but its concentration in β-cells relative to nonsusceptible pancreatic endocrine cells is not known. Low concentrations of GSH could make the β-cell more vulnerable to oxidative attack from the free-radical species of oxygen that result from alloxan exposure. Another relevant fact is that alloxan reacts with GSH and other thiol-containing compounds (30). It is not known whether alloxan reduces GSH levels in pancreatic β-cells, but we have reported that exposure of isolated hepatocytes to alloxan produces a depletion of GSH and subsequent cytotoxicity (31). The entrance of alloxan into the β-cell, therefore, may also deplete GSH. It is necessary to investigate the role of GSH in β-cells exposed to alloxan along with the roles played by other endongenous substances that have been shown to interfere with the islet cell toxicity of this diabetogenic compound.

Sugars and Protection from Alloxan-Induced Cellular Damage

Alloxan may selectively damage pancreatic β-cells because they contain a unique functional or structural system that makes them susceptible to damage. Because the β-cell responds to glucose with insulin release and because glucose can protect β-cells from alloxan-induced damage, it has been postulated that alloxan may act near a specific glucose receptor that is involved in insulin secretion (32). A glucose receptor unique to the β-cell has not been found, but the structural requirements for glucose protection from alloxan is consistent with the existence of such a receptor. For example, D-glucose and 3-O-methylglucose are protective, but D-galactose and D-fructose have little protective capacity (9). Mannoheptulose, an antagonist of glucose transport and metabolism, is capable of eliminating the protective effect of glucose (32). In general, hexoses that are potent in eliciting insulin release are more effective in protecting β-cells from alloxan.

The well-known capacity of D-glucose to protect pancreatic islets from alloxan coupled with knowledge that ·OH may be involved in alloxan action prompted us to determine whether D-glucose could protect islets from free radicals produced by sources other than alloxan. Autoxidizing dihydroxyfumarate was used as a source of O_2^- and ·OH in an isolated pancreatic islet system as described above. It was found that the presence of D-glucose in high concentration (5 mg/ml) protected isolated islets from the insulin inhibitory effects normally produced by dihydroxyfumarate exposure (19). In the same series of experiments it was found that D-galactose was ineffective in protecting β-cells. These results are identical to those found using alloxan (9) and suggest the dihydroxyfumarate and alloxan damage islets via similar mechanisms. These results also suggest that glucose may not protect pancreatic islets from alloxan through a receptor-based mechanism. It seems unlikely, because of structural dissimilarities, that alloxan and dihydroxyfumarate would attack the β-cell at the same site, presumably at or near a glucose receptor. It seems more likely that each of these substances can damage pancreatic islets through the generation of free-radical forms of oxygen and that the presence of a high glucose concentration in some way alters the toxic process.

A mechanism for alloxan cytotoxicity based solely on the generation of toxic free-radical species of oxygen should allow damage to any type of cell that has been isolated and exposed to an adequate concentration of alloxan. In addition, if glucose can protect pancreatic β-cells from alloxan-induced injury through a process that is not unique to those cells, then the hexose should protect any cell type. In our most recent studies with alloxan, we have studied the susceptibility of freshly isolated rat hepatocytes to alloxan-induced cytotoxicity and the capacity of D-glucose to protect those cells. Hepatocyte preparations were chosen for these experiments because they consist mainly of a single cell type, parenchymal cells, and because a high yield of viable cells can be readily obtained. In addition, indices of hepatocyte damage are well known (33). Although alloxan has not been reported to cause liver damage *in vivo*, we expected that damage to isolated hepatocytes would occur at sufficiently high concentrations of alloxan.

Freshly isolated rat hepatocytes were exposed to various concentrations of alloxan, and the leakage of intracellular components (lactate dehydrogenase and K^+) was measured as an index of cell damage. In addition, the glutathione content of the cells was measured because loss of this peptide can result in, or act as a signal for, cell damage (34). The data shown in Fig. 4 are typical of the results we have obtained from hepatocytes incubated with alloxan. There is a rapid, concentration-dependent drop in cellular glutathione followed by a decrease in intracellular K^+ and

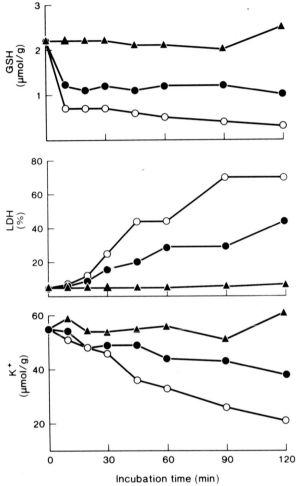

Fig. 4. Damage to freshly isolated rat hepatocytes caused by incubation of the cells with various concentrations of alloxan. Alloxan was added to produce initial concentrations of 0 mM (▲), 3.5 mM (●), and 7.0 mM (○). The time course for changes in glutathione and potassium content per gram wet weight of tissue and the percentage leakage of lactate dehydrogenase (LDH) from cells were followed for 120 min.

and increase in the leakage of lactate dehydrogenase. From these data it is apparent that alloxan concentrations of 3.5 mM and above can produce damage to hepatocytes, causing the plasma membrane to become permeable to intracellular components. These concentrations of alloxan are about five times greater than those needed to produce functional damage to pancreatic endocrine cells. Various substances are being tested for their capacity to protect hepatocytes from damage caused by alloxan exposure. The results in Table II show that D-glucose and D-mannitol can protect hepatocytes from alloxan. L-Glucose, however, is not protective.

It appears that hepatocytes, like pancreatic β-cells, are susceptible to injury caused by exposure to alloxan. Studies are continuing to characterize this damage and to examine whether various agents that protect the pancreatic islet system can also protect hepatocytes. At this time we are not certain whether a hydroxyl radical mechanism is responsible for alloxan-induced injury to hepatocytes. However, it seems likely that these radicals are involved because of their documented production in oxygenated biological systems containing alloxan (4). The protection provided by mannitol, a scavenger of ·OH, also supports this mechanism for a cytotoxic action of alloxan in hepatocytes. A similar mechanism for alloxan action in hepatocytes and pancreatic β-cells is suggested by the capacity of D-glucose but not L-glucose to protect cells. The protective effect of glucose in hepatocytes does not support a mechanism for glucose protection of pancreatic β-cells that involves a specialized glucose receptor unique to the β-cell. D-Glucose may act as a radical scavenger in this system, but this remains to be documented. At this time the mechanism by

TABLE II

Protection of Hepatocytes by Sugars from Alloxan-Induced Leakage of Lactate Dehydrogenase[a]

Treatment	Lactate dehydrogenase (% leakage)[b]
Alloxan (control)	31 ± 6
D-Glucose + alloxan	15 ± 1[c]
L-Glucose + alloxan	31 ± 8
D-Mannitol + alloxan	13 ± 1[c]

[a] Isolated hepatocytes were preincubated with the sugar (100 mM) for 10 min at 37°C before the addition of alloxan to produce a concentration of 7 mM. Further incubation was carried out for 60 min, after which time lactate dehydrogenase (LDH) activity in the media and in the cells was determined.

[b] Data are expressed as mean $\pm$ SE for four different experiments. Percent leakage is the fraction of total LDH activity that resides in the cell-free media after incubation of hepatocytes with alloxan.

[c] Significantly different from alloxan alone (control).

which D-glucose protects cells from alloxan remains obscure. A clearer picture of the mode of protection provided by D-glucose may emerge when the results of testing a large variety of hexoses in the hepatocyte and pancreatic islet systems can be compared.

CONCLUSIONS

There is evidence to support the hypothesis that free-radical species of oxygen are involved in the damage produced by alloxan in insulin-secreting cells of the pancreas. Results from studies *in vivo* and *in vitro* point to the very reactive ·OH as the ultimate toxic substance when cells are exposed to alloxan or its reduction product dialuric acid. The subcellular site of attack of these radicals is not clear. When cells are exposed to solutions containing alloxan, it seems likely that ·OH is produced extracellularly and that plasma membrane damage can result. The protection provided by superoxide dismutase, catalase, and DETAPAC in *in vitro* systems probably occurs because of a reduction in the formation of oxygen free radicals in the extracellular space. This is suggested because these protective substances probably do not readily enter cells. Because alloxan can enter pancreatic islet cells, it is also possible that O_2^- and ·OH can be generated inside the cell. More studies directed toward answering the questions surrounding the site of action of alloxan-generated oxygen free radicals are necessary.

An important part of the mechanism by which alloxan damages insulin-producing cells remains to be elucidated because the reasons for the cell-selective action of alloxan *in vivo* are not known. If alloxan is not concentrated at or within the β-cells, these cells must contain unique amounts of a substance or substances that can account for their susceptibility. It is not clear whether alloxan is concentrated in β-cells relative to other cells in the body. Even if alloxan were concentrated in these cells, the difficult question of whether this accumulation results in a greater production of toxic free radicals would remain unanswered. A unique feature of the β-cell is its capacity to produce insulin, and more attention should be given to a possible link between insulin production and alloxan toxicity. The stimulation of insulin secretion by glucose via a specialized receptor that is vulnerable to alloxan has been considered, but we have provided some evidence throwing doubt on this mechanism. More data are needed to implicate a glucose and/or alloxan receptor in the mechanism for alloxan cytotoxicity. Finally, we can speculate that there may be as yet unrecognized processes occurring within the β-cell that are responsible for its susceptibility. It is also possible that unchanged alloxan acts in concert with oxygen free radicals generated from the autoxidation of dialuric acid to produce damage to β-cells. The complexity of the mechanism for alloxan provides a great challenge and an important opportunity to understand how chemicals can exhibit cell-specific damage through a mechanism involving free-radical species of oxygen.

ACKNOWLEDGMENT

Research on alloxan in this laboratory was supported by USPHS, NIH Grant GM-12675.

REFERENCES

1. Rerup, C. C. (1970). Drugs producing diabetes through damage of the insulin secreting cells. *Pharmacol. Rev.* **22:**485–517.
2. Fischer, L. J., and Rickert, D. E. (1975) Pancreatic islet-cell toxicity. *CRC Crit. Rev. Toxicol.* **3:**231–263.
3. Cohen, G., and Heikkila, R. E. (1974). The generation of hydrogen peroxide, superoxide radical and hydroxyl radical by 6-hydroxydopamine, dialuric acid and related cytotoxic agents. *J. Biol. Chem.* **249:**2447–2452.
4. Heikkila, R. E., Winston, B., and Cohen, G. (1976). Alloxan-induced diabetes—evidence for hydroxyl radical as a cytotoxic intermediate. *Biochem. Pharmacol.* **25:**1085–1092.
5. Heikkila, R. E., and Cabbat, F. (1978). Protection against alloxan-induced diabetes in mice by the hydroxyl radical scavenger dimethylurea. *Eur. J. Pharmacol.* **52:**57–60.
6. Heikkila, R. E. (1977). The prevention of alloxan-induced diabetes by dimethylsulfoxide. *Eur. J. Pharmacol.* **44:**191–193.
7. Schauberger, C. W., Thies, R. L., and Fischer, L. J. (1977). Mechanism of protection from alloxan diabetes provided by *n*-butanol. *J. Pharmacol. Exp. Ther.* **201:**450–455.
8. Bhattacharya, G. (1954). On the protection against alloxan diabetes by hexoses. *Science* **120:**841–843.
9. Tomita, T., Lacy, P. E., Matchinsky, F. M., and McDaniel, M. L. (1974). Effect of alloxan on insulin secretion in isolated rat islets perifused *in vitro*. *Diabetes* **23:**517–524.
10. Borg, L. A. H., Eide, S. J., Andersson, A., and Hellerström, C. (1979). Effects *in vitro* of alloxan on glucose metabolism of mouse pancreatic B-cells. *Biochem. J.* **182:**797–802.
11. Niki, A., Niki, H., Miwa, I., and Lin, B. (1976). Interaction of alloxan and anomers of D-glucose on glucose-induced insulin secretion and biosynthesis *in vitro*. *Diabetes* **25:**574–579.
12. Fischer, L. J., and Hamburger, S. A. (1980). Inhibition of alloxan action in isolated pancreatic islets by superoxide dismutase, catalase and a metal chelator. *Diabetes* **29:**213–216.
13. Czapski, G., and Ilan, Y. (1978). On the generation of the hydroxylation agent from superoxide radical. Can the Haber–Weiss reaction be the source of ˙OH radicals. *Photochem. Photobiol.* **28:**651–653.

14. Borg, D. C., Schaich, K. M., Elmore, J. J., and Bell, J. A. (1978) Cytotoxic reactions of free radical species of oxygen. *Photochem. Photobiol.* **28:**887–907.
15. Lacy, P. E., and Kostionovsky, M. (1967). Method for the isolation of intact islets of Langerhans from the rat pancreas. *Diabetes* **16:**35–39.
16. Fischer, L. J., and Hamburger, S. A. (1980). Dimethylurea: A radical scavenger that protects isoslated pancreatic islets from the effects of alloxan and dihydroxyfumarate exposure. *Life Sci.* **26:**1405–1409.
17. Grankvist, K., Marklund, S., Sehlin, J., and Täljedal, I. (1979). Superoxide dismutase, catalase and scavengers of hydroxyl radical protect against the toxic action of alloxan on pancreatic islet cells *in vitro. Biochem. J.* **182:**17–25.
18. Halliwell, B. (1977). Generation of hydrogen peroxide, superoxide and hydroxyl radicals during the oxidation of dihydroxyfumarate by peroxidase. *Biochem. J.* **163:**441–448.
19. Fischer, L. J., and Hamburger, S. A. (1981). Impaired insulin release after exposure of pancreatic islets to dihydroxyfumarate. *Endocrinology* **108:**2331–2335.
20. Dunn, J. J., and McLetchie, N. G. B. (1943). Experimental alloxan diabetes in the rat. *Lancet* **2:**384–387.
21. Pagliara, A. S., Stillings, S. N., Zawalich, W. S., Williams, B. S., and Matchinsky, F. M. (1977). Glucose and 3-O-methylglucose protection against alloxan poisoning of pancreatic alpha and beta cells. *Diabetes* **26:**973–979.
22. Hammarström, L., and Ullberg, S. (1966). Specific uptake of labelled alloxan in the pancreatic islets. *Nature (London)* **212:**708–709.
23. Landau, B. R., and Renold, A. E. (1954). The distribution of alloxan in the rat. *Diabetes* **3:**47–50.
24. Janes, R. G., and Winnick, T. (1953). Distribution of C^{14}-labeled alloxan in the tissues of the rat and its mode of elimination. *Proc. Soc. Exp. Biol. Med.* **81:**226–229.
25. Weaver, D. C., McDaniel, M. L., and Lacy, P. E. (1978). Alloxan uptake by isolated rat islets of Langerhans. *Endocrinology* **102:**1847–1855.
26. Crouch, R. K., Gancy, S. E., Kimsey, G., Galbraith, R. A., Galbraith, G. M. P., and Buse, M. (1981). The inhibition of superoxide dismutase by diabetogenic drugs. *Diabetes* **30:**235–241.
27. McCord, J. M., and Fridovich, I. (1969). Superoxide dismutase: An enzymic function for erythrocuprein (hemocuprein). *J. Biol. Chem.* **244:**6049–6055.
28. DelRio, L. A., Ortega, M. G., López, A. L., and Gorgé, J. L. (1977). A more sensitive modification of the catalase assay with the Clark oxygen electrode. *Anal. Biochem.* **80:**409–415.
29. Ammon, H. P. T., Akhtar, M. S., Grimm, A., and Niklas, H. (1979). Effect of methylene blue and thiol oxidants on pancreatic islet GSH/GSSG ratios and tolbutamide mediated insulin release *in vitro. Naunyn-Schmiedeberg's Arch. Pharmacol.* **307:**91–96.
30. Lazarow, A., Patterson, J. W., and Levey, S. (1948). The mechanism of cysteine and glutathione protection against alloxan diabetes. *Science* **108:**308–309.
31. Harman, A. W., and Fischer, L. J. (1981). Protection from alloxan toxicity in isolated hepatocytes by sugars. *Biochem. Pharmacol.,* in press.
32. Scheynius, A., and Täljedal, I. B. (1971). On the mechanism of glucose protection against alloxan toxicity. *Diabetologia* **7:**252–255.
33. Baur, H., Kasperek, S., and Pfaff, E. (1976). Criteria of viability of isolated liver cells. *Hoppe-Seyler's Z. Physiol. Chem.* **356:**827–838.
34. Mitchell, J. R., Jollow, D. J., Potter, W. Z., Gillette, J. R., and Brodie, B. B. (1973). Acetaminophen-induced hepatic necrosis. IV. Protective role of glutathione. *J. Pharmacol. Exp. Ther.* **187:**211–217.

Chapter 17

Clinical Use of Superoxide Dismutase and Possible Pharmacological Approaches

A. M. MICHELSON

INTRODUCTION

Since the identification of superoxide dismutase in 1969 by McCord and Fridovich (1), the fundamental physiological roles of the superoxide anion and the various superoxide dismutases have been explored and defined with astonishing rapidity. This chapter presents various aspects that we have developed, or that are currently under investigation, in Paris. In some sections we describe completed work, whereas in others we present preliminary results in which the connection between the biochemical description and clinical meaning in terms of human pathology is incompletely understood as yet. In some instances, we found it difficult to procure samples of normal human tissues for direct comparison with abnormal samples.

ALTERED SUPEROXIDE DISMUTASE CONTENT ASSOCIATED WITH VARIOUS HUMAN DISORDERS

We have previously described variations of erythrocyte copper–zinc-containing superoxide dismutase (CuSOD) obtained from human beings

277

PATHOLOGY OF OXYGEN
Copyright © 1982 by Academic Press, Inc.

suffering from a variety of pathological conditions (2). This work has since been extended by the studies described in the following subsections.

Chronic Schizophrenia

The concentration of erythrocyte CuSOD was estimated in 17 selected adult schizophrenics aged 21–50 years (2 women, 15 men) and compared with the values for 14 controls aged 32–63 years (3 women, 11 men). A statistically significant increase ($p < .02$) of 13.6% was observed (3) in the patients (520.2 ± 17.1 μg CuSOD per gram hemoglobin; SD 69.8) compared with the normal subjects (458 ± 18.6 μg CuSOD per gram hemoglobin; SD 70.5). These results confirmed earlier observations (2) obtained with a mixed population of patients with various mental disorders. There was no difference in the level of erythrocyte glutathione peroxidase (GPX) from normal values.

Autic Children

Infantile development psychoses are precociously expressed in the first months or years after birth. The characteristics are (a) an autism with respect to surrounding persons, (b) an absence of verbal communication, and (c) stereotyped behavior. Although such cases are relatively rare, we were able to examine 36 children and young adults (aged 4–19 years) who were rigorously selected at the clinical level for the above three characteristics and who exhibited no neurological or electroencephalographic anomalies and absence of psychotropic chemotherapy. These were compared with a control population (21 subjects aged 5–18 years). In addition to the content of CuSOD (located on chromosome 21 in human beings) and GPX (chromosome 3) in erythrocytes, we examined the content of these two enzymes as well as that of manganese superoxide dismutase (MnSOD) (chromosome 6) in fractionated blood platelets, since these offer a convenient metabolic reflection of synapses (4–6).

A significantly greater concentration of CuSOD was present in the erythrocytes and platelets of the autic subjects than in those of the normal subjects, whereas the content of platelet MnSOD was unchanged. No difference in platelet GPX levels was observed, whereas markedly less GPX was found in the erythrocytes of autic subjects than in those of normal subjects. These changes contrast with those found in adult schizophrenics. The ratio of [CuSOD] to [GPX] was twofold higher in erythrocytes of the autic children tested. Indeed, 23 of the 24 psychotic subjects tested showed a ratio greater than the mean normal value.

We have previously discussed possible biochemical mechanisms involving an alteration of the metabolism of certain neuromediators due to perturbation of the major enzymes that provide protection against activated oxygen species (2). Whether this is a cause or a consequence of the cerebral dysfunction leading to infantile development psychoses remains to be established. It is nevertheless clear that the intermediary metabolism of molecular oxygen plays an important role in mental pathology.

Diabetics

In collaboration with Dr. J. C. Bonneau (Centre de Transfusion Sanguine et de Génétique Humaine de Bois-Guillaume) erythrocyte CuSOD, catalase, and GPX were measured in a group of diabetic patients (7). The CuSOD content was higher by about 14% in the diabetic subjects, whereas the GPX level showed a significant decrease to almost half the normal value, suggesting an interdependent control and regulation of these two enzymes. In contrast, the catalase level did not change significantly although a slight increase was noted.

Hepatic Disorders

Numerous erythrocyte anomalies have been observed in various cirrhoses and hepatic diseases, which are often accompanied by a lower content of GPX. Diminished GPX levels have been reported in cases of transitory hemolytic anemia in newborn children (8), in a single case of chronic hemolytic anemia (9), and in a cirrhotic subject during severe hemolytic anemia (10). In collaboration with Dr. A. Najman (Hopital St. Antoine, Paris) erythrocyte CuSOD and GPX levels were examined in patients with a variety of hemolytic anemic and cirrhotic disorders (11). The concentration of erythrocyte CuSOD was slightly higher than normal, but the values were much more dispersed compared with the controls. The concentration of GPX, however, was very significantly decreased. A bimodal distribution of erythrocyte GPX values in the patients was observed, suggesting that at least two biochemical mechanisms may be involved in the pathology, which may be the result of the diversity of clinical symptoms. As observed with diabetic patients, erythrocyte catalase was unchanged. Three patients were examined after successful treatment of liver disease, and analysis in each case revealed a decrease of 5–10% in CuSOD and a marked increase in GPX (values of 1.81, 3.78, and 1.79 increased to 7.03, 11.21, and 3.96 nmol NADPH oxidized each minute per milligram hemoglobin, respectively). These results also provide a strong indication that superoxide dismutase and GPX are interdependent, although the respective genes are located on different chromosomes.

Breast Cancer

We previously described protection of cultured mammalian cells against irradiation by exogenous superoxide dismutase (12). It was thus of interest to determine whether the radiosensitivity or radioresistance of human breast cancers may be correlated with the superoxide dismutase content of the tumors. Various reports have described a lower than normal content or a total absence of MnSOD in tumor cells [13–17; see also references cited by Michelson (18)]. A lower than normal concentration of mitochondrial CuSOD in tumor cells was also reported (19). However, in general, cultured cell systems were used, and isolated cells can display remarkable differences when compared with tissue *in vivo*. The superoxide dismutase content in samples of different types of human tumors was measured (20), but in these studies a rather unreliable assay system (epinephrine oxidation) was used. The data showed an extremely wide variation from 0.23 to 160.5 units/g tumor (700-fold difference between maximal and minimal).

With the collaboration of Dr. H. Magdelenat, Dr. C. Bidron, and Dr. C. Rothmeyer (Service de Radiopathologie, Dr. H. Jammet, Institut Curie, Paris) we obtained a number of breast tumor samples taken from patients before radiotherapy. These samples either have been, or are, in the process of being examined (21). The content of CuSOD and MnSOD was determined, as was that of the estrogenic receptor. The results for superoxide dismutase to date for 36 patients are shown in Fig. 1. The dispersion of values for CuSOD activity was much greater than in erythrocytes (normal values and distribution were observed in erythrocytes of cancer patients). The significance of these results is not yet clear because of the difficulty of obtaining normal breast tissue for comparative purposes.

Variations of superoxide dismutase content may reflect tumor type and growth. It is possible that this difference affects radioresistance, but the correlation can be made only after the time necessary to determine the value of tumor regression after radiotherapy. So far, two cases have shown a total disappearance of the tumor. These cases presented the two *lowest* values for CuSOD, which is suggestive of an association.

Since obtaining these data, we have developed an ultrasensitive radioimmunochemical technique (using antigens radiolabeled at approximately 1500 Ci/mM) for determining the protein content of human CuSOD and MnSOD (22) which has provided a sensitive measure in addition to

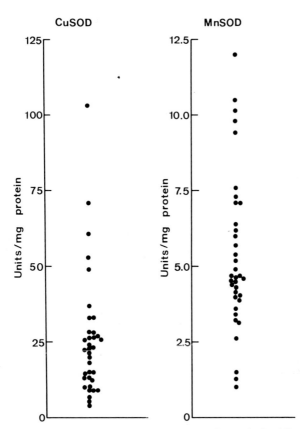

Fig. 1. Superoxide dismutase activity in breast tumor tissue obtained from 36 patients. The data are given as individual values expressed as luminol units per milligram protein. Normal tissue in three cases had values of 27.6, 4.4, and 14.5 units of CuSOD per milligram protein and 3.3, 2.5, and 12.0 units of MnSOD, respectively. For comparison purified CuSOD has a specific activity of 50 units/μg.

enzymatic assay. Measurements will be made to determine both the quantity and specific activity of the two enzymes. If indeed loss of superoxide dismutase activity occurs in human tissue as a consequence of tumor formation, this should clarify whether there is a loss or degradation of enzyme protein or production of an inhibitor of CuSOD, MnSOD, or both.

A correlation between CuSOD activity and the estrogenic receptor may also exist. In all cases, when the activity of CuSOD was less than 10 units/mg protein, the receptor was absent. However, in the absence of a suitable number of normal breast samples for estimation, this correlation must remain uncertain.

In a related study, erythrocyte superoxide dismutase was measured in four surviving members of a family that had received massive doses of irradiation (^{60}Co). We observed very low levels of erythrocyte CuSOD (396–448 μg CuSOD per gram hemoglobin compared with normal values of 500–700 μg CuSOD per gram hemoglobin); GPX values were elevated (closely grouped at an average of 11.5 units compared with normal values of 7–8 units). This family is being followed during their recovery, since they represent another example of superoxide dismutase and GPX interrelationships.

Results from Other Laboratories

No significant differences in CuSOD or MnSOD were found (23) in erythrocytes and lymphocytes from patients with juvenile neuronal ceroidlipofuscinosis (Spielmeyer–Vogt–Batten's disease) compared with healthy adults. The activity of both enzymes was normal in cultured skin fibroblasts taken from patients with ataxia-telangiectasia (chromosomal breakage syndromes) (24) and in erythrocytes from patients with β-thalassemia (25). The erythrocyte superoxide dismutase content in rheumatoid arthritis patients was found to be normal (26) but was decreased in polymorphonuclear leukocytes of children with rheumatoid arthritis (27). The content of GPX, however, was normal. A low superoxide dismutase level is also associated with hyperbilirubinemia (28), and a deficiency of MnSOD has been observed in patients with Dugin–Johnson–Sprinz syndrome (29).

PHARMACOLOGICAL APPLICATION

The above survey indicates that either high or low levels of superoxide dismutase can be associated with certain pathological states. Biochemically, this enzyme is necessary to maintain a low steady-state cellular concentration of O_2^-. High levels of this radical, either locally or in the total organism, lead to membrane damage and inflammation, among other possibilities. Abnormally high concentrations of superoxide dismutase, however, can interfere with certain normal metabolic oxidative processes and may even increase oxidation rates by reducing the concentration of O_2^-, which can act as a free-radical chain terminator or may block the production of extremely toxic hydroxyl radicals by reaction of an organic free radical with H_2O_2 [see Michelson (18) for discussion].

$$RH + H_2O_2 \rightarrow R + H^+ + HO^- + HO^-$$

In pathological cases in which the level of superoxide dismutase is lower than normal, possible pharmacological approaches can be envisioned which involve the administration of exogenous superoxide dismutase. Such proposals have already received considerable study (30,31). The pharmacological application of superoxide dismutase is governed by a number of parameters, including circulation lifetime, penetration into cells, organ specificity, and intracellular localization of the exogenous enzyme.

Cell Penetration

Since superoxide dismutases are proteins with molecular weights ranging from 33,000 to 96,000, cellular penetration does not readily occur. Nevertheless, administration by various techniques (intravenous, intraperitoneal) does afford a certain degree of protection against high-energy radiation (32) and is effective against various acute and chronic inflammatory conditions such as rheumatoid arthritis and osteoarthritis (31). It is likely that, in such cases, superoxide dismutase is effective in reducing extracellular levels of O_2^- produced during phagocytosis or by other means.

In recent years, the possible application of liposome-packaged material has received considerable attention. It was thus of interest to study the cellular penetration of diverse superoxide dismutases and the corresponding liposomal preparations. As a model cell we used human erythrocytes. Various forms of superoxide dismutase were chosen which ranged in pI from 4.4 to 8.7 (selected with a view to the charge characteristics of the erythrocyte). These were obtained from both prokaryote and eukaryote sources and contained either copper, manganese, or iron as the metal prosthetic group (hence covering the three major classes of superoxide dismutases). The enzymes used were bovine CuSOD (pI = 4.9), human CuSOD (pI = 4.6), bacterial (*Photobacterium leiognathi*) CuSOD (pI = 8.7), human MnSOD (pI = 7.8 and 8.3), and bacterial (*P. leiognathi*) FeSOD (pI = 4.4).

Since radioactively labeled superoxide dismutases were necessary for this work, we decided to use a general method useful with all superoxide dismutases which caused no degradation and yielded a stable marker. Iodination (^{125}I) has frequently been used, but we found that after injection of the enzyme into animals very rapid liberation of the radioactive iodine occurred *in vivo* with concentration of the radioactive label (but not the enzyme) in the thyroid. (This invalidates certain studies on the metabolism of superoxide dismutase.) We found the best approach to be preparation of the apoenzyme by removal of the metal (Cu, Mn, or Fe) followed by reconstitution with radioactive cobalt (^{60}Co or [57]Co). This gave extremely high yields of incorporation of radioactivity (essentially 95–100%) using a slight excess of apoenzyme, and the enzyme thus radiolabeled was stable. Carrier-free radioactive cobalt was diluted with native enzyme.

Liposomes were prepared by standard techniques. Electron microscopy showed that the liposomes were polydisperse, ranging from 60 to 460 nm in diameter. Filtration of the liposomes on Millipore filters ranging from 0.45 to 8 μm confirmed this result since essentially all the material passed a filter of 1.2 μm. Human erythrocytes were incubated with free superoxide dismutase or the various liposome preparations. The vesicles were well washed and lysed, and the released superoxide dismutase was partially purified by treatment with chloroform/ethanol to remove the hemoglobin. Radioactivity of the partially purified superoxide dismutase was measured by scintillation counting. Alternatively, direct counting of the washed erythrocytes was employed. The degree of penetration of human erythrocytes by the free enzymes and by anionic and cationic liposomes (dipalmitoyllecithin) containing the superoxide dismutases is shown in Table IA for prewashed erythrocytes and for whole blood. Very low levels of penetration occurred with the free enzymes (from 100 to 3460 molecules per erythrocyte). In general, the penetration was higher with washed erythrocytes than when the enzyme was diluted by plasma proteins. Contrary to expectations, no correlation of pI of the enzyme and penetration capacity was observed. This may be a consequence of pI dependence on total basic or acidic amino acid content of the protein, whereas for effective binding of the enzyme to the outer membrane of the erythrocyte only external lysine amino groups are presumably involved. Penetration of enzymes encapsulated in negatively charged dicetyl phosphate liposomes was not much greater than that of the free enzymes. This could result from the negative charge of the outside of the erythrocyte membrane. The most striking results are seen with stearylamine liposomes. Erythrocyte penetration is more efficient in whole blood than with washed cells, and a large increase in cellular superoxide dismutase is obtained. With the homologous system, human erythrocuprein liposomes and human erythrocytes, the content can be tripled (204% increase in superoxide dismutase). The type of superoxide dismutase used influences penetration since liposomes containing acidic superoxide dismutases (human and bovine CuSOD and bacterial FeSOD) are more efficient than those containing basic superoxide dismutases (human MnSOD and bacterial CuSOD). This can be explained in terms of total liposome structure and composition if it is assumed that more stearylamine is incorporated per liposome with the acidic superoxide dismutases than with those char-

TABLE IA

Penetration of Erythrocytes[a] by Native Superoxide Dismutases and by Superoxide Dismutases Encapsulated in Liposomes

Enzyme[b]	Free SOD		SOD in dicetyl phosphate liposome		SOD in stearylamine liposome	
	Molecules per erythrocyte	% of endogenous enzyme	Molecules per erythrocyte	% of endogenous enzyme	Molecules per erythrocyte	% of endogenous enzyme
Bovine CuSOD						
Washed erythrocytes	2,236	0.79	2,904	1.03	399,635	141.58
Total blood	150	0.05	938	0.33	489,585	173.45
Human CuSOD						
Washed erythrocytes	720	0.26	3,033	1.07	515,542	182.64
Total blood	100	0.04	—	—	576,194	204.13
Bacterial CuSOD						
Washed erythrocytes	460	0.16	3,315	1.17	158,826	56.27
Total blood	130	0.05	23,130	8.19	247,491	87.68
Human MnSOD						
Washed erythrocytes	2,520	0.89	—	—	—	—
Total blood	1,460	0.52	10,895	3.86	263,445	93.3
Bacterial FeSOD						
Washed erythrocytes	460	0.16	7,170	2.54	—	—
Total blood	3,460	1.22	20,565	7.29	436,310	154.57

[a] The human blood used in these experiments contained 5.88×10^9 erythrocytes per milliliter; 92.5 μg CuSOD per milliliter (approximately 280,000 molecules of SOD per erythrocyte). Cells were incubated with an approximately sixfold excess of SOD (free or in liposomes) compared with the endogenous enzyme.

[b] All forms of SOD contained ^{60}Co or ^{57}Co, which replaced the normal metal prosthetic group in the native enzymes. The source of each enzyme used is described in the text.

acterized by a high pI value, thus giving liposomes with better penetration characteristics.

The effects of modifying the lecithin component in liposome preparations on their capacity to penetrate human erythrocytes are shown in Table IB. With fully saturated lecithins, chain length has an effect, with a marked optimum at fatty acid esters of 16 carbon atoms and both shorter or longer chain lengths giving liposomes that are less efficient. The ester linkage can be replaced by an ether linkage (dihexadecyllecithin) with a slight improvement over the dipalmitoyllecithin. However, when an unsaturated residue is introduced, for example, when a palmitoyl residue is replaced by oleoyl (9,10 double bond), a large decrease in penetration capacity is observed. This is even more marked if both chains are unsaturated (dioleoyllecithin) since penetration is now essentially abolished. These results show the striking biological effects that result from relatively minor changes in liposome membrane structure due to the more open conformation imposed by a single double bond in the fatty acid residues.

Circulation Lifetime

This problem has been pursued with considerable success by McCord and co-workers using superoxide dismutase coupled to polymers such as polyethylene glycol, dextran, or Ficol. We polymerized the superoxide

TABLE IB

Effect of Composition of Liposomal Lecithin on Penetration of Washed Erythrocytes with Bovine CuSOD Encapsulated in Stearylamine[a]

	SOD in stearylamine liposome	
Lecithin	Molecules per erythrocyte	% of endogenous SOD
Dihexadecyl ether	509,747	180.6
Dilauroyl (12)[b]	279,997	99.2
Dimyristoyl (14)	270,469	95.8
Dipalmitoyl (16)	420,135	148.8
Distearoyl (18)	155,174	55.0
Dioleoyl (18)	3,266	1.16
Oleoyl, palmitoyl	129,796	46.0

[a] Experimental parameters were the same as those described in Table IA.

[b] Number of carbon atoms.

dismutase itself after treating it with methyl 4-mercaptobutyrimidate to give a superoxide dismutase in which lysine ϵ-amino groups were substituted by thiobutanol residues. About 70% of the enzymatic activity was retained. In aerobic, aqueous solutions the substituted superoxide dismutase polymerized (by formation of —S—S— links) to a solid gel. This is readily reversed by treatment with mild reducing agents such as mercaptoethanol to give the monomer enzyme. Studies are in progress to determine the circulating lifetime of this modified superoxide dismutase.

Organ Specificity

Since the efficiency of action of superoxide dismutase administered as a pharmacological agent is a function of (a) the rate of excretion from the entire organism (either as the native molecule or via proteolytic degradation), (b) the concentration of superoxide dismutase localized in a specific organ of particular interest and its lifetime in this organ, and (c) the time of circulation in the blood system, it was of interest to examine these parameters with the various forms of superoxide dismutase and liposome preparations containing superoxide dismutase. Two animals, the rat and the rabbit, were chosen for study. The CuSOD content of rat erythrocytes is very similar to that of human erythrocytes (261,000 molecules per erythrocyte, compared with an average value of 260,000 for human beings). The rabbit is sufficiently large to be a convenient model for certain hospital techniques such as scintillography.

Rat Studies

Carrier-free [57]Co-labeled superoxide dismutase (see page 283 for a description of the specific forms of the enzyme used) diluted with cold native enzyme and the corresponding liposomal preparations were administered to rats by intravenous injection in the vein of the penis. Each rat received 5×10^5 cpm per injection, corresponding to about 10 μg of superoxide dismutase. After suitable time intervals the rats were killed, and blood and various organs were removed. Samples of each organ were then weighed and counted directly in a γ counter. The maximum percent incorporation of the original injection is given for different organs (per gram of tissue) in Table II. Maxima were attained in general within the first time interval, but with certain preparations and certain organs from 1 to 6 hr were required. In view of the limited number of rats used for each point, this could reflect individual differences among the animals, but because of the remarkable linearity of exponential decay observed for cer-

TABLE II

Maximum Incorporation of Superoxide Dismutase per Gram Tissue[a,b]

Form of SOD	Liver	Kidney	Spleen	Lung	Erythrocyte
Bovine CuSOD	0.55	11.22	0.14	0.26	0.15
Cationic liposome					
Dipalmitoyl	2.27	7.75	0.54	3.35	0.19
Dihexadecyl	1.71	6.05	1.19	7.90	0.07
Sphingomyelin	2.10	4.37	2.41	2.18	0.17
Anionic liposome					
Dipalmitoyl	2.82	4.19	1.30	0.34	0.16
Dihexadecyl	2.27	2.38	0.68	0.33	0.06
Human CuSOD	0.41	14.75	0.21	0.23	0.14
Dipalmitoyl					
Cationic liposome	2.07	16.47	0.63	3.15	0.08
Anionic liposome	2.78	8.78	0.94	0.73	0.06
Bacterial CuSOD	0.54	10.92	0.18	0.31	0.97
Dipalmitoyl					
Cationic liposome	2.12	5.82	1.89	3.96	0.07
Anionic liposome	2.93	8.39	2.00	0.56	0.07
Bacterial FeSOD	0.36	12.46	0.15	0.39	0.12
Dipalmitoyl					
Cationic liposome	1.58	10.65	1.43	3.28	0.13
Anionic liposome	1.48	5.31	2.01	0.41	0.08
Human MnSOD	0.46	0.88	0.37	1.40	0.79
$^{57}Co^{2+}$	0.09	1.14	0.05	0.23	0.03
Total organ weight (g)	12.8	2.1	2.3	2.7	17

[a] Percentage per gram organ weight.

[b] Superoxide dismutase was injected (iv) into rats as either the purified enzyme or incorporated into liposomes. Samples were taken at 20 min, 1, 3, 6, 24, and 48 hr after injection and the maximum value reported. Tail vein blood samples were obtained 5 min after injection.

tain organs this is unlikely, particularly since similar observations were made using rabbits. It is more likely that this represents a normal physiological accumulation rate. This is despite the fact that the total blood content of the injected superoxide dismutase dropped to 2.5–5.6% at 1 hr and to 1.3% at 6 hr (mean values).

The highest concentrations of the enzyme (per gram of tissue) occurred in the kidney, as might be expected. Except for human MnSOD, all the free superoxide dismutase preparations showed this organ specificity. Lung tissue appeared to concentrate human MnSOD most efficiently (3.8% per total organ). The liver is also selective (but less so than the kidneys) for the free enzyme. The liposome-encapsulated superoxide dismu-tases were concentrated largely in the liver (19–37.5% per whole organ), particularly with anionic liposomes, which were also selected by the spleen to a greater extent than cationic liposomes. The latter, however, were specific for the lungs, with values up to 21% of the initial input for the entire organ. There was a high concentration of sphingomyelin cat-ionic liposomes in the spleen.

Close examination of Table II shows that the concentration of enzyme in a particular organ is modified by (a) the nature of the superoxide dismu-tase encapsulated, (b) the ionic character of the liposome, and (c) the composition of the lecithin. For example, 24 times more bovine CuSOD contained in the stearylamine dihexadecyl lecithin (ether rather than ester linkages) liposome was incorporated into the lung than bovine CuSOD contained in the dicetyl phosphate dihexadecyllecithin liposome. (All cat-ionic liposomes contained stearylamine, which was replaced by dicetyl phosphate in the anionic liposomes.) These differences may be compared with those previously described for the penetration of erythrocytes.

The question of whether organ specificity is a result of differences in cell penetration or of structural factors involving the entire organ will be resolved by comparative studies of the penetration of enzyme into iso-lated human cells (liver, kidney, lung, etc.) in culture.

Analysis of the decay time of enzymes in each organ indicated that the rate of decay was not a simple exponential function but showed a rapid phase followed by a much slower rate of loss. In some cases this could reflect rates of intracellular destruction of the liposome, liberating free su-peroxide dismutase. It is evident that if a liposome can enter the cell it can also leave, whereas if free protein is liberated inside the cell its exit will be more difficult. Rate of decay was a function of the organ, the nature of the superoxide dismutase encapsulated, and the composition of the liposome. Thus, 50% lifetimes in the spleen were 30-fold greater for bovine CuSOD in the cationic dihexadecyllecithin liposome (60 hr) than for the enzyme in the anionic dipalmitoyllecithin liposome (2 hr). This cationic liposome also had a maximal half-life in the liver (40 hr) and in the lung (8 hr). Renal excretion was, in general, largely complete in 24 hr. Among the unencap-sulated superoxide dismutases, human MnSOD was most rapidly lost from the liver but was retained longest in the blood plasma (50% time, 1.67 hr), whereas bacterial CuSOD (even more basic than MnSOD) showed decay characteristics similar to those of the acidic superoxide dis-mutases such as bovine CuSOD and bacterial FeSOD. Values for the in-jection of the same quantity of free $^{57}Co^{2+}$ as used in the superoxide dis-mutase injections are given in Table II to indicate that leakage of the radioactive label does not occur.

Rabbit Studies

In collaboration with B. Perdereau, H. Magdelénat, and C. Barbaroux of the Service de Médecine Nucléaire (Dr. R. Gongora), Institut Curie, Paris, we were able to examine the organ distribution of bovine superoxide dismutase in rabbits by using a scintograph coupled to a computer (33). The representative scintograph image in Fig. 2 clearly shows the kidneys and the cardiovascular and pulmonary systems. The bladder is weakly visible wth the beginning of excretion. With cationic liposomal bovine CuSOD, high concentration in the lungs was observed 15 min after injection. Fifteen minutes after injection of anionic liposomal bovine CuSOD, the enzyme was concentrated in the liver and there were traces in the kidneys and bladder. Cationic liposomal bacterial CuSOD was highly concentrated in the lungs 31 min after injection. Injection of anionic liposomal human CuSOD resulted in concentration in the liver, kidneys, and bladder 31 min after injection. A very marked asymmetry in the kidneys was clearly visible (Fig. 3), suggesting renal hypertrophy. To verify this, the same rabbit was injected 1 month later with 150 μCi of ^{99}Tc-labeled dimercaptosuccinic acid (routinely used for kidney examination in human beings) and reexamined. Both kidneys were normal in this image, however, and showed identical integrated counts. Since it is highly unlikely that a renal perturbation of the amplitude indicated in Fig. 3 would be sponstaneously rectified in 1 month, this suggests that such liposomal preparations could be useful in the evaluation of defective kidney function by analysis of the retention of liposomes ($\leq$ 1μm in diameter) as a complement to examination with small molecules. In this respect it is of interest that the total counts of the two kidneys of the rabbit in Fig. 3 were essentially identical with those of a normal rabbit, suggesting renal compensation for a defective kidney, which is not unusual. Variation in organ mass, e.g., depth of the organ, is automatically corrected by computer analysis.

Reduced zone ratios of the relative concentrations of superoxide dismutase in rabbit kidney, liver, and lungs following administration of the different preparations indicated the dependence of organ distribution on the type of superoxide dismutase used and the form in which it was administered (Table III). Analysis of organ ratio of radiolabeled superoxide dismutase as a function of time indicated relative metabolic stabilities or clearance rates of the enzyme that in many ways paralleled observations in rats with respect to physiological properties of the various preparations (data not shown).

The kinetics of incorporation and of decay for the enzyme preparations

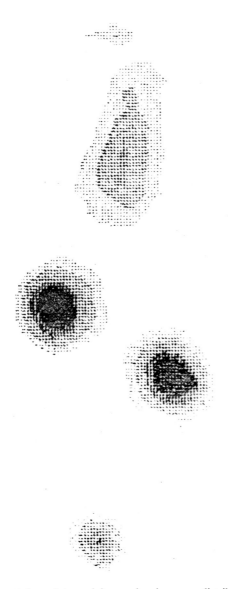

Fig. 2. Representative scintograph image showing organ distribution of injected radiolabeled superoxide dismutase. A preparation containing 35 μCi of [57]Co-labeled bovine CuSOD (approximately 145 μg protein) was injected into the ear vein of a rabbit (3.0–3.5 kg body weight). The image was recorded 15 min after injection.

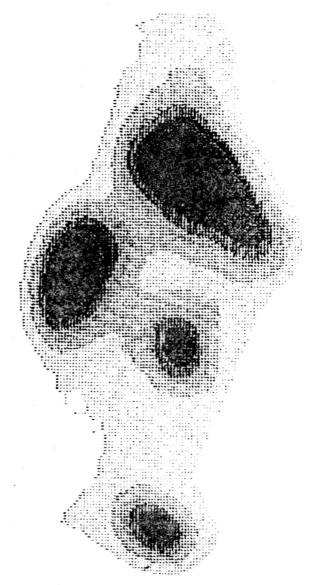

Fig. 3. Representative scintograph image showing organ distribution of injected radiolabeled liposome-incorporated superoxide dismutase. Experimental conditions were the same as described in Fig. 2 except that ^{57}Co-labeled human CuSOD was incorporated into anionic dicetyl phosphate liposomes before injection and the image was recorded 31 min after injection. Note the pronounced renal hypertrophy.

TABLE III

Reduced Zone Ratios[a]

Form of SOD	Kidney	Liver	Lung	Urinary elimination
CuSOD				
Bovine	100	13.3	21.7	+
Human	100	13.9	—	+
Bacterial	100	20.8	7.9	+++
Cationic liposomes				
Bovine	50	9.1	100	+
Human	100	33.3	100	+
Bacterial	40	50	100	++
Anionic liposomes				
Bovine	33.3	100	10 − 5	+
Human	100	100	10	++
Bacterial	50	100	100	+

[a] Values were obtained from scintograph recordings at 1 hr (or time of achievement of maximal ratio) after rabbits were injected with radiolabeled SOD in the form indicated.

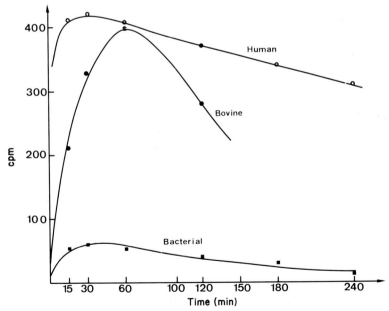

Fig. 4. Rate of incorporation and decay of free ^{57}Co-labeled CuSOD in rabbit kidney. Data are given per total organ. For experimental details see Table IA.

are shown in terms of total organ counts in Figs. 4–6. For each type of superoxide dismutase administration, the highest concentration of labeled superoxide dismutase was chosen to be depicted. It is of interest that, whereas maximal kidney concentration of the various forms of free superoxide dismutase requires from 30 min to 1 hr, retention of the liposomal preparations in lung is very efficient and is virtually complete in 15 sec, that is, with a single circulation of the blood system.

Very approximate decay times of radiolabeled CuSOD to 50% of maximal activity are given in Table IV, as are the exponential half-lives (t_1 and t_2). All liposome injections in rabbits involved dipalmitoyllecithin and stearylamine (or dicetyl phosphate) liposomes. Other variations, such as a dihexadecyllecithin, have not yet been examined.

Although slight differences in response occur between rats and rabbits, it is clear that, depending on the availability of suitable packaging, superoxide dismutases can be introduced with a relatively high degree of selection at reasonable concentrations into different organs of animals and presumably also in man.

Intracellular Localization

Although we have begun experiments in this laboratory to study the intracellular localization of administered superoxide dismutase, no data were available at the time of this writing.

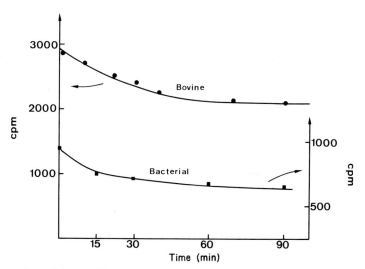

Fig. 5. Rate of decay of ^{57}Co-labeled CuSOD (in cationic liposomes) in rabbit lung. Data are given per total organ. For experimental details see Table IA.

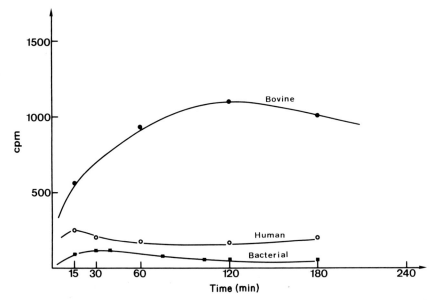

Fig. 6. Rate of incorporation and decay of [57]Co-labeled CuSOD (in anionic liposomes) in rabbit liver. Data are given per total organ. For experimental details see Table IA.

MEDICAL APPLICATIONS OF SUPEROXIDE DISMUTASE

As mentioned earlier in this chapter, certain illnesses are associated with a low level of superoxide dismutase—for example, in polymorphonucleophiles of rheumatoid arthritis patients (children). It was therefore

TABLE IV

Approximate Time of Decay of Administered [57]Co-labeled CuSOD to 50% of Original Activity

Type of SOD	Free SOD, kidney	Cationic liposomes, lung	Anionic liposomes, liver
Bovine	8.0 hr	1 hr, 20 min (t_1 7 min; t_2 3 hr)	5 hr, 30 min (t_1 14 min; t_2 6 hr)
Human	10.0 hr	1 hr	12 hr
Bacterial	7.0 hr	2 hr, 40 min (t_1 2 min; t_2 5 hr)	No measurable decay

of interest to examine the possible beneficial action of some of the preparations described above. In collaboration with Dr. J. P. Camus (Hopital Tenon, Paris) we are following the effects of the direct injection of superoxide dismutase preparations into the knee joints of adult rheumatoid arthritis patients. After administration of the enzyme as either human superoxide dismutase or bovine CuSOD, fluid was withdrawn at intervals to determine the content of superoxide dismutase by the highly sensitive and specific radioimmunological techniques developed in this laboratory.

In a more general sense a wide range of autoimmune diseases are of considerable interest with respect to O_2^- and superoxide dismutases as a result of the pioneering work of Ingrid Emerit and co-workers (Laboratory of Cytogenetics, Institut Biomèdical des Cordeliers, Paris). Autoimmune diseases generally involve increased chromosome breakages—for example, in diffuse scleroderma and systemic sclerosis (34–36). Anomalous chromosome breakage is observed in patients with ulcerative colitis (37) and diverse collagen diseases (38), as well as Crohn's disease (39). In the case of increased chromosome breakage in patients with progressive systemic sclerosis, lupus erythematosus, and rheumatoid arthritis a serum factor present in the patients' blood was observed (40–43). Dr. I. Emerit and co-workers, in collaboration with J. Maral and A. M. Michelson, have partially purified this clastogenic factor (to the point where no UV or visible absorption or fluorescence is observed with the quantities available). The factor has a molecular weight of about 5000. The addition of this factor produces chromosome breaks in lymphocytes of normal subjects. Activated oxygen species (O_2 and HO·) are thought to play a major role in initiating inflammatory response. For this reason we studied the role of free radicals in the origin of chromosome breakage in the above-cited diseases. The breakage rate in lymphocyte cultures of patients and the action of their ''breakage factor'' on control cells were considerably reduced by the radical-scavenging enzyme superoxide dismutase (Table V). Similar protective effects of superoxide dismutase on spontaneous chromosome breaks in cultured lymphocytes from patients with Werner's syndrome (44) or Fanconi's anemia (45) as well as on radiation-induced breaks (46) have been reported. A clastogenic factor similar to that described above may well be present in the serum of patients with Bloom's syndrome (47), an autosomal human disorder characterized by growth retardation, sunlight-induced skin eruptions, and a high incidence of cancer. In addition to the indirect evidence for the association of O_2^- with chromosome breakage, i.e., the action of exogenous superoxide dismutase, we have also shown that chromosome breaks and rearrangements are produced in lymphocyte cultures if O_2^- is generated in the medium by photoreduction of FMN with near-UV light (48).

TABLE V

Rate of Chromosomal Breakage in Lymphocytes

| | Lymphocyte cultures of patients | | | | | | Lymphocyte cultures of healthy subjects treated with clastogenic factor from patients | | | |
| | Progressive systemic sclerosis (3)[a] | | Rheumatoid arthritis (2)[a] | | Systemic lupus erythematosus (1)[a] | | Progressive systemic sclerosis (3)[a] | | Systemic lupus erythematosus (1)[a] | |
Additions	None	SOD[b]	None	SOD[b]	None	SOD[b]	None	SOD[b]	None	SOD[b]
Total mitoses studied	116	131	84	100	50	50	150	143	50	50
Total chromosome aberrations	38	6.9	22.6	4.0	24.0	6.0	18.0	4.2	60.0	2.0

[a] Numbers in parentheses indicate number of subjects.
[b] 10 μg/ml.

Normal human lymphocytes produce a very low level of O_2^-, but when they are stimulated by phytohemoglutinin an increase in O_2^- production is observed. The purified clastogenic factor of I. Emerit also stimulates production of O_2^-, which is inhibited by exogenous superoxide dismutase. A possible molecular explanation of the various autoimmune diseases thus lies in an increased production of O_2^- (or secondarily of HO· radicals) induced in certain maladies by a specific serum clastogenic factor or by other intracellular processes (such as reduced superoxide dismutase content or increased O_2^- concentration due to diverse perturbations of oxidative metabolism). Activated oxygen species attack the chromosomes, leading to breakage, and at the same time modify the DNA such that it becomes antigenic, perhaps by partial denaturation (49), thus giving rise to anti-DNA antibodies.

L-Cysteine also inhibits the aberration rate induced by the clastogenic factor on normal lymphocytes (41), as does D-penicillamine (48). Indeed, the use of D-penicillamine in the treatment of Crohn's disease has been extensively developed by Dr. Jacques Emerit (Hôpital de la Salpêtrière, Paris) with remarkable success (50,51).

In view of the above discussion of autoimmune diseases in terms of molecular biology, it was of interest to examine the action of superoxide dismutase in specific cases. J. Emerit treated a patient suffering from Crohn's disease with an external application of a liposomal preparation of superoxide dismutase with remarkable results. Reduction of inflammation was seen in a few hours, and after 2–3 weeks of treatment with two applications per day the amelioration of the clinical symptoms was indeed striking (see color plate). This improvement was particularly impressive with respect to lesions of the anal and vulval regions since, in general, fistulas in these areas are never cured.

Equally striking clinical amelioration was observed upon treatment with the same preparation of a patient suffering from dermatomyositis (J. Emerit). This type of treatment will be extended to other diseases such as sclerodermias, lupus erythematosus, progressive chronic polyarthritis, and hemorrhagic rectocolitis, as well as to other cases of Crohn's disease and dermatomyositis. It will be of considerable interest to determine whether a decline in the level of anti-DNA antibodies occurs in certain cases during the treatment.

Cancer

As we have previously mentioned (2), injection of superoxide dismutase into transplanted melanoma tumors in hamsters causes tumor regression and an increase in survival time. We have begun to investigate

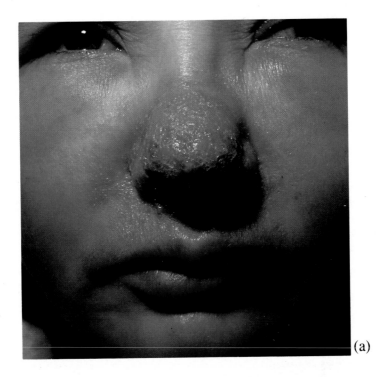

(a)

Patient with Crohn's disease. (a) Facial lesion before treatment. (b) Facial area following treatment with SOD. The right side of the face was treated with a topical application of SOD liposomes. The left side was untreated. The photograph was taken after 36 hr. Note the diminished swelling, the improvement around the eye on the right side. (c) Following the initial partial treatment, both sides of the face were treated with SOD liposomes. The photograph was taken after 25 days of treatment. (d) Anal fistulas (after rectal ablation) before treatment. (e) Anal region following 11 days of topical treatment with liposome SOD. (f) Vulval fistulas before treatment. (g) Vulval region following 18 days of topical treatment with SOD liposomes. Very marked improvement can be seen in both the ulcerations and the edema.

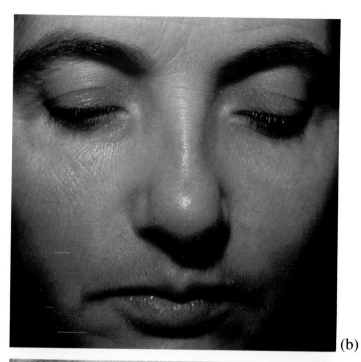

(b)

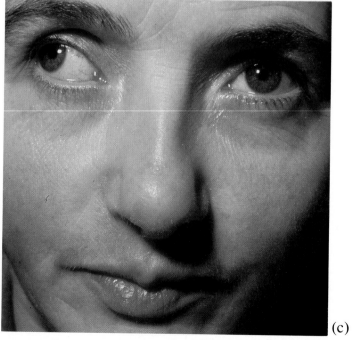

(c)

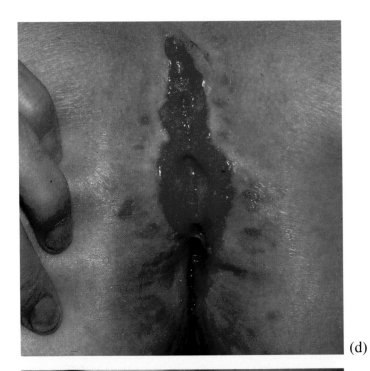

(d)

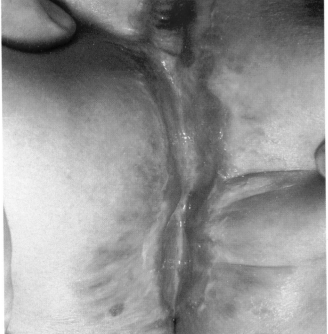

(e)

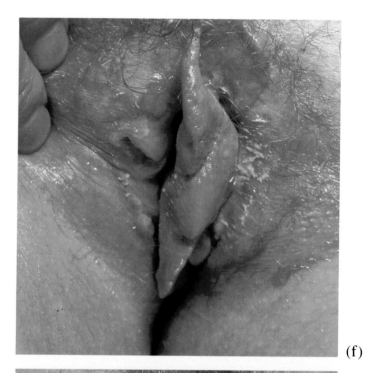

(f)

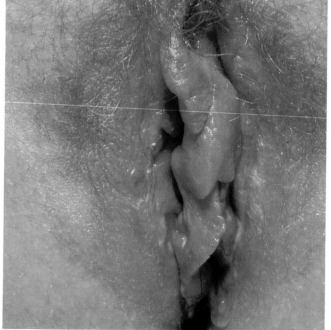

(g)

the action of the various liposomal preparations on different cancers in animals.

Other Possibilities

The treatment of burn traumas with superoxide dismutase should be of interest, as should the application of liposomal superoxide dismutase to mosquito bites. It is the author's opinion that a concerted (perhaps international) effort be made to develop the possible medical applications of superoxide dismutases.

ACKNOWLEDGMENTS

The studies described in this chapter represent the work of a number of collaborators. In particular, I would like to acknowledge the contributions of K. Puget and P. Durosay. Financial support was obtained from the CNRS (E.R. 103), INSERM (contract no. 77.4.0842), DGRST (contract no. 77.7.0280), and Fondation pour la Recherche Mèdicale Francaise.

REFERENCES

1. McCord, J. M., and Fridovich, I. (1969). Superoxide dismutase. An enzymatic function for erythrocuprein (hemocuprein). *J. Biol. Chem.* **244**:6049.
2. Michelson, A. M., Puget, K., Durosay, P., and Bonneau, J. C. (1977). Clinical aspects of the dosage of erythrocuprein. *In* "Superoxide and Superoxide Dismutases" (A. M. Michelson, J. M. McCord, and I. Fridovich, eds.), p. 467. Academic Press, New York.
3. Golse, B., Debray, Q., Puget, K., and Michelson, A. M. (1978). Superoxide dismutase I and glutathione peroxidase levels in erythrocytes of adult schizophrenics (Letter). *Nouv. Presse Med.* **7**:2070.
4. Golse, B., Debray-Ritzen, P., Puget, K., and Michelson, A. M. (1977). Analysis of platelet superoxide dismutase I in the development of childhood psychoses (Letter). *Nouv. Presse Med.* **6**:2449.
5. Golse, B., Debray-Ritzen, P., Puget, K., and Michelson, A. M. (1978). Erythrocyte and platelet levels of superoxide dismutases (1 and 2) and glutathione peroxidase in developmental child psychoses (Letter) *Nouv. Presse Med.* **7**:1952.
6. Golse, B., Debray-Ritzen, P., Durosay, P., Puget, K., and Michelson, A. M. (1978). Alterations in two enzymes: Superoxide dismutase and glutathione peroxydase in developmental infantile pychosis (infantile autism). *Rev. Neurol.* **134**:699.
7. Puget, K., Durosay, P., Michelson, A. M., and Bonneau, J. C. (1979) unpublished.
8. Necheles, T. F., Bole, S., and Allen, D. M. (1968). Erythrocyte glutathione-peroxidase deficiency and hemolytic disease of the newborn infant. *J. Pediatr.* **72**:319.
9. Necheles, T. F., Maldonado, N., Barquet-Chediak, A., and Allen, D. M. (1969). Homozygous erythrocyte glutathione-peroxidase deficiency: Clinical and biomedical studies. *Blood* **33**:164.

10. Najman, A., Lichtenstein, H., Buc, H., and Gorin, N. C. (1974). Deficit en glutathion peroxydase, acanthocytose et anémie hemolytique au cours d'une cirrhose. *Sem. Hop.* **50**:3127.
11. Najman, A., Fraitag, B., Puget, K., Lichtenstein, H., Bodin, P., Gorin, N. C., Michelson, A. M., Conte, M., and Duhamel, G. (1980). Anémie hémolitique avec acanthacytose et déficit en glutathion peroxydase erythrocytaire au cours des maladies hépatiques sévères: Etude de 5 cas. *La Nouvelle Presse Médicale* **9**:161.
12. Michelson, A. M., and Buckingham, M. E. (1974). Effects of superoxide radicals on myoblast growth and differentiation. *Biochem. Biophys. Res. Commun.* **58**:1079.
13. Oberley, L. W., Bize, I. B., Sahu, S. K., Leuthauser, S. W. H. Chan, F. H. and Gruber, H. E. (1978). Superoxide dismutase activity of normal murine liver, regenerating liver, and H6 hepatoma. *JNCI, J. Natl. Cancer Inst.* **61**:375.
14. Yamanaka, N., and Deamer, D. (1974): Superoxide dismutase activity in WI-38 cell cultures: Effects of age, trypsinization and SV-40 transformation. *Physiol. Chem. Phys.* **6**:95.
15. Sahu, S. K., Oberley, L. W., Stevens, R. H., and Riley, E. F. (1977). Superoxide dismutase activity of Ehrlich ascites tumor cells. *JNCI, J. Natl. Cancer Inst.* **58**:1125.
16. Peskin, A. V., Zbarskii, I. B., and Konstantinov, A. A. (1976). Issledovanie superoksiddismutaznoi aktivnosti v opukholerykh tkaniakh. *Dokl. Akad. Nauk SSSR* **229**:751.
17. Petkau, A., Monasterski, L. G., Kelly, K., and Friesen, H. G. (1977). Modification of superoxide dismutase in rat mammary carcinoma. *Commun. Chem. Pathol. Pharmacol.* **17**:125.
18. Michelson, A. M. (1978). Biological aspects of superoxide dismutase. *In* "Frontiers in Physical Chemical Biology" (B. Pullman, ed.), p. 309. Academic Press, New York.
19. Peskin, A. V., Loen, Ya. M., and Zbarskii, I. B. (1977). Superoxide dismutase and glutathione peroxidase activities in tumors. *FEBS Lett.* **78**:41.
20. Sykes, J. A., McCormack, F. X., Jr., and O'Brien, T. J. (1978). A preliminary study of the superoxide dismutase content of some human tumors. *Cancer Res.* **38**:2759.
21. Michelson, A. M. (1979). Superoxide dismutases. *In* "Metalloproteins, Structure, Molecular Function and Clinical Aspects" (U. Weser, ed.), p. 88. Thieme Verlag, Stuttgart.
22. Baret, A., Michel, P., Imbert, M. R., Morcellet, J. L., and Michelson, A. M. (1979). A radioimmunoassay for copper containing superoxide dismutase. *Biochem. Biophys.Res. Commun.* **8**:337.
23. Marklund, S., and Plum, C. M. (1978). Superoxide dismutase in juvenile neuronal ceroid-lipofuscinosis (Spielmeyer–Vogt–Batten's disease). *J. Neurochem.* **31**:521.
24. Abeliovich, D., and Cohen, M. M. (1978). Normal activity of nucleoside phosphorylase, superoxide dismutase and catalase in skin fibroblasts cultured from ataxia-telangiectasia patients. *Isr. J. Med. Sci.* **14**:284.
25. Concetti, A., Massei, P., Rotilio, G., Brunori, M., and Rachmilewitz, E. A. (1976). Superoxide dismutase in red blood cells: Method of assay and enzyme content in normal subjects and in patients with beta-thalassemia (major and intermedia). *J. Lab. Clin. Med.* **87**:1057.
26. Scudder, P., Stocks, J., and Dormandy, T. L. (1976). The relationship between erythrocyte superoxide dismutase activity and erythrocyte copper levels in normal subjects and in patients with rheumatoid arthritis. *Clin. Chim. Acta* **69**:397.
27. Rister, M., Bauermeister, K., Gravert, U., and Gladtke, E. (1978). Superoxide-dismutase deficiency in rheumatoid arthritis (Letter). *Lancet* **1**:1094.
28. Rotilio, G., Rigo, A., Bracci, R., Bagnoli, F., Sargentini, I., and Brunori, M. (1977). Determination of red blood cell superoxide dismutase and glutathione peroxidase in newborns in relation to neonatal hemolysis. *Clin. Chim. Acta* **81**:131.

29. Peters, T. J., and Seymour, C. A. (1978). The organelle pathology and demonstration of mitochondrial superoxide dismutase deficiency in two patients with Dubin–Johnson–Sprinz syndrome. *Clin. Sci. Mol. Med.* **54**:549.
30. Huber, W., and Saifer, M. G. P. (1977). Orgotein, the drug version of bovine Cu-Zn superoxide dismutase. I. A summary account of safety and pharmacology in laboratory animals. *In* "Superoxide and Superoxide Dismutases" (A. M. Michelson, J. M. McCord, and I. Fridovich, eds.), p. 517. Academic Press, New York.
31. Menander-Huber, K. B., and Huber, W. (1977). Orgotein, the drug version of bovine Cu-Zn superoxide dismutase. II. A summary of chinical trials in man and animals. *In* "Superoxide and Superoxide Dismutases" (A. M. Michelson, J. M. McCord, and I. Fridovich, eds.), p. 537. Academic Press, New York.
32. Petkau, A., Chelack, W. S., and Pleskach, S. D. (1976). Letter: Protection of post-irradiated mice by superoxide dismutase. *Int. J. Radiat. Biol.* **29**:297.
33. Michelson, A. M., Puget, K., Perdereau, B., and Barbaroux, C. (1981). Scintigraph studies on the localisation of liposomal superoxide dismutase injected into rabbits. *Mol. Physiol.* **1**:71.
34. Emerit, I., Housset, J., deGrouchy, J. P. and Camus, J. P. (1971). Chromosomal breakage in diffuse scleroderma, a study of 27 patients. *Rev. Eur. Etud. Clin. Biol.* **16**:684.
35. Emerit, I., Feingold, J., and Housset, E. (1976). Chromosomal breakage and scleroderma: Studies in family members. *J. Lab. Clin. Med.* **88**:81.
36. Emerit, I. (1976). Chromosomal breakage in systemic sclerosis and related disorders (Editorial). *Dermatologica* **153**:145.
37. Emerit, I., Emerit, J., Tosoni-Pittoni, A., Bousquet, O., and Sarrazin, A. (1972). Chromosome studies in patients with ulcerative colitis. *Humangenetik* **16**:313.
38. Emerit, I., Feingold, J., Camus, J. P., and Housset, E. (1974). Etude chromosomique des maladies du collagene. *Ann. Genet.* **17**:251.
39. Emerit, J., Emerit, I., Levy, E., and Loygue, J. (1978). La D-pénicillamine est-elle efficace dans la maladie de Crohn? *Gastroenterol. Clin. Biol.* **2**:114.
40. Emerit, I., and Marteau, R. (1971). Chromosome studies in 14 patients with disseminated sclerosis. *Humangenetik* **13**:625.
41. Emerit, I., Levy, A., and Housset, E. (1974). Breakage factor in systemic sclerosis and protector effect of L-cysteine. *Humangenetik* **25**:221.
42. Emerit, I., Levy, A., and Housset, E. (1973). Sclérodermie généralisée et cassures Chromosomiques mise en évidence d'un facteur cassant dans le sérum des malades. *Ann. Genet.* **16**:135.
43. Emerit, I., and Michelson, A. M. (1980). Chromosome instability in human and murine auto-immuno disease. Anticlastogenic effect of superoxide dismutase. *Acta Physiol Scand.* **492**:59.
44. Nordenson, I. (1977). Chromosome breaks in Werner's syndrome and their prevention *in vitro* by radical-scavenging enzymes. *Hereditas* **87**:151.
45. Nordenson, I. (1977). Effect of superoxide dismutase and catalase on spontaneously occurring chromosome breaks in patients with Fanconi's anemia. *Hereditas* **86**:147.
46. Nordenson, I., Beckman, G., and Beckman, L. (1976). The effect of superoxide dismutase and catalase on radiation-induced chromosome breaks. *Hereditas* **82**:125.
47. Tice, R., Windler, G., and Rary, J. M. (1978). Effect of cocultivation on sister chromatid exchange frequencies in Bloom's syndrome and normal fibroblast cells. *Nature (London)* **273**:538.
48. Emerit, I., Keck, M., Levy, A., Feingold, J., and Michelson, A. M. (1982). Activated oxygen species at the origin of chromosome breakage and sister chromatid exchanges. *Mutation Research* **103**:165.

49. Lacour, F., Nahon-Merlin, E., and Michelson, A. M. (1973). Immunological recognition of polynucleotide structure. *Curr. Top. Microbiol. Immunol.* **62**:1.
50. Emerit, J., and Michelson, A. M. (1981). Crohn's Disease. *In* "Developments in Gastro-enterology. Vol. I. Recent Advances in Crohn's Disease" (A. S. Pena, I. T. Weterman, C. C. Booth, and W. Strober, eds.), p. 486. Martinus Nijhoff, The Hague/Boston/London.
51. Emerit, J., Camus, J. P., and Michelson, A. M. (1980). Treatment of autoimmune diseases with superoxide dismutase and D-penicillamine. *In* "Biological and Clinical Aspects of Superoxide and Superoxide Dismutase" (W. H. Bannister and J. V. Bannister, eds.), p. 381. Elsevier/North Holland, New York/Amsterdam/Oxford.

DISCUSSION

FRIDOVICH: How was the ^{57}Co associated with the superoxide dismutase, and how can you be sure that the Co remained bound to the enzyme *in vivo?*

MICHELSON: Apoenzymes were prepared by withdrawal of the metal (Cu, Mn, or Fe) and replacement by carrier-free ^{57}Co. The radioactive protein was then heavily diluted with the native nonradioactively labeled enzyme. That the Co^{2+} does not leak was shown by parallel studies in which the same amount of ^{57}Co was injected into the animal. Parallel *in vitro* studies also showed that the Co label was as stable as the original metal in the protein.

McLENNAN: Does CuZnSOD (bovine) cross the blood–brain barrier? This question has some relevance considering the differences noted at this meeting in the failure of superoxide dismutase to modify neurobiological models of inflammation in contrast to models of inflammation outside of the central nervous system.

MICHELSON: No superoxide dismutase in any of the preparations described crossed the blood–brain barrier in rats or rabbits. We tried using a sphingomyelin liposome, but this also failed to cross the barrier.

McLENNAN: One way to test the hypothesis regarding the value of superoxide dismutase in immunological diseases is to study the New Zealand B/W hybrid mouse, which is a model of immune complex disease. Have you had any experience with this model?

MICHELSON: Dr. I. Emerit has considerable experience with the New Zealand B/W hybrid mouse and has described this work in several publications.

Chapter 18

Superoxide Dismutase Treatment of Myelosuppression Resulting from Cancer Chemotherapy

ROY P. VILLASOR

INTRODUCTION

Myelosuppression is a common, well-documented undesirable side effect of cancer chemotherapy. The resulting leukopenia requires a reduction of the dose of the chemotherapeutic agent, an increase in the time between injections, or a termination of the therapy, all of which may jeopardize the effectiveness of chemotherapy. When the leukocyte count falls below 1000/mm³ of blood, there is danger of severe infection, which may lead to death. This critical situation may require placing the patient in a germ-free or sterile environment. In addition, the most effective antibiotics must be administered and other measures taken to prevent and control infection while the bone marrow recovers.

Chemotherapists, therefore should be interested in all possible means of protecting the bone marrow and of hastening its recovery from myelosuppression. If successful, such measures would not only prevent unnecessary fatalities from chemotherapy, but would also allow the administration of higher tumorcidal doses or the continuation of the therapy beyond the usual limits of tolerance. From the immunological standpoint, the protection and rapid recovery of the bone marrow could enhance the immunological defenses, which are usually suppressed by aggressive chemotherapy.

PATHOLOGY OF OXYGEN
Copyright © 1982 by Academic Press, Inc.
All rights of reproduction in any form reserved.
ISBN 0-12-068620-1

It was surmised from studies on the biological effects of ionizing radiation (1) as well as the protection against radiation damage afforded by administered superoxide dismutase (2) that the myelosuppression following chemotherapy may also be caused by the enhanced production of superoxide radicals by the propagation of free radical chain reactions. Hence, in 1976, pilot studies were begun to assess the potential usefulness of superoxide dismutase in the treatment of myelosuppression associated with the chemotherapy of cancer.

CANCER CHEMOTHERAPY

The first case of leukopenia resulting from cancer chemotherapy and radiation to be treated with superoxide dismutase occurred in Manila in December 1977. A patient with metastatic breast cancer developed severe leukopenia for the second time following combination chemotherapy and radiation. When her leukocyte count dropped to 600/mm³ of blood, she became seriously ill with an infection from *Pseudomonas* and β-hemolytic *Streptococcus*. In addition, she had two carbuncles, one below the right eye and another on the right thigh. Adrenocorticotropin (ACTH), given successfully for severe leukopenia (250/mm³ of blood) 1 month previously, did not provide a sufficiently rapid effect when used a second time. However, upon the administration of superoxide dismutase (orgotein, Diagnostic Data, Inc.), the leukocyte count rose rapidly and exceeded the normal level in just 3 days (Fig. 1A).

A rapid and dramatic resolution of the carbuncles occurred following a combined intralesional and intramuscular injection of superoxide dismutase. In a few days, the inflamed areas shrank to small necrotic cores, which were easily removed. Rapid healing followed.

Many factors influence the reaction of the blood count to chemotherapy and to measures against leukopenia. Among them are the following:

1. Age. Patients older than 65 years are more likely to develop severe myelosuppression than younger patients and also have a poorer chance of recovery.

2. The extent or stage of cancer. Patients with metastatic disease and with poor performance status according to the Karnofsky scale are poor responders when leukopenia supervenes. This is particularly true when there is previous liver damage and when the bone marrow is invaded by the tumor growth.

3. Immunological status.

4. Previous chemotherapy or radiation.

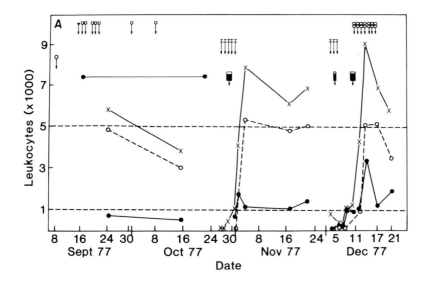

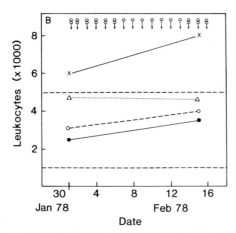

Fig. 1. (A) Comparison of the effects of treatment with ACTH and superoxide dismutase (orgotein) on the depression of leukocyte count (severe leukopenia) resulting from radiation therapy for cancer. The patient was a 41-year-old woman, with metastatic breast cancer. She received cobalt therapy (4500 rads) from September 16 to October 20 (●——●). Blood cells are designated as follows: total leukocytes (x——x), absolute segmenters (○-----○), lymphocytes (●——●). Therapy is indicated as follows: exploratory laparotomy, bilateral oophorectomy (⚲); endoxan, 200 and 500 mg (⊽); Acthar gel, 2 ml ACTH (∓); superoxide dismutase, 10 mg (⚲); blood transfusion (1 unit, ▯) (2 units, ▮). (B) Effect of intravenously administered superoxide dismutase on the depressed leukocyte count of an 80-year-old woman with basal ganglia degeneration. Blood cells are designated as follows: total leukocytes (x——x), absolute segmenters (○-----○), lymphocytes (●——●). Hemoglobin is represented by △-----△. Therapy is indicated as follows: superoxide dismutase, 5 mg (⚲), 10 mg (⚲).

5. The chemotherapeutic agent used, as well as the dosage and the timing or schedule.

6. The use of other adjuvants to prevent and minimize myelosuppression and promote rapid recovery. This includes the use of corticosteroids, blood transfusion, intravenous iron preparations, inosine compounds, bacillus Calmette–Guerin vaccine and other immunostimulants, and immunopotentiators such as leyamisole and methisoprinol.

Because so many factors are involved and because the number of patients with cancer-chemotherapy-associated leukopenia available to us is limited, we were unable to conduct a controlled randomized study. We therefore developed a pilot study that utilized mainly cases of leukopenia following cyclophosphamide treatment. This anticancer drug is the most extensively studied chemotherapeutic agent. Several dosage schedules or regimens of this drug have been used. Cyclophosphamide has a platelet-sparing effect, and the recovery from myelosuppression is rapid enough to allow for a shorter time period for the follow-up evaluation.

In order to maximize the potential effect of superoxide dismutase, the enzyme was administered intravenously in all but three cases in a dose of from 5 to 20 mg. The 10 mg dose was the most commonly used. Superoxide dismutase was also administered to patients with medical conditions other than cancer to ascertain its effect on the blood cell count.

In an 80-year-old woman suffering from chronic intention tremors due to basal ganglia degeneration, superoxide dismutase had a definite stimulating effect on the bone marrow, as reflected by the increase to high normal values of total leukocyte, absolute segmenter, and absolute lymphocyte counts. The hemoglobin level in this patient was not affected (Fig. 1B).

In various studies of leukopenia following cyclophosphamide treatment (3), the average response to a large single dose of 1000 mg, or about 20 mg/kg, administered intravenously was a maximum depression of leukocyte count occurring between the seventh and thirteenth day after treatment (Fig. 2). Most investigators report a return to normal values at about 10 days after the minimum leukocyte count occurs. The values in Fig. 2 serve as a baseline for comparison with the effect of superoxide dismutase on leukopenia produced by different dosage schedules of cyclophosphamide and other drugs.

Cyclophosphamide is frequently given in massive daily doses of 30 mg/kg per day for 5 days for difficult, rapidly progressing, or threatening cancer, such as bronchogenic carcinoma with superior vena caval syndrome, brain metastases, or generalized metastatic breast cancer. In the case of a 71-year-old woman treated for metastatic breast cancer accord-

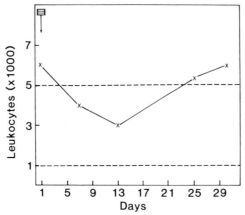

Fig. 2. Leukocyte count following a single treatment with cyclophosphamide. Total leukocytes (x——x), cyclophosphamide, 1000 mg (⊟).

ing to the above-described schedule, the leukocyte count dropped rapidly to a point of apparent irreversibility in 9 days (Fig. 3A). The patient subsequently died of infection. Among patients given this high-dose regimen, the minimum leukocyte count, usually below 1000/mm³, at which life is threatened is reached between the second and ninth day following the fifth intravenous injection of cyclophosphamide.

A 56-year-old man with bronchogenic carcinoma (small cell type) with metastases to the brain and skull was treated with a high-dosage regimen of cyclophosphamide with a resulting depression of leukocyte count (Fig. 3B). Superoxide dismutase given intravenously in an average dose of 10 mg daily dramatically raised the leukocyte level to normal in 3–8 days. The safe level of 1000/mm³ of blood was reached within 3 days following this treatment. No infection was observed in this patient.

It was previously noted that in patients with advanced cancer already under chemotherapy, particularly patients who are weak and have had previous radiation treatment and/or chemotherapy, superoxide dismutase if given early, before the onset of leukopenia, can prevent this side effect from occurring. This appeared to be the case with a 52-year-old woman suffering from terminal cancer of the cervix uteri with frozen pelvis (Fig. 4A). Superoxide dismutase also apparently allowed the continuation of chemotherapy in an even higher dosage and in combination with cobalt therapy in the case of a 36-year-old woman with terminal adenocarcinoma (primary unknown) with metastases to the bones and lungs (Fig. 4B).

Leukopenia produced by other anticancer drugs, such as methotrexate, nitrogen mustard, vincristine, 5-fluorouracil, and phthorafur, is also ap-

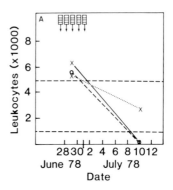

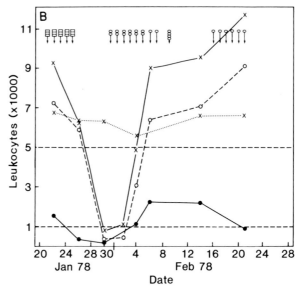

Fig. 3. (A) Depression of leukocyte count following a single treatment with cyclophos-phamide (30 mg/kg daily for 5 days) for metastatic breast cancer. The patient was a 71-year-old woman. Blood cells are designated as follows: total leukocytes (x——x), absolute seg-menters (O-----O). Hemoglobin is represented by x·····x. Therapy is indicated as follows: endoxan, 2000 mg (⊟). (B) Effect of intravenous administration of superoxide dismutase on leukopenia following high-dose chemotherapy (30 mg/kg daily for 5 days). The patient was a 56-year-old man with bronchogenic carcinoma including small cell-type metastases to the brain and skull. Blood cells are designated as follows: total leukocytes (x——x), absolute segmenters (O-----O), lymphocytes (●——●). Hemoglobin is represented by x·····x. Ther-apy is designated as follows: endoxan, 1500 mg (⊟); superoxide dismutase, 5 mg (♀), 10 mg (♀), 20 mg (♀).

parently reversed by superoxide dismutase treatment with the same degree of effectiveness as seen with cyclophosphamide. The expected drop in leukocyte count after a combination nitrogen mustard–vincristine regimen was seen in a 72-year-old man suffering from a histiocytic type of malignant lymphoma with metastases to the lungs and liver. The nadir of 180 leukocytes per cubic millimeter of blood was reached in 9 days despite transfusion of 4 units of whole blood. Following the regular administration of superoxide dismutase with increased dose to 20 mg/day given

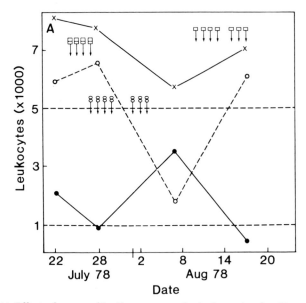

Fig. 4. (A) Effect of superoxide dismutase on the leukopenia of a 52-year-old woman with terminal cancer of the cervix uteri with metastases. Blood cells are designated as follows: total leukocytes (x———x), absolute segmenters (O-----O), lymphocytes (●———●). Therapy is indicated as follows: endoxan, 500 mg (⊟), 1000 mg (⊟); superoxide dismutase, 10 mg iv (⦶). (B) Effect of superoxide dismutase on white blood cell count during extended high-dose cancer therapy. The patient was a 36-year-old woman with terminal, metastasizing adenocarcinoma. Blood cells are designated as follows: total leukocytes (x———x), absolute segmenters (O-----O), lymphocytes (●———●). Hemoglobin is represented by x·····x. Therapy is designated as follows: cobalt therapy (●———●) from January 1 to February 10; 5-fluorouracil, 500 mg (⦶), 750 mg (⦶); FT 207,800 mg (▮); superoxide dismutase 10 mg iv (⦶). (C) Effect of increased dose of superoxide dismutase on the depressed leukocyte count in a cancer patient treated with chemotherapy. The patient was a 72-year-old man with a malignant lymphoma and metastases to the lungs and liver. Blood cells are designated as follows: total leukocytes (x———x), absolute segmenters (O-----O), lymphocytes (●———●). The therapy is indicated as follows: HN₂ vincristine (↓); blood transfusion, 4 units (▮); superoxide dismutase, 10 mg (⦶), 20 mg (⦶).

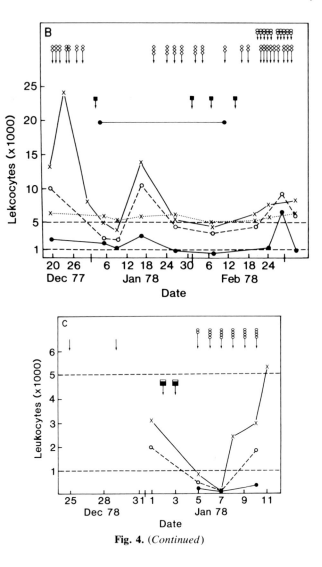

Fig. 4. (*Continued*)

intravenously, the leukocyte count rose to a safe level of 1000/mm³ in 2 days and to the normal level of 5000/mm³ in 4 days (Fig. 4C).

MISCELLANEOUS CASES

Myelosuppression unrelated to cancer chemotherapy was treated with superoxide dismutase. A 71-year-old woman with a case of chronic sideroblastic anemia accompanied by severe myelosuppression did not respond to treatment with prednisone and frequent blood transfusions. Following the administration of superoxide dismutase, the total leukocyte count was elevated. When assessed individually, the segmenters and lymphocytes were beyond the normal level. This increase, however, occurred after approximately 1 month (Fig. 5A).

An opposite effect on leukocyte level was observed in a patient with an

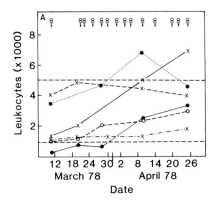

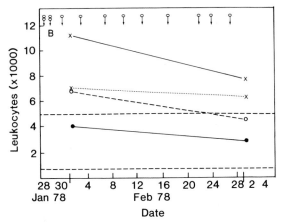

Fig. 5. (A) Effect of superoxide dismutase administration in severe myelosuppression associated with sideroblastic anemia. The patient was a 71-year-old woman. Blood cells are designated as follows: total leukocytes (x——x), platelets (●-----●), absolute segmenters (○-----○), absolute lymphocytes (●——●), reticulocytes (x·······x). Hemoglobin is represented by x·····x. Therapy is designated as follows: superoxide dismutase, 10 mg (♀). (B) Effect of superoxide dismutase on the leukocyte count in a 49-year-old woman with acute osteoarthritis. Blood cells are designated as follows: total leukocytes (x——x), absolute segmenters (○-----○), lymphocytes (●——●). Hemoglobin is represented by x·····x. Therapy is designated as follows: superoxide dismutase, 5 mg (♀), 10 mg (♀).

initial high leukocyte count. Acute osteoarthritis of the knee in a 49-year-old woman was unresponsive to oral antirheumatic medications and to intraarticular corticosteroid injections. The leukocyte count remained high. The response to superoxide dismutase administration, however, was a decrease to low normal leukocyte values (Fig. 5B).

EVALUATION

Thirty-two consecutive cases of leukopenia treated with superoxide dismutase either during or after chemotherapy for cancer were included in this study. Seven were treated with ACTH before superoxide dismutase became available for treatment. Twenty-three cases were treated with superoxide dismutase. Two were treated with a combination of ACTH and superoxide dismutase.

Superoxide dismutase was given intravenously in a routine dose of 10 mg/day in most cases. There were no observed adverse reactions to this treatment when given by any route. In all cases in which the superoxide dismutase was given early enough and the patient was not too critically ill with cancer, there was a fairly rapid recovery of the leukocyte count, which was much faster than expected from treatment with other agents.

Of the 32 patients studied, 17 had leukopenia with cell counts below $1000/mm^3$ of blood. Thirteen of these patients were treated with superoxide dismutase and 4 with ACTH. Of the 13 superoxide dismutase-treated patients, 3 died, 2 of terminal disease and 1 of infection, the superoxide dismutase treatment having been started too late because of an error in the assessment of the leukocyte count. In the superoxide dismutase-treated group, the full restoration of the leukocyte count to normal took from 3 to 11 days, or an average of 4.7 days (Table I). However, partial recovery to the safe level of 1000 cells/mm^3 of blood and higher took from 0.5 to 6.5 days, or an average of 3 days. In the ACTH-treated patients, full recovery took from 5 to 11 days, or an average of 6.7 days. Thus, in severe leukopenia, superoxide dismutase treatment resulted in a faster recovery of the leukocyte count to normal than did ACTH treatment.

Of the 13 patients with leukocyte counts above $1000/mm^3$, the full recovery of 3 patients in the ACTH-treated group varied from 1 to 6 days, or an average of 2.7 days, whereas in the 10 superoxide dismutase-treated patients, full recovery took 2–16 days, or an average of 8 days. In patients with mild to moderate leukopenia, full recovery of the leukocyte count was faster with ACTH than with superoxide dismutase (Table I).

The observed difference in the time required to reach the normal leuko-

TABLE I

Recovery of Leukocyte Number after treatment of Patients with ACTH and with Superoxide Dismutase

Leukocyte count after chemotherapy	Recovery[a] (days)	
(per mm³ blood)	ACTH	Superoxide dismutase
>1000	2.7	8.0
<1000	6.7	4.7

[a] Average value; calculated from the number of patients observed, as well as the number of days required for recovery.

cyte count of 5000/mm³ may be due to the different mechanisms of action of ACTH and superoxide dismutase. Both superoxide dismutase and corticosteroids appear to have membrane-stabilizing capabilities (4), which prevent the leakage of hydrolytic enzymes from lysosomes, thus sparing to some extent the leukocyte population from the destructive action of chemotherapy. The main action of antiinflammatory steroids, however, is the immediate mobilization of the white blood cells from the marginal reserve pool into the blood circulation. Superoxide dismutase, however, catalyzes the destruction of the free radicals of oxygen or superoxide, with apparent detoxifying effects. This may prevent further destruction of bone marrow and allow the proliferation and rapid recovery of the leukocytes.

In severe leukopenia, when the marginal reserve pool of leukocytes is severely depleted, the response to ACTH becomes slower and the drug may not be effective in the long run. Superoxide dismutase seems to provide immediate protective action by detoxifying the superoxide free radical, the presence of which can result in destructive free-radical chain reactions. Superoxide dismutase has another very important characteristic in cancer therapy that ACTH does not have: It does not interfere with the developing delayed hypersensitivity reaction (5) and may actually potentiate cell-mediated immune response. In contrast, by increasing the production of corticosteroids, ACTH suppresses immunity.

ACKNOWLEDGMENTS

Appreciation is expressed for the hard work and assistance of Susan S. Wong and Antonio Tan in collecting and presenting the data on which this study is based.

REFERENCES

1. Behar, D., Czapski, G., Dorfman, L. M., Rabani, J., and Schwarz, H. A. (1970). The acid dissociation constant and decay kinetics of the perhydroxyl radical. *J. Phys. Chem.* **74:**3209.
2. Petkau, A., Chelack, W. S., and Peskach, S. D. (1978). Protection by superoxide dismutase of white blood cells in X-irradiated mice. *Life Sci.* **22:**867.
3. Stoll, B. A., and Matar, J. H. (1961). Cyclophosphamide in advanced breast cancer. *Br. Med. J.* **2:**283.
4. Huber, W., and Saifer, M. G. P. (1977). Orgotein, the drug version of bovine Cu-Zn superoxide dismutase. I. A summary account of safety and pharmacology in laboratory animals. *In* "Superoxide and Superoxide Dismutase" (A. M. Michelson, J. M. McCord, and I. Fridovich, eds.), p. 517. Academic Press, New York.
5. Menander-Huber, K. B., and Huber, W. (1977). Orgotein, the drug version of bovine Cu-Zn superoxide dismutase. II. A summary account of clinical trials in man and animals. *In* "Superoxide and Superoxide Dismutase" (A. M. Michelson, J. M. McCord, and I. Fridovich, eds.), p. 537. Academic Press, New York.

DISCUSSION

McGINNESS: How did the subpopulations of leukocytes respond to the treatment, and how long did the elevated levels of leukocytes persist?

VILLASOR: I have charted only the total white blood cells/leukocytes (WBC's), absolute segmenters, and absolute lymphocytes. The effect on the latter two are variable depending on many factors. In noncancer cases, there is a normalizing effect on these three parameters. (The hemoglobin is not affected.) In most cancer cases, the absolute lymphocyte and absolute segmenter numbers follow the rise of the total WBC's. In others, the absolute lymphocyte number goes down. I did not chart the monocytes.

ŌYANAGUI: What is the clinical effect of superoxide dismutase on tumor cell metastasis?

VILLASOR: It would not be possible to determine such an effect clinically because of the means of treatment. I do not think that superoxide dismutase has a direct antitumor effect, but then I am studying very advanced cases of cancer with so many variables that any specific antitumor therapy is bound to fail. I find I have to resume chemotherapy in many cases in order to maintain control of tumor growth.

Chapter 19

Superoxide Dismutase Efficacy in Ameliorating Side Effects of Radiation Therapy: Double-Blind, Placebo-Controlled Trials in Patients with Bladder and Prostate Tumors

FOLKE EDSMYR

INTRODUCTION

CuZn-Superoxide dismutase is an enzyme that has the properties of an antiinflammatory drug. It differs from many other antiinflammatory agents presently being used (1) in that it apparently is free of serious side effects and is very safe when administered to man and animals (2). It is a stable, soluble metalloprotein of molecular weight about 32,000 found intracellularly in liver, kidney, red blood cells, and other tissues in various amounts (3). Both the amino acid sequence of the two subunits and the structural features of the protein have been determined, so that the essential molecular features of the molecule are well understood (4,5).

In nature, CuZnSOD occurs in all cells of oxygen-consuming organisms, where it catalyzes the dismutation of superoxide anions (O_2^-), which can be formed by a host of intracellular autoxidations (6). When it is generated extracellularly, O_2^-, described as an active radical, can be a

315

PATHOLOGY OF OXYGEN

threat to the integrity of living systems, since the concentration of superoxide dismutases in mammalian plasma is very low (about 10 ng/ml). It has been shown that exogenous superoxide dismutase *in vitro* inhibits the cytotoxic effects of the superoxide anion generated by phagocytosing neutrophils and macrophages (7). That irradiation results in cell death with subsequent invasion of phagocytosing cells has long been established (8). The undesirable side effects of radiation therapy are at least partly due to such phenomena.

We initiated our studies in Stockholm in 1973 on the basis of the belief that superoxide dismutase could reduce inflammatory side effects in patients receiving high-dose irradiation for the treatment of pelvic tumors. Since the destruction of malignant cells by high-energy radiation is largely a direct-hit nuclear event that occurs in the presence of a relatively high concentration of superoxide dismutases in the cytosol, we believed that there would be no interference with the tumorolytic events by extracellular superoxide dismutase. That this is true is supported by *in vitro* as well as *in vivo* animal experiments (Tables I and II), which document the absence of any superoxide dismutase effect on tumor tissue for various radiation regimens, for intratumor injections, and for systemic injections of up to 400 mg/kg.

CLINICAL TRIALS

For our clinical trials we selected two types of pelvic tumors: urinary bladder carcinoma and prostatic carcinoma. These provided useful parameters for evaluating the effect of superoxide dismutase during and after irradiation of the localized tumor. The tumors were all classified before the therapy according to the UICC TNM system. Histological grading followed the World Health Organization system. In our studies, the tumors fell into stages T_2-T_4 and malignancy grades 1–3. The studies were designed as double-blind, placebo-controlled with the code system retained in the United States and unknown to us.

Four or 8 mg of either superoxide dismutase (administered as orgotein, Diagnostic Data, Inc.) or a placebo dissolved in approximately 1 ml of saline solution (USP) were injected deeply, subcutaneously, 15–30 min after the completion of each daily radiation session.

All patients received high-energy radiation with 6 MV X rays delivered by a linear accelerator using a three-field technique (10). Patients received antibacterial therapy throughout the trial and were permitted to use one

TABLE I

Effects of Superoxide Dismutase Administration on Tumor Growth and Radiotherapy in Mice

Test system	Species (number)	Irradiation[a]	Superoxide dismutase[b] (dose and time)	Effects
KHT sarcoma[c]	Mice (8)	300 × 10, 2 weeks	4 and 40 mg/kg, sc (5 times/week for 4 weeks)	None
L$_1$A$_2$ cell line,[d] C$_3$H mouse lung	Mice, tissue culture[e] (3)	200, 400, 600, 800, 1000, respectively, to culture (300–400 cells)	200 μg in 10 ml (3 hr before or ½ hr after irradiation)	None
Jejunal crypt cells *in vivo*[d]	Mice (4)	100, 200, 400, 600, 800, 1000, respectively to gut	50 mg/kg, ip; 2 mg/ml (2 hr before or ½ hr after irradiation)	None
13762 mammary adeno-carcinoma transplants	Rats (10)	None	250 μg/4 sites intratumor (days 13–17, 19–23)	None
Walker carcinoma	Rats (6)	None	1.6 mg/kg intratumor (7 days)	None

[a] 250 KV, 15 mA, rads.
[b] Administered as orgotein, Diagnostic Data, Inc.
[c] R. P. Hill, personal communication.
[d] See Overgaard *et al.* (9).
[e] BME (GIBCO C-14) + 10% fetal calf serum.

specified antidiarrheal agent as needed. No other antiinflammants in addition to superoxide dismutase were permitted.

The effects of the experimental medication were assessed using the following parameters: pain, dysuria, maximum voided volume, interval between voidings during day and night, severity of diarrhea, and amount of medication needed to control diarrhea. The patients were evaluated at regular intervals after entry into the trial. One visit always coincided with the termination of therapy. Follow-up evaluations were done at least at about 4 months and 2 years thereafter. Hematology and urinalysis were performed at each visit, and clinical chemistry was carried out at the beginning and end of the treatment.

TABLE II

Effects of Superoxide Dismutase on Tumors from Different Systems

Tumor system (species)	Superoxide dismutase		Other treatment	Effect on tumor
	Dosage (mg/kg)	Route of administration		
Mammary adenoma carcinoma (rat, $n = 10$)	0.25 (× 10)	Intratumor	—	No change in growth pattern
Mammary adenoma carcinoma (rat, $n = 10$)	0.30 (×55)	sc	Estradiol alkylating agent	No change in growth pattern
Lymphocytic leukemia L-1210 (mice, $n = 454$)	0.02–400	sc	—	No change in growth pattern
Melanocyte carcinoma B-16 (mice, $n = 100$)	25–400 (×9)	ip	—	No change in growth pattern
Lymphocytic leukemia P-338 (mice, $n = 30$)	25–400 (×9)	ip	—	No change in growth pattern
Lewis lung carcinoma (mice, $n = 50$)	25–400 (×9)	ip	—	No change in growth pattern
Lymphocytic leukemia L-1210 (mice, $n = 200$)	0.025–0.4	sc	Cyclophosphamide	No change in growth pattern
Lymphocytic leukemia L-1210 (mice, $n = 250$)	0.025–0.4	sc	Nitrogen mustard	No change in growth pattern
Lymphocytic leukemia L-1210 (mice, $n = 400$)	0.025–0.4	sc	BCNU	Increase in survival time
KHT sarcoma (mice, $n = 30$)	0.4–40 (×20)	so	Radiation	No change in growth pattern
KHT sarcoma (mice, $n = 30$)	0.4–40 (×1)	sc	Radiation	No change in growth pattern

TREATMENT OF BLADDER CARCINOMA

In the first double-blind, placebo-controlled study on 42 patients with urinary bladder carcinoma, superoxide dismutase (4 mg) and placebo medication were randomly distributed among the patients. Twenty-one patients received superoxide dismutase, and 21 received the placebo. The patients entering the trial were randomly assigned to either 6400 or 8400 rads given during 2 months. In the first group, a calculated tumor dose of 200 rads was given once per day, 5 days weekly. In the second group, a calculated tumor dose of 100 rads was given three times daily with 4-hr intervals. Both groups received treatment 5 days/week with a rest of 2 weeks following the first 3 weeks of treatment.

The efficacy of superoxide dismutase when compared with the placebo is summarized in Table III, which shows that in six of seven parameters evaluated superoxide dismutase was significantly ($p < .05 – .001$) more effective in reducing signs and symptoms in both the bladder and the bowel (11). This indicates that superoxide dismutase provides a therapeutic regimen for control of these side effects.

Follow-up evaluations, after the termination of radiation therapy, at 4 months and 2 years, have now been completed for the patients in this trial. All 35 patients meeting the selection criteria of the protocol (20 patients who had received superoxide dismutase and 15 patients who had

TABLE III

Efficacy of Superoxide Dismutase Compound Compared with Placebo: Amelioration of Side Effects of Radiation Therapy for Bladder Carcinoma[a]

Parameter	Level of statistical significance (p)
Maximum voided volume of urine >200 ml	$<.05$[b]
Interval between voidings during day	$<.05$[b]
Interval between voidings during night	NS[c]
Severity of signs and symptoms from bladder	$<.05$[b]
Percentage of diarrhea complaints (visits to physician)	$<.025$[b]
Percentage of diarrhea complaints requiring medication	$<.001$[b]
Dose of antidiarrheal medication	$<.0025$[b]

[a] See Edsmyr et al. (11).
[b] Chi-square test.
[c] Not significant.

received placebo) were alive at the 4-month posttreatment evaluation. At that time, the amelioration of radiation-induced side effects in the bladder and bowel by superoxide dismutase compared with placebo was even more pronounced than at the termination of therapy. For example, 4 of 15 patients in the placebo group still had symptoms of proctitis, whereas all patients in the group treated with superoxide dismutase were free of it (12). At the 2-year follow-up, however, only 9 of the 35 patients were still alive (5 patients who had received superoxide dismutase and 4 who had received the placebo). This number was too small for statistical evaluation of ameliorative effects at this stage. It appears, however, that superoxide dismutase treatment concurrent with radiation therapy did not influence patient survival time or tumorolytic efficacy of irradiation. Therefore, because of the high death rate due to tumor recurrence, the late side effects of radiation treatment for bladder tumors could not be analyzed accurately.

TREATMENT OF PROSTATE CARCINOMA

In a second double-blind, placebo-controlled trial, 8 mg of superoxide dismutase or placebo per injection was administered to 50 patients receiving radiation therapy (5400 rads per 7 weeks) for poorly differentiated prostate carcinomas (Table IV). The administration of medication and evaluation of patients were performed as described above. In this study, radiation-induced side effects were seen in considerably fewer patients than expected from prior clinical experience. This is not an unusual effect. The mean calculated tumor dose including the bladder is 1000 rads lower in the group of prostatic carcinomas than in the group of bladder

TABLE IV

Parameters of Superoxide Dismutase Efficacy in Ameliorating Side Effects of Radiation Therapy for Prostatic Tumors

Patients selected	Diagnosed prostate tumors: T2–T4
Number of patients	50
Dosage: superoxide dismutase (orgotein) or placebo	8 mg administered subcutaneously after completion of daily radiation therapy
Radiation dosage	5400 rads in 7 weeks
Signs and symptoms	Maximal voiding volume; voiding frequency (bowel, bladder); pain; antidiarrheal medication: requirement and dosage

carcinomas. In the patients experiencing radiation-induced side effects, parameters lending themselves to analysis included change in overall signs and symptoms in bowel and bladder and change in voiding frequency of bowel and bladder, both during the day and at night. As shown in Figs. 1–6, superoxide dismutase therapy ameliorated side effects more effectively than placebo. In addition, the only patient who required surgery as a result of radiation-induced injury to the bowel belonged to the placebo-treated group. In view of the low overall frequency of serious, radiation-induced side effects, the differences between superoxide dismutase and placebo treatments were only occasionally statistically significant.

The two trials concluded so far show that, with the administration of superoxide dismutase, a single-drug therapeutic treatment of radiation-induced side effects could replace the currently used symptomatic treatment with anticholinergic drugs, analgesics, and opiates. An additional and more challenging aspect of these studies is the potential for using concomitant superoxide dismutase treatment in order to employ higher radiation doses, which might provide better therapeutic results (Table V). In a first attempt to explore this, we are now conducting a double-blind, placebo-controlled trial in patients suffering from poorly differentiated prostate carcinomas. The patients receive a radiation regimen of 5000 rads for

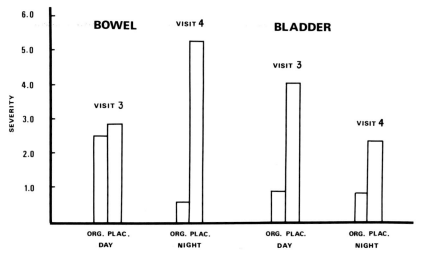

Fig. 1. Effect of placebo (PLAC.) and superoxide dismutase (ORG.) treatment on the severity of the side effects of radiation therapy on bowel and bladder function. Descriptions of the patients, details of treatment, and the signs and symptoms used for this evaluation are listed in Table IV. Signs and symptoms were evaluated for both the day and the night, as indicated.

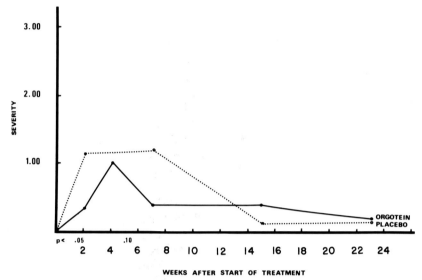

Fig. 2. Effect of prolonged treatment with placebo or superoxide dismutase (orgotein) on the severity of the side effects of radiation therapy on bowel function. The change in the severity of symptoms was evaluated.

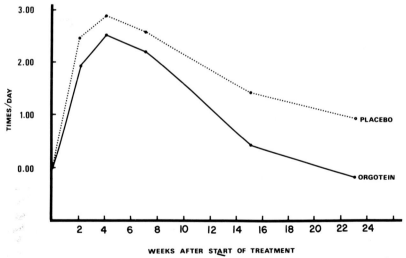

Fig. 3. Effect of prolonged treatment with placebo or superoxide dismutase (orgotein) on the frequency of bowel function following radiation therapy. Change in daytime frequency only was recorded.

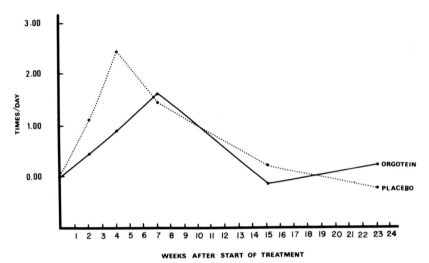

Fig. 4. Effect of prolonged treatment with placebo or superoxide dismutase (orgotein) on the frequency of bladder function following radiation therapy. Change in nighttime frequency only was recorded.

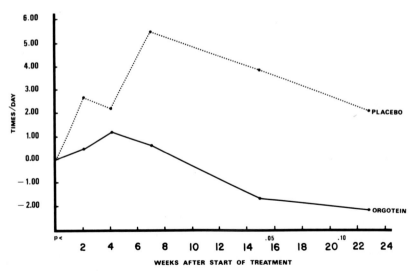

Fig. 5. Effect of prolonged treatment with placebo or superoxide dismutase (orgotein) on the frequency of bowel function following radiation therapy. Change in nighttime frequency only was recorded.

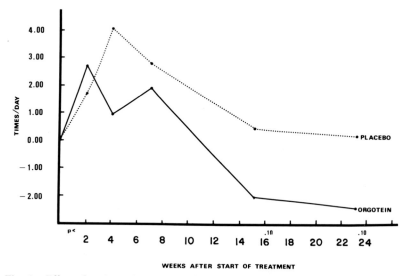

Fig. 6. Effect of prolonged treatment with placebo on superoxide dismutase (orgotein) on the frequency of bladder function following radiation therapy. Change in daytime frequency only was recorded.

7 weeks, which is directed at the prostatic gland as well as the surrounding lymph nodes. This includes a considerable volume of the body. After a 2-week rest interval a booster dose of 2000 rads is given for 2 weeks and is directed at the prostate only. Superoxide dismutase (16-mg doses) or the placebo is injected after each individual irradiation session and also daily

TABLE V

Parameters of Superoxide Dismutase Efficacy in Ameliorating Side Effects of Large-Field Radiation Therapy for Prostate Tumors and Adjacent Lymph Nodes

Patients selected	Diagnosed prostate tumors: T2–T4
Number of patients	50
Dosage: superoxide dismutase (orgotein) or placebo	16 mg administered subcutaneously after completion of daily radiation therapy and during rest period
Radiation	≥6 MV X irradiation, 5000 rads in 7 weeks to prostate and lymph nodes; 2 weeks rest, followed by 2000 rads as a booster for 2 weeks to prostate alone
Signs and symptoms	Maximal voiding volume; voiding frequency (bowel, bladder); pain; anti-diarrheal medication, requirement and dosage

during the 2-week rest period. For this clinical trial procedure, therefore, a total dose of 7000 rads is directed at the prostate, whereas a larger area, including the lymph nodes adjacent to the prostate, is exposed to a total dose of 5000 rads.

CONCLUSIONS

The contention that extracellularly administered superoxide dismutase does not interfere with tumor destruction caused by radiation therapy is now supported by *in vitro* and *in vivo* experiments with tumors in animals or animal cells, as well as by the clinical results obtained to date from patients treated for bladder malignancy. In these patients, superoxide dismutase administration concomitant with radiation therapy did not influence tumorolytic efficacy during the irradiation regimen or until the time of the final assessment 2 years after treatment.

The two double-blind, placebo-controlled trials completed thus far (for bladder and for prostate tumors) show that with superoxide dismutase administration a *therapeutic,* single-drug treatment of radiation-induced side effects is possible and could replace symptomatic treatment with anticholinergic drugs, analgesics, and opiates.

The preliminary results reported here indicate that concomitant administration of superoxide dismutase may make it possible for an irradiated patient to tolerate higher radiation doses. The administration of a higher radiation dosage with ameliorated adverse side effects may result in better tumor therapy. The validity of this premise is presently being explored in another double-blind, placebo-controlled trial in patients with prostatic carcinoma treated with an irradiation regimen in which a total dose of 7000 rads is directed at the prostate and a total dose of 5000 rads is directed at a larger area, including the lymph nodes adjacent to the prostate.

REFERENCES

1. Fridovich, I. (1975). A free radical pathology: Superoxide radical and superoxide dismutases. *Annu. Rep. Med. Chem.* **10**:257–264.
2. Carson, S., Vogin, E. E., Huber, W., and Schulte, T. L. (1973). Safety tests of orgotein, an antiinflammatory protein. *Toxicol. Appl. Pharmacol.* **26**:184.
3. Fridovich, I. (1975). Superoxide dismutases. *Annu. Rev. Biochem.* **44**:147.
4. Steinman, H., Naik, V., Abernethy, J., and Hill, R. (1974). Bovine erythrocyte superoxide dismutase. Complete amino acid sequence. *J. Biol. Chem.* **249**:7326.

5. Richardson, J., Thomas, K., Rubin, B., and Richardson, D. (1975). Crystal structure of bovine Cu-Zn superoxide dismutase at 3Å resolution: Chain tracing and metal ligands. *Proc. Natl. Acad. Sci. U.S.A.* **72:**1319.
6. Fridovich, I. (1975). A free radical pathology: Superoxide radical and superoxide dismutases. *Annu. Rep. Med. Chem.* **10:**257.
7. Salin, M. L., and McCord, J. M. (1975). Free radicals and inflammation. Protection of phagocytosing leukocytes by superoxide dismutase. *J. Clin. Invest.* **56:**1319.
8. Moss, W. T., and Ackermann, L. V., ed. (1965). "Therapeutic Radiology, 2nd ed. Mosby, St. Louis, Missouri.
9. Overgaard, J., Nielsen, O. S., Overgaard, M., Steenholdt, S., Jakobsen, A., and Sell, A. (1979). Studies on the possible radiation protective effect of orgotein in normal and malignant cells. *Acta Radiol.* **18:**305.
10. Littbrand, B., Edsmyr, F., and Revesz, L. W. (1975). A low dose fractionation scheme for the radiotherapy of carcinoma of the bladder. *Bull. Cancer* **62:**241.
11. Edsmyr, F., Huber, W., and Menander, K. B. (1976). Orgotein efficacy in ameliorating side effects due to radiation therapy. I. Double-blind, placebo-controlled trial in patients with bladder tumors. *Curr. Ther. Res.* **19:**198.
12. Menander-Huber, K. B., Edsmyr, F., and Huber, W. (1978). Orgotein (superoxide dismutase): A drug for the amelioration of radiation-induced side effects. A double-blind, placebo-controlled study in patients with bladder tumors. *Urol. Res.* **6:**255.

DISCUSSION

FRIDOVICH: How are you able to present data from your study when the code of the double-blind, placebo-controlled study has not yet been broken?

EDSMYR: We can present these data because the code identifying which individual is receiving the treatment and which is receiving the placebo is stored in a computer code in the United States. I have the coded clinical records in Stockholm, and from these files I can read all clinical and laboratory observations without knowing which individual patient is receiving the superoxide dismutase and which is receiving only placebo. The information identifying each patient is available only in the computer code. If I had the code, I would not be able to present these results in an objective manner because my clinical observations would be directed by my knowledge of the treatment of specific patients.

Chapter *20*

Superoxide Dismutase: A New Drug for the Treatment of Peyronie's Disease

GEORGE BARTSCH AND H. MARBERGER

INTRODUCTION

Despite the use of a wide variety of methods of treatment, both systemic and local, no satisfactory therapy for Peyronie's disease has yet been found (1,2). The search for an effective treatment, therefore, is still proceeding. Clinical studies have indicated the potential usefulness of superoxide dismutase in various urological disorders, especially in the treatment of radiation cystitis (3,4). This chapter presents the results obtained on the long-term superoxide dismutase treatment of 23 patients with Peyronie's disease.

PATIENTS

All 23 patients were diagnosed as showing the signs and symptoms of Peyronie's disease and were under treatment at the Department of Urology of the University of Innsbruck. All gave their informed consent before entering the study. The patients were instructed to return for regular checkups and to report immediately any adverse reactions or complications during treatment.

327

PATHOLOGY OF OXYGEN
Copyright © 1982 by Academic Press, Inc.
All rights of reproduction in any form reserved.
ISBN 0-12-068620-1

CLINICAL METHODS

Superoxide dismutase, a water-soluble metalloprotein, in contrast to other antiinflammatory agents, combines efficacy with substantial safety. Its pharmacodynamic effects were discovered in 1965 and first described in 1968 (5). The enzyme has since been shown to be effective in several animal models of induced inflammation and clinically in degenerative joint disease of man, as well as in a variety of disorders in several species of animals (6–9). Its toxicological, teratological, and immunological safety has been documented (10). Intravenous, intraarterial, intramuscular, subcutaneous, intraurethral, intramural, intrathecal, subconjunctival, and intraarticular routes of administration have all been utilized with complete safety (9). Except for a few cases of mild rash and occasional pain at the injection site, no adverse reactions have been noted in clinical investigations.

Superoxide dismutase (orgotein, Diagnostic Data, Inc.) was provided as a sterile, nonpyrogenic, lyophilized powder in single-use vials, each containing 2 or 4 mg drug stabilized with 4 or 8 mg sucrose, respectively. These preparations have a superoxide dismutase activity of at least 3000 units/mg protein. For administration, the contents were dissolved in sodium chloride injection, USP (pH 6.5–7.0). Individual doses were prepared by combining the contents of a sufficient number of superoxide dismutase vials of final concentration 1–2 mg/ml saline. Injections were given under general anesthesia, using a special syringe (Fig. 1). In this way, the solution could be deposited by manual pressure (Fig. 2) into the pathologically altered area of the indurated plaques.

Individual doses and dose regimen are listed in Table I. The mean total intraplaque dose was 35.8 mg, and the mean dose per injection was ap-

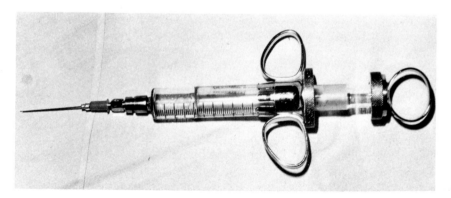

Fig. 1.   Special syringe for depositing the enzyme intraplaqueally.

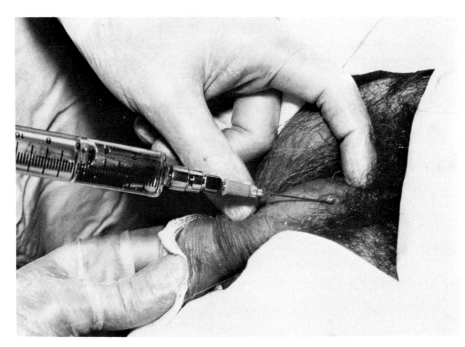

Fig. 2. Deposition of the enzyme under manual pressure into the pathologically altered area of the indurated plaques.

proximately 8.2 mg. Initially, all patients received three intraplaque injections at monthly intervals. The patients who required more than three injections received additional therapy at approximately monthly intervals. Depending on the clinical improvements, therapy thereafter was administered when needed. The patients were instructed to observe and regard any adverse reactions during treatment and to pay particular attention to any sensitization reactions.

EVALUATION

The same investigator conducted the evaluation of treatment for all of the patients. The following parameters were used: overall clinical status, pain without erection, pain on erection, deviation of the penis, induration size, and induration consistency. The pain status and the degree of penis deviation were determined using a five-point scale of increasing severity as follows: 0, none; 1, slight; 2, moderate; 3, severe; 4, very severe. In-

TABLE I

Cumulative Intraplaque Superoxide Dismutase Dose with Successive Treatment (mg)

Patient	Visit 1	2	3	4	5	6	7	8	9	10	11	12	13	Total visits—last
A.F.	5	15	25	35	45	45	55	65	69	69	69			69
B.B.	10	20	30											20
C.C.	10	20	30	30	40	50	60							50
D.F.-1	10	20	30											20
D.F.-2	10	20	30	40										40
G.A.	5	10	10	20	30	30	40							30
G.E.	10													10
G.P.	10	20	30	40										30
H.A.	10	20	30											20
H.M.	10	20	20											20
H.R.	10	20	20	30										20
K.A.	6	12	18	24	30	35	40	45	55	65	65			65
K.E.	10	20	30	40	44									40
K.H.	10	20	30											20
K.J.	5	10	20	20										20
K.W.	10	20	20	20										20
L.J.	10	20	30	30	40									30
S.E.	5	10	15	20	25	30	40	50	50					50
S.F.	5	10	15	25	35	45	55							45
S.K.	10	20	25											20
S.T.	10	18	28	38	48	58	68							58
U.A.	8	18	28	32	36	40	45	50	55	60	65	70	78	70
W.J.	5	10	15	15	25	35	45	55						45
W.S.	5	10	15	25	25									25
Total	189	363	514	444	423	368	448	265	229	194	199	70	78	20–70
Mean	8.23	16.5	23.4	27.8	35.3	40.9	49.8	53.0	57.3	64.7	66.3	70	78	35.8
n	24	23	23	17	12	4	9	5	4	3	3	1	1	24

duration consistency was evaluated using the following five-point scale: 0, normal; 1, soft; 2, semisoft; 3, starting to soften; 4, hard. At each visit a composite score was prepared from the individual readings. All of the data included in Tables I–VI are based on this analysis and are expressed in terms of mean scores and ranges of all visits for each patient, with the score at the last visit also listed.

RESULTS

The observations made during this study are presented in Tables I–VI and describe the response to treatment with superoxide dismutase in terms of signs and symptoms (pain on erection, pain without erection, deviation of penis, induration size, and induration consistency). The number

TABLE II

Effect of Superoxide Dismutase[a] on Pain with Erection

Patient	0	1	2	3	4	5	6	7	8	9	10	11	12	13
					Evaluation score at successive visits									
A.F.	2	1	1	0	0	0	0	0	0	0	0			
B.B.	3	2	0	0										
C.C.	1	0	0	0	0	0	0							
D.F.-1	3	0	1											
D.F.-2	3	0	0	0	0									
G.A.	3	0	0	0	0	0	0							
G.E.	2													
G.P.	3	0	0	0										
H.A.	3	1	0	0										
H.M.	2	1	0											
H.R.	3	1	0	1										
K.A.	2	2	1	0	0	0	0	0	0	0	0	0		
K.E.	2	0	0	0	0	0								
K.H.	3	1	0											
K.J.	2	0	0	0	0									
K.W.	1	1	0	0	0									
L.J.	3	3	2	1	0									
S.E.	3	1	0	0	0	0	0	0	0	0				
S.F.	2	1	1	0	0	0	0							
S.K.	3	2	1											
S.T.	3	3	0	0	0	0	1	1						
U.A.	3	1	1	0	0	0	0	0	0	0	0	0	0	0
W.J.	2	1	0	0	0	0	0	0	0					
W.S.	3	1	0	0	0	0								
Mean	2.5	1.0	0.35	0.11	0	0	0.11	0.17	0	0	0	0	0	0
n	23	22	23	19	15	11	9	6	5	4	3	2	1	1
Mean dose (mg)		8.23	16.5	23.4	27.8	35.3	40.9	49.8	53.0	57.3	64.7	66.3	70.0	78.0

[a] Intraplaque administration.

of injections required to produce and maintain clinical benefit ranged between 4 and 7. Twenty patients experienced improvement and loss of pain on erection with 1 or 2 injections. Only four patients required 9, 11, or 13 injections to maintain clinical benefit (Table I). In general, a dose of 10 mg per injection produced the desired response.

Clinical benefit, as measured by all the parameters of evaluation, generally become noticeable after the first injection. The parameter that changed first and most extensively was the loss of pain on erection after treatment (Table II). This loss of pain on erection was observed in almost all patients after the first injection of the protein. At the third visit, only two patients (H. R. and L. J.) complained of a small degree of pain on erection (Table II). The mean composite score of all patients before therapy was 2.5. In all patients, the degree of positive response noted in sub-

TABLE III

Effect of Superoxide Dismutase[a] on Pain without Erection

Patient[b]	Evaluation score at successive visits													
	0	1	2	3	4	5	6	7	8	9	10	11	12	13
B.B.	1	0	0	0										
G.A.	2	0	0	0	0	0	0							
H.A.	1	0	0	0										
K.H.	3	0	0											
L.J.	1	1	0	0	0									
S.T.	2	2	0	0	0	0	0	0						
U.A.	1	0	0	0	0	0	0	0	0	0	0	0	0	0

[a] Intraplaque administration.
[b] Only those patients reporting pain without erection were evaluated in this study.

TABLE IV

Effect of Superoxide Dismutase[a] on Induration Size

Patient	Approximate size of plaque(s) at successive visits (cm²)													
	0	1	2	3	4	5	6	7	8	9	10	11	12	13
A.F.	8.0	8.0	8.0	8.0	3.0	1.0	0.25	0.25	0.25	0	0			
B.B.	4.0	4.0	4.0	4.0										
C.C.	8.0	8.0	8.0	7.0	7.0	7.0	6.0							
D.F.-1	6.0	6.0	6.0											
D.F.-2	5.2	5.4	5.0	3.6	1.5									
G.A.	1.0	1.0	1.0	1.0	1.0	0.75	0.75							
G.E.	2.0													
G.P.	2.0	2.0	1.5	1.5										
H.A.	3.0	3.0	3.0	3.0										
H.M.	3.0	3.0	2.3											
H.R.	3.0	3.0	0.3	0.3										
K.A.	5.0	4.5	4.5	3.8	3.8	3.8	3.8	2.5	2.5	2.5	2.5	0		
K.E.	6.0	6.0	6.0	6.0	4.5	0.5								
K.H.	8.0	8.0	8.0											
K.J.	1.5	1.5	1.1	1.1	1.1									
K.W.	15.0	15.0	15.0	15.0										
L.J.	6.0	6.0	6.0	5.0	4.5									
S.E.	4.0	4.0	4.0	3.0	3.0	2.0	2.0	2.0	1.0	1.0				
S.F.	2.0	2.0	2.0	2.0	2.0	1.5	0.2							
S.K.	3.5	3.5	3.5											
S.T.	4.0	4.0	4.0	4.0	4.0	3.0	3.0	3.0						
U.A.	10.0	10.0	7.5	7.5	7.5	7.5	7.5	7.5	7.5	5.0	5.0	1.0	1.0	0.5
W.J.	3.75	3.75	3.75	2.8	2.8	2.1	2.1	1.6	1.6					
W.S.	2.0	2.0	2.0	1.5	1.1	1.1								
Mean	4.82	4.92	4.61	4.25	3.34	2.75	2.84	2.82	2.58	2.13	2.50	0.50	1.0	0.5
n	24	23	23	19	14	11	9	6	5	4	3	2	1	1

[a] Intraplaque administration.

TABLE V

Effect of Superoxide Dismutase[a] on Deviation of the Penis

Patient	Evaluation score at successive visits													
	0	1	2	3	4	5	6	7	8	9	10	11	12	13
A.F.	4	3	3	2	2	2	1	1	1	0	0			
B.B.	4	3	3	2										
C.C.	4	4	2	1	0	0	0							
D.F.-1	3	2	2											
D.F.-2	4	3	2	2	1									
G.A.	2	2	2	2	1	1	1							
G.E.	3													
G.P.	4	3	4	4										
H.A.	4	3	3	3										
H.M.	3	2	1											
H.R.	3	2	1	1										
K.A.	3	3	3	2	2	2	2	1	1	1	1	0		
K.E.	3	3	3	2	0	0								
K.H.	4	3	3											
K.J.	3	3	2	2	1									
L.J.	4	4	4	3	2									
S.E.	3	3	3	1	1	1	0	0	0	0				
S.F.	3	3	3	3	3	1	0							
S.K.	3	3	3											
S.T.	3	3	3	3	2	1	1	1						
U.A.	3	3	3	2	2	2	2	2	2	2	1	0	0	0
W.J.	4	4	4	3	3	2	2	2	2					
W.S.	3	3	3	2	2	2								
Mean	3.32	2.95	2.73	2.28	1.57	1.27	1.00	1.16	1.20	0.75	0.67	0.50	0.50	0
n	23	22	22	18	14	11	9	6	5	4	3	2	1	1

[a] Intraplaque administration.

TABLE VI

Effect of Superoxide Dismutase[a] on Induration Size

	Reduction from baseline size			
	67–100%	34–66%	1–33%	0%
Time (months)	23.8	14.2	12.7	8.5
Superoxide dismutase (mg)	51.1	35.0	26.9	23.3
Number of patients	7	2	7	6

[a] Intraplaque administration.

sequent visits was striking. The mean score of all patients after the first treatment reached 1.0 and dropped to zero after the third visit, showing that with only two exceptions all patients were free of pain on erection.

Achievement of relief from pain without erection showed a similar response after treatment. Only 7 of the 23 patients complained of pain without erection before treatment (Table III). After the initial treatment time of 3 months, all 7 of these patients had gained relief from pain without erection. The rate of changes in the induration size upon treatment differed with the changes in clinical signs. The mean approximate plaque size was estimated to be 4.8 cm² before therapy (Table IV). A reduction in the size of fibrotic plaques was observed after 12–15 months of treatment. Nine patients were followed for more than 15 months (more than five visits) and showed a significant decrease in the amount of fibrotic plaques. In the case of the patients for whom no reduction of the induration size was observed, no long-term observations were made (e.g., B.B., D.F.-1, H.A., K.H., K.W.). Except for these patients, all those treated showed a reduction in the induration size to different degrees (Table VI).

Values for the changes in deviation before, during, and after treatment were compiled for 22 patients (Table V). The results are similar to the changes in induration size following treatment. A statistically significant reduction in the degree of deviation occurred after 12–15 months. A score of 2 or less was observed in all patients who were evaluated for five successive periods (Table V). Clinical evidence was collected for more than 15 months (after the fifth visit) for seven patients. Deviation of the penis was completely relieved in all patients in this group.

No adverse effects of superoxide dismutase injection were observed in this study. No immunological reactions were seen. None of the patients reported pain directly after injection, in contrast to intraplaqueal administration of other drugs.

CONCLUSIONS

Peyronie's disease is a plastic induration of the penis that is usually seen in men of middle age. It is characterized by a fibrous infiltration of the intercavernous septum of the penis. The fibrosis results in the formation of a cordlike structure varying in length and breadth. These pathological changes are called plaques and cause curvature of the penis on erection. The degree of curvature depends on the extent of fibrosis.

To treat this disease, a wide spectrum of drugs as well as surgical treatment has been used over the years. Conservative treatment has included the administration of vitamin E, cortisone, or *p*-aminobenzoic acid potassium. Treatment with deep roentgen therapy and radium packs has also been used. Surgical treatment involves excision of the fibrotic plaques. The latter treatment results in a high percentage of impotence. Both drug and surgical therapy have proved to be unsatisfactory and often have severe side effects.

The results of this trial using superoxide dismutase for the treatment of Peyronie's disease are very encouraging. The drug was effective and outstandingly safe. No immunological reactions were seen. None of the patients reported pain in the penis following intraplaqueal administration of superoxide dismutase. The special syringe shown in Fig. 1 appears to be ideal for intraplaque injection, so that the drug can be deposited directly into the pathologically altered tissue. In contrast to patients treated with other therapeutic modalities, these patients experienced an immediate loss of pain after treatment. In nearly all patients, subjective complaints, such as pain both with and without erection, were diminished or disappeared after the first injection. The patients who were observed for more than 12–15 months showed statistically significant improvement in clinical status regarding reduction of induration size and penis deviation on erection.

The rate of response to this therapy varied among patients, although during the course of treatment all patients eventually improved with successive injections. The majority of the patients had relief from pain on erection after one to two injections of 10 mg of superoxide dismutase. The first clinical response was the loss of pain both with and without erection. Induration size and degree of deviation of the penis became significantly reduced in patients who underwent long-term treatment of more than 12–15 months. In the majority of patients, however, a reduction of the induration size of different degrees was observed.

The mechanism of action of superoxide dismutase in Peyronie's disease is not yet fully known. Observations from *in vitro* experiments demonstrate that the enzyme protects lysosomes against damage caused by heat or enzymatic action (4). Superoxide dismutase is now known to control the mobilization of polymorphonuclear leukocytes (PMN's) into the circulation after subcutaneous injection and also to protect phagocytosing PMN's against breakdown caused by the release of superoxide radical (11), which is generated by phagocytosing PMN's. The amount of superoxide radical released into the extracellular environment is sizable (12,13). In 1971, a positive identification was made between the commercial product, orgotein, and the enzyme superoxide dismutase discovered by McCord and Fridovich (14). Whether the overall efficacy of the superoxide dismutase preparation in the treatment of Peyronie's disease is a result of the oxygen-radical-scavenging activity of the enzyme and, if so, to what extent and how this is accomplished remain to be determined.

In conclusion, the results of this study indicate that superoxide dismutase is a valuable therapeutic drug for the treatment of Peyronie's disease. In terms of the lack of observable side effects, this agent is clearly superior to other available drugs. Local intraplaqueal administration appears to be the route of choice since it allows one to deposit the enzyme directly into the pathologically altered tissue.

REFERENCES

1. Hasche-Klünder, R. (1970). Zur Behandlung der Induratio penis plastica. *Urologe A* p. 335.
2. Hasche-Klünder, R. (1978). Zur Behandlung der Induratio penis plastica mit para-amino-benzosaurem Kalk (P ABK). *Urologe A* **17:**224.
3. Marberger, H., Huber, W., Bartsch, G., Schulte, T. L., and Swoboda, P. (1974). Orgotein, a new antiinflammatory metalloprotein drug. Evaluation of clinical efficacy and safety in inflammatory conditions of the urinary tract. *Int. Urol. Nephrol.* **6:**61.
4. Marberger, H., Bartsch, G., Huber, W., Menander, K. B., and Schulte, T. L. (1976). Orgotein, a new drug for the treatment of radiation cystitis. *Curr. Ther. Res.* **19:**198.
5. Huber, W., Schulte, T. L., Carson, S., Goldhamer, R. E., and Vogin, E. E. (1968). Some chemical and pharmacological properties of a novel anti-inflammatory protein. *Toxicol. Appl. Pharmacol.* **12:**308.
6. Breshears, D. E., Brown, C. D., Riftel, D. M., Cobble, R. J., and Cheesman, S. F. (1974). Evaluation of orgotein in treatment of locomotor dysfunction in dogs. *Mod. Vet. Pract.* **55:**85.
7. Cushing, L. S., Decker, W. E., Santos, F. K., Schulte, T. L., and Huber, W. (1973). Orgotein therapy for inflammation in horses. *Mod. Vet. Pract.* **54:**17.
8. Decker, W. E., Edmondson, A. H., Hill, H. E., Holmes, R. A., Padmore, C. L., Warren, H. H., and Wood, W. C. (1974). Local administration of orgotein in horses. *Mod. Vet. Pract.* **55:**773.
9. Lund-Oleson, K., and Menander, K. B. (1974). Orgotein, a new anti-inflammatory metalloprotein drug; preliminary evaluation of clinical efficacy and safety in degenerative joint disease. *Curr. Ther. Res.* **16:**706.
10. Carson, S., Vogin, E. E., Huber, W., and Schulte, T. L. (1973). Safety tests of orgotein, an anti-inflammatory protein. *Toxicol. Appl. Pharmacol.* **26:**184.
11. Salin, M. L., and McCord, J. M. (1975). Free radicals and inflammation: Protection of phagocytosing leukocytes by superoxide dismutase. *J. Clin. Invest.* **56:**1319.
12. Babior, B. M., Kippnes, R., and Curnutte, J. (1973). Biological defense mechanisms: The production by leukocytes of superoxide: a potential bactericidal agent. *J. Clin. Invest.* **52:**741.
13. Johnston, R. B., Keele, B. B., Misra, H. P., Webb, L. S., Leymeyer, J. E., and Rajagopalan, K. V. (1975). Superoxide anion generation and phagocytic bactericidal activity. *In* "The Phagocytic Cell in Host Resistance" (J. A. Bellanti and D. H. Dayton, eds.), p. 61. Raven, New York.

14. McCord, J. M., and Fridovich, I. (1969). An enzyme function for erythrocuprein. *J. Biol. Chem.* **244**:6049.

DISCUSSION

JONES: Have you tried routes of injecting superoxide dismutase other than the intraplaque route?

BARTSCH: No, we have not.

Chapter 21

Superoxide Dismutase Therapy in Degenerative Joint Disease

KNUD LUND-OLESEN

INTRODUCTION

The therapeutic potential of Cu/Zn-superoxide dismutase first came to the attention of Danish researchers in early 1971 when it was realized that the protein preparation orgotein (Diagnostic Data, Inc.), which had been the subject of many animal experimental studies and some human trials, was identical to superoxide dismutase (1). The following characteristics of the agent were of particular interest.

1. It produces no significant toxic effects in clinically acceptable doses (2).
2. It is a natural rather than synthetic substance (3).
3. It is found in all aerobic organisms with an oxidative metabolism (4).
4. It protects membranes from damage by oxygen radicals (5), which is significant since oxygen radicals are an important part of the inflammatory process.
5. It inhibits the production of a chemotactic factor that brings polymorphonuclear leukocytes (PMN's) to the site of infection (6).
6. When it is administered exogenously and is therefore present in the joint fluid, it allows PMN's to leave the joint cavity alive following phagocytosis since it protects the cells from radical-induced injury (7).
7. Although it might be expected to cause an allergic reaction, it has

339

PATHOLOGY OF OXYGEN
Copyright © 1982 by Academic Press, Inc.
All rights of reproduction in any form reserved.
ISBN 0-12-068620-1

not been associated with such a reaction when administered in purified form. On the contrary, the compound provided protection to guinea pigs sensitized with horse serum when they were given challenge doses of horse serum followed by superoxide dismutase (2).

8. It is a poor antigen since it must be administered together with Freund's adjuvant in order to produce antibodies to the protein.

Taking these points into consideration, it would appear that superoxide dismutase would be suitable for the treatment of most inflammatory diseases, as well as conditions in which oxygen toxicity is a potential danger. The ideal route of administration would, of course, be oral, but there is no doubt that a protein having a molecular weight of approximately 32,000 would be catalytically degraded by proteolytic enzymes before being absorbed in the intestine. Thus, the form of administration of the agent is currently limited to injections, either subcutaneous, intramuscular, or other. In Ringe, Denmark, a number of noncontrolled and controlled trials have been carried out with the enzyme using different routes of administration in the treatment of a variety of diseases generally associated with inflammatory processes.

Theoretical Considerations

The process of inflammation has not yet been fully elucidated. However, there is considerable evidence to suggest that inflammation, like many other reactions in the human body, is one of action and counteraction. It may be presumed that certain diseases or pathological states such as polyarthritis, osteoarthritis, and hypoxia initiate inflammation in the joints. In rheumatoid arthritis is has been demonstrated that the oxygen tension of synovial fluid can drop to almost zero (8). It has been reported that hypoxia is followed by the release of lysosomal enzymes (9). The action of these enzymes causes death and produces cell debris. The debris must be removed, and for this purpose phagocytosing PMN's are essential. Increased vascularization follows, and PMN's fill the joint fluid. The metabolic activation that follows the stimulation of PMN's by particulate matter results in the production of O_2^- and other oxygen-derived radicals. The PMN's cannot leave the joint fluid and die as a result of free-radical attack. Lysosomal enzymes are then released from the damaged and dead cells, and destruction of the cartilage and bone follows. Superoxide dismutase, which catalytically removes O_2^-, is known to stabilize membranes and thus can protect the integrity of PMN's. Viable PMN's are capable of leaving the joint, thus preventing the further release of lysosomal enzymes. By its catalytic action, which includes the oxidation to molecular oxygen of partially reduced oxygen radicals, superoxide dismutase actually increases oxygen tension in the joints. Superoxide dismutase, therefore, can be viewed as enhancing the resistance of the joint to hypoxia, which can be caused both by increased oxygen consumption in conditions of limited oxygen supply and by the well-known vasculitis in the affected joint in rheumatoid arthritis (10). In the osteoarthritic joint, low oxygen tension (and poor circulation) is caused by hindrance of venous drainage from the subchondral bone. The arteriovenous pressure difference is very low and has been described as "the intraosseous engorgement pain syndrome" (11).

DEGENERATIVE JOINT DISEASE

The first actual clinical trial of superoxide dismutase at Ringe was carried out in 1972 (12). The study included 22 patients, all suffering from degenerative joint disease, and involved the intraarticular administration of the protein. Degenerative joint disease was chosen for study because the evaluation of osteoarthritic knee joints is easier than that of rheumatoid knee joints, although both diseases, in my judgment, involve inflammation and respond well to superoxide dismutase. Between 1 and 15 injections were given. The total amount of superoxide dismutase injected into the joints varied considerably, due mainly to the type of patient and the general treatment each patient was undergoing (e.g., long-term rehabilitation). The schedule of treatment is shown in Table I. In some cases the treatment was restricted to a single dose of 2 mg, whereas in other cases it was possible to continue treatment for a considerable time, a total of 30 mg being administered. The longest period of treatment was 9 months. The results of this open trial were very positive. A definite improvement in the condition of the joint was observed for periods of more than 90 days after the last injection in 16 of the 19 patients monitored after treatment. Because of the encouraging response, a double-blind trial was undertaken using superoxide dismutase versus a placebo.

The second clinical investigation was designed as a 22-week double-blind, placebo-controlled study of the efficacy and long-term safety of superoxide dismutase when injected intraarticularly into elderly patients with active inflammatory osteoarthritis of the knees. The object of the investigation, briefly stated, was to determine (a) whether intraarticular injections of superoxide dismutase could be safely used for an extended period of time, (b) whether the route of administration was acceptable to

TABLE I

Summary of Treatment with Superoxide Dismutase of Patients with Rheumatoid Arthritis[a]

1. *Dosage*

Route	Dose range (mg)	Number of injections	Total dose (mg)
Subcutaneous	2–4	544	1227
Intraarticular	2–10	282	651
Intrathecal	4	2	8

2. *Dosage per patient*

Route	Number of injections	Dose (mg)
Subcutaneous	1–86	2–207
Intraarticular	1–75	2–166
Intrathecal	2	8

3. *Location of intraarticular injections (282)*

	Knee	Hip	Elbow	Wrist	Shoulder
Number of injections	148	42	37	32	21

[a] Patients studied over the period 1971–1976.

both patient and physician, (c) whether the agent would produce allergic reactions (this could be best accomplished by the injection of superoxide dismutase every 2 weeks), and (d) whether a placebo effect occurred (which was determined by giving intraarticular injections for nearly 6 months). In retrospect, this extended protocol was wise since a surprisingly good placebo effect lasted almost halfway through the investigation.

Four parameters were employed in the evaluation of the efficacy:

1. *Pain.* Day and night pain, as well as pain on walking, was evaluated using a five-point scale: 1, none; 2, mild; 3, moderate; 4, severe; 5, very severe.

2. *Circumference.* The knee joint was measured in centimeters with a flexible tape.

3. *Function.* This was evaluated as follows:

Use of aids: 1, cane for long walks only; 2, cane; 3, crutch; 4, two canes; 5, two crutches.

Limp: 1, none; 2, mild; 3, moderate; 4, severe; 5, very severe.

Maximal distance walked without stopping: 1, 500 meters; 2, 300–500 meters; 3, 100–300 meters; 4, 50–100 meters; 5, indoors only.

Ability to climb stairs: 1, normal; 2, normal with help of banister; 3, with cane or crutch; 4, with assistance; 5, impossible.

4. *Use of analgesics:* Each patient's diary of drug scheduling was monitored.

In addition, the judgments of the physician and patient were used to evaluate the quality of the therapeutic response. All of the patients were carefully observed for any adverse reactions to the treatment. Forty-five patients were originally included in the investigation; however, the final analysis included only 31 patients, 14 having been excluded for various reasons (Table II).

For analysis, the scores for all pain parameters were added together, since not all patients had day pain, night pain, and pain on walking together at all times. The patients treated with superoxide dismutase experienced much greater pain relief than patients treated with placebo throughout the trial. The difference in pain scores showed statistical significance immediately after the first injection ($p < .05$). After the fourth injection, the statistically significant difference remained throughout the trial, with a p value of $< .0025$ at week 22.

The measurement of circumference was carried out according to the above-described procedure. Since many of the patients were grossly overweight, however, accurate measurements were impossible, and therefore the results were considered too unreliable to be included in the final evaluation.

For analysis, the scores of the individual functional parameters (use of aids, limp, maximal distance walked without stopping, and ability to climb stairs) were added together, since not all patients suffered from all of the listed functional losses at all times during the trial. After the fourteenth week, recovery of function in the group receiving superoxide dismutase became more pronounced than in the group receiving placebo, the difference becoming increasingly greater throughout the trial. The differ-

TABLE II

Patients Excluded from the Final Analysis of the Study[a]

	Treatment	
Reason for exclusion	Superoxide dismutase	Placebo
No roentgenological evidence of osteoarthritis	1	3
Inactive disease	1	—
Drug treatment excluded by protocol	1	2
Transient adverse reactions	6	—
Total	9	5

[a] Original number, 45.

ences reached statistical significance at week 20 ($p < .05$) and increased in significance at week 22 ($p < .01$).

At the start of the trial, the placebo patients used significantly fewer analgesics (Pyramidon, Dextropropoxifen, or salicylamide) than the superoxide dismutase patients. Patients in both groups used only one of the three analgesics listed. The marked relief from pain experienced by the patients on superoxide dismutase therapy was accompanied by a decrease in the use of analgesics, which became more pronounced with time and was near statistical significance at the end of the trial ($p < .10$). The results of the trial are summarized in Table III. It should be noted that three patients were excluded from this analysis, two because of surgery before week 22, and one because of an injection administered in addition to the scheduled protocol at week 10. Furthermore, six patients in the group treated with superoxide dismutase had concomitant active osteoarthritis of the hip, which was not specifically treated. These patients were included in the analysis even though their hip disease may have skewed the results of the functional parameters against superoxide dismutase treatment. It can be seen, however, from Table III that superoxide dismutase was significantly more effective ($p < .001$) than placebo in the treatment of long-standing osteoarthritis.

It should be mentioned at this point that transient adverse reactions were noted early in the trial. These consisted of redness, swelling, and pain of the joint after injection, although all of the symptoms disappeared rapidly. It was found that, although the superoxide dismutase administered as orgotein (kindly donated by Diagnostic Data, Inc.) complied with the pyrogenic quality assurance parameters established by the U.S. Food and Drug Administration, it contained sufficient endotoxin to produce side effects severe enough to require cessation of the treatment in six patients, four of whom had generalized reactions. After this the protein was further purified by the manufacturer. When the purified product was ad-

TABLE III

Evaluation of Patients with Osteoarthritis Treated with Superoxide Dismutase or Placebo

Treatment	Worse	No change	Improved	Greatly improved
Superoxide dismutase				
Physician evaluation	0	1	8	7
Patient evaluation	0	1	6	10
Placebo				
Physician evaluation	2	7	2	0
Patient evaluation	2	6	2	1

ministered, the mild side effects observed were of the same frequency as those occurring after the use of placebo. Some of the localized reactions may have been caused by bleeding or damage due to joint puncture, which also took place in the placebo-treated patients.

In this investigation the best results appeared to be obtained in joints where the morphological changes had not reached an irreversible stage; that is, the poorest results were seen in joints where severe destructive changes had caused incorrect positioning of the joint and incorrect loading. This result had not been foreseen in the protocol. It should also be noted that, although the author was responsible for the collection of the clinical data, the final evaluation and statistical analysis were conducted independently in the United States.

In summary, it can be said that there was considerable improvement in the majority of the patients after 22 weeks of treatment with superoxide dismutase. This improvement was gradual and progressive during the whole period of treatment and led finally to these patients being considered almost free of symptoms. The results of these two trials, the open and double-blind, have since been confirmed by other investigators (13–15). Very good results were also obtained in many single cases in which therapy consisted of a combination of superoxide dismutase (2–4 mg) and a microcrystalline steroid (Lederspan) given as an intraarticular injection. It is possible to predict that superoxide dismutase counteracts the adverse effects of the steroid.

MULTIPLE SCLEROSIS

Multiple sclerosis is considered by some investigators to be an infectious condition caused by some exogenic factor and an endogenic immune defect leading to a "slow virus disease." If this is correct, then the possibility of improving the condition of patients suffering from multiple sclerosis by the administration of superoxide dismutase definitely exists. This was attempted in Ringe in an uncontrolled open trial with 58 patients (32 women and 26 men). The superoxide dismutase was administered both subcutaneously and intrathecally.

The evaluation of results from a trial such as this is extremely difficult, but since the intrathecal route is not an easy route of administration and far from pleasant for the patient one may safely assume that patients who return for additional injections definitely consider the treatment to be of value. This was the case with 26 of the patients. In addition, a large number returned for intramuscular treatment over a longer period of time.

Upon questioning, the returning patients stated that the treatment with superoxide dismutase was beneficial.

Initially, all the patients were treated by means of subcutaneous and then intramuscular injections, but it was the opinion of the author that the enzyme was not reaching the central nervous system because it could not cross the blood–brain barrier (16). The entire regime, therefore, was revised so that all of the patients received the superoxide dismutase intrathecally. A total of 92 intrathecal injections were given. Thirty-two patients received one, 21 received two, 4 received three, and 1 received six intrathecal injections. Injections were given with a range of superoxide dismutase: 8 mg (25 cases), 4 mg (41 cases), 2 mg (24 cases), and 3 mg (2 cases). No less than 45% of the patients returned for intrathecal treatment until the use of the agent was discontinued owing to the introduction of new regulations in Denmark regarding the use of unregistered drugs.

Spinal fluids from 15 patients were analyzed for superoxide dismutase content at Diagnostic Data, Inc., U.S.A. and found to contain significantly less than spinal fluids from persons without neurological disease (to be published). All patients were, in addition, receiving the drug either intramuscularly or subcutaneously.

The results of this uncontrolled investigation indicate that a controlled long-term trial of superoxide dismutase treatment of multiple sclerosis would be of value.

NEUROLOGICAL CONDITIONS

Superoxide dismutase has also been used in the same manner in the attempted treatment of a number of neurological disorders. The group of patients in this study was composed of six women and six men. The results, as might be expected, were somewhat inconclusive, due mainly to the small number of patients participating.

BACK PAIN AND HEADACHE

Superoxide dismutase treatment was used on six male and three female patients, all complaining of "back pain." Again, the results were difficult or impossible to interpret because of the small number of cases and the variety of causes of back pain.

A mixed group of patients was treated intraspinally with superoxide dismutase. The group consisted of a woman with headache due to iodine allergy, a woman with headache of unknown origin, and a man suffering from rheumatoid arthritis. A man with arachnoiditis was also treated with the agent. The results were as varied as the composition of the group. In two patients, the woman with the iodine allergy and the man with arachnoiditis, the results were excellent. In the other two cases, no conclusions could be drawn.

The two cases in which the results were excellent are described here in more detail. The patient suffering from arachnoiditis was admitted to the hospital in May 1972 at the age of 53 years. Physical examination revealed partial paralysis of the legs, and the patient complained of continuous severe back pain. Since very little can be done to help such patients, it was considered that an attempt to treat the condition by the administration of superoxide dismutase would be fully justified. However, since it had been shown in animal experiments that the enzyme does not cross the blood–brain barrier (16), the decision was made to administer superoxide dismutase intrathecally. This patient was the first to be given an intrathecal injection of superoxide dismutase. The first injection contained 2 mg and was followed by 4 mg given as a muscular infiltration on the same day. Approximately 1 month later the patient was given 2 mg intraarticularly in the right knee to treat osteoarthritis. This treatment was followed 7 days later by another injection of 4 mg intramuscularly. Finally, an additional 2 mg of superoxide dismutase was injected 1 week later into the same joint. The general condition of the patient improved, and his low back pain, as well as the paralysis of the legs, disappeared. He was discharged from the hospital in August 1972 and recommended for a disability pension. However, we have been informed that this patient resumed his former employment as a night watchman and bicycled approximately 20 km per night without any ill effects. It would, of course, be unscientific to attribute the improvement in this patient's condition to the superoxide dismutase treatment but, on the other hand, there are few other ways to explain such impressive results.

The second patient in whom superoxide dismutase treatment produced striking results was the woman suffering from iodine allergy. The 64-year-old patient, a former nurse, suffered from low back pain and lumbago and after being admitted to the hospital, was subjected to high myelography with Duroliopaque in June 1975. A severe, almost intractable headache rapidly developed, and in July 1975 the patient was admitted to the Ringe Rehabilitation Centre with Duroliopaque allergy and still suffering from among other things a continuous headache. She was treated on admission with Ledercort (4 mg three times daily for 2 days, followed by 2 mg three times daily for 2 days, and then 2 mg morning and evening for another 2 days) and 2 mg of superoxide dismutase subcutaneously twice daily for 8 days (a total of 16 mg superoxide dismutase). The headache gradually disappeared. In September, 1 month and 5 days after the initial treatment, the patient was readmitted due to a recurrence of the headache. She was then given 4 mg superoxide dismutase intraspinally in 4 ml NaCl, following which the headache progressively disappeared; the patient was completely free of the headache 4 days after the treatment. Another recurrence occurred in December, when the patient had been completely free of this symptom for slightly more than 2 months. She was again given 4 mg superoxide dismutase intraspinally and 2 days later was again free of headache. In January of the following year (1976) the patient was again admitted to the hospital suffering from headache and given 8 mg of superoxide dismutase intraspinally in 5 ml NaCl. The headache disappeared the following day. The patient was again free of the headache for a period of just over 2 months, only to develop a headache again in late March. Another intraspinal injection of 8 mg superoxide dismutase produced substantial improvement in the condition, although a relapse occurred a few days later, in all probability due to psychological stress. However, another injection of 6 mg of superoxide dismutase intraspinally produced good effects, and the patient was discharged. Readmitted to the hospital in April and in June 1976, again because of headache, she was given 8 mg of superoxide dismutase intraspinally on both occasions with a favorable effect. The patient has not been seen since June 1976, although her private practitioner has indicated that the headache has completely disappeared. During the course of the superoxide dismutase treatment the patient had received a total of 16 mg of superoxide dismutase subcutaneously and 46 mg intraspinally. It would appear that the latter route was the most effective in this case because the drug does not pass the blood–brain barrier, as mentioned above.

MISCELLANEOUS CONDITIONS

It is very difficult at the Rehabilitation Centre in Ringe to carry out well-planned clinical trials because the normal work of the center is directed toward the rehabilitation of patients after long-term treatment in other hospitals. However, occasionally a patient is admitted who is definitely a candidate for superoxide dismutase treatment. Unfortunately, under these circumstances the agent can be tested only in an open trial on one patient. Such a patient was admitted to the center in February 1972, suffering from a number of complaints, including gangrene of the big toe of the right foot. It should be noted here that the patient's lower left leg had been amputated some time earlier due to gangrene. The decision was made to test the effect of intraarterial superoxide dismutase on this patient in an attempt to confine the gangrene to the toe and thus avoid further amputation. The injections were given in the femoral artery.

A large area of the lateral surface of the toe was black and necrotic, although the necrosis had not gone as far down as the bone. Approximately 10 days after admission, the patient was given the first intraarterial injection of 2 mg of superoxide dismutase in 5 ml NaCl. This treatment was repeated 13 times at intervals of between 3 and 6 days, after which it was supplemented by the subcutaneous injection of 2 mg superoxide dismutase at intervals of approximately 2–3 days until the patient had received a total of 28 mg intraarterially and 36 mg subcutaneously. Throughout the period, the condition of the necrotic area was surprisingly unchanged, although at times the patient complained of pain in the area of the necrosis. From June 22 until November 29, 1972, the patient received an additional 305 mg of superoxide dismutase subcutaneously, which presumably kept the necrosis under control. Attempts were made throughout this period to discontinue the superoxide dismutase treatment; however, the patient immediately complained of almost unbearable pain, and the treatment was therefore resumed. On November 29, 1972, the superoxide dismutase treatment was discontinued since by this time the patient had occupied a hospital bed for 9 months and had to be discharged. Following discontinuation of the treatment, the pain became intolerable to the patient and he requested amputation. The amputation was carried out on January 16, 1973. During the operation both arteries were found to be completely occluded by atheromatous plaques.

Although this is only a single case, it is rather striking in its course inasmuch as necrosis of the toes in patients of this type usually progresses so rapidly that amputation becomes essential within a month or so, and in this case it was possible, presumably because of the superoxide dismutase treatment, to maintain a status quo condition of the necrotic toe for a period of 7 months. Had the patient not been subjected to amputation, it was our impression that the condition could have been kept in check for an even longer period of time by means of the superoxide dismutase injections. This case suggests not only that superoxide dismutase may be of value in the treatment of gangrene, but that it can safely be administered intraarterially without any side effects.

SUMMARY OF CLINICAL EFFECTS

During the first trial period in which superoxide dismutase was used in the treatment of a wide variety of diseases, it became clear that this agent could be administered by almost all routes of injection without serious side effects. Unfortunately, side effects were noted first in the double-blind trial, but these were virtually eliminated by the additional purification of the product by the manufacturer.

Because of the large geographic area served by the Rehabilitation Centre in Ringe and the large patient load, patients are often discharged as early as possible. Therefore, necessary follow-up to treatment is almost impossible unless the patient is readmitted to the hospital at a later date. Thus, apart from the patients in the two trials completed on the treatment of osteoarthritis, one an open trial and the other a double-blind placebo trial, the great majority of the patients treated with superoxide dismutase have had a variety of diseases. This situation allows for no firm conclusions as to the efficacy of superoxide dismutase but only suggests that further work should be undertaken.

Nonetheless, it is our general impression that the enzyme is highly effective in the treatment of degenerative diseases of the joints, although it is obvious that the best results can be obtained in such patients at an early stage. Furthermore, the agent is effective in the treatment of a wide variety of inflammation diseases including rheumatoid arthritis, as well as those in which oxygen toxicity is an important component. On the whole it can safely be said that superoxide dismutase constitutes a much required addition to our armory of drugs for combating inflammatory disease. Moreover, it is just as effective, if not more effective, than the corticosteroids and is totally without the adverse side effects of steroids. In summary, it is a compound that can be administered with considerable safety and without the occurrence of the dramatic side effects associated with other antiinflammatory drugs.

Finally, it is worth noting that following the injection of the compound, particularly intramuscularly, not only myself, but also the great majority of patients, remarked spontaneously that the injection produced a feeling of animation, inasmuch as muscular fatigue disappeared for a considerable amount of time.

FUTURE USE OF SUPEROXIDE DISMUTASE

One of the difficulties following the use of extracorporal circulation during surgery of the heart is the damage that occurs after normal circulation is reestablished. During the use of extracorporal circulation, the heart is subjected to a warm ischemic phase, during which there is an oxygen deficit. This oxygen deficit produces the release of lysosomal enzymes in the heart muscle, causing damage to the cells. The presence of exogenic superoxide dismutase inhibits this process because of its membrane-stabilizing effect. After normal circulation is reestablished, there is a burst of metabolic activity, including increased oxygen consumption by heart cells. This process produces a large quantity of superoxide radical. Although superoxide dismutase is an intracellular constituent, the hypoxic cells might have a compromised synthesis or an inadequate content during the warm ischemic phase, leading to a superoxide dismutase deficiency. Such a deficiency would leave the cells vulnerable to radical attack. Treatment of a patient with superoxide dismutase before, during, and after the use of extracorporal circulation would appear to be rational, inasmuch as the agent would first minimize the liberation of lysosomal enzymes during the warm ischemic phase and in addition would catalyze the transformation of the toxic radical (O_2^-) to oxygen and hydrogen peroxide, once again reducing the damage to the heart muscle. The rationale for this intervention is supported by recently reported results indicating protection of the vascular system from oxygen radical attack by the administration of exogenous superoxide dismutase (17,18). If the above considerations are correct, superoxide dismutase would be equally effective in transplantation surgery since it would protect the transplant both during the warm ischemic phase, to which all transplants are subjected, during transportation, as well as during the phase in which normal circulation is reestablished.

There are a number of interesting facts regarding muscle fatigue and the level of superoxide dismutase in tissue. (a) Experiments have shown that "after running in place for 20 seconds as violently as possible the person goes into debt to the amount of 5.5 litres of oxygen, and that it takes 14 minutes to recover" (19). (b) The level of superoxide dismutase in the lungs of rats is related to the oxygen pressure of the atmosphere (20). (c) Only if the rat is adapted can it tolerate 1 atmosphere of pure oxygen, and adapted rats have a higher level of superoxide dismutase in their lungs (20,21).

From the above it can be argued that the normal muscle cell has a certain content of superoxide dismutase that is sufficient to remove a certain amount of superoxide radical generated under normal metabolism. However, when the muscle is exposed to excessive stress (for example, "violent" running) the amount of superoxide dismutase present is inadequate to cope with the excess O_2^- produced. This condition, perhaps in association with increased production of lactate, produces muscle fatigue. The injection of exogenous superoxide dismutase can increase the effective level of superoxide dismutase in the muscle tissue, thus providing a means of removing oxygen radicals before fatigue develops. If these speculations are correct, then the use of superoxide dismutase in the training of athletes, for example, might increase performance level. Such an approach could be useful in many other cases in which excessive muscular performance is essential.

In conclusion, although superoxide dismutase is of great interest to biochemists on theoretical grounds, it has another rather surprising (as a protein) potential use—that of a new drug. This discovery points the way for further clinical studies and introduces new aspects in the management of human metabolism both in illness and in health.

ACKNOWLEDGMENTS

The author wishes to thank Diagnostic Data, Inc., California, U.S.A. for generously supplying the orgotein (ontosein®). Dr. Wolf Huber and Dr. Kerstin Menander-Huber have been extremely helpful. The ethical and clinical aspects involved in the trial of this new drug have presented many difficulties.

REFERENCES

1. Huber, W., and Saifer, M. G. P. (1977). Orgotein, the drug version of bovine Cu-Zn superoxide dismutase. I. A summary account of safety and pharmacology in laboratory animals. *In* "Superoxide and Superoxide Dismutases" (A. M. Michelson, J. M. McCord, and I. Fridovich, eds.), pp. 518–23. Academic Press, New York.
2. Carson, S., Vogin, E. E., Huber, W., and Schulte, T. L. (1973). Safety tests of orgotein, an anti-inflammatory protein. *Toxicol. Appl. Pharmacol.* **26**:184–202.
3. McCord, J. M., and Fridovich, I. (1969). An enzymic function for erythrocuprein (hemocuprein). *J. Biol. Chem.* **244**:6049–6055.
4. Fridovich, I. (1977). Oxygen is toxic. *BioScience* **27**:462–466.
5. Lynch, R. E., and Fridovich, I. (1978). Effects of superoxide on the erythrocyte membrane. *J. Biol. Chem.* **253**:1838–1845.
6. McCord *et al.,* this volume.
7. Salin, M. L., and McCord, J. M. (1977). Free radicals in leukocyte metabolism and inflammation. *In* "Superoxide and Superoxide Dismutases" (A. M. Michelson, J. M. McCord, and I. Fridovich, eds.), pp. 262–268. Academic Press, New York.
8. Lund-Olesen, K. (1970). Oxygen tension in synovial fluids. *Arthritis Rheum.* **13** (6):769–776.
9. DeDuve, C. (1964). Lysosomes and cell injury. *In* "Symposium on Injury, Inflammation and Immunity" (L. Thomas, J. W. Uhr, and L. Grant, eds.), pp. 292–300. Williams and Wilkins, Baltimore.
10. Bywaters, E. G. L. (1957). Peripheral vascular obstructions in rheumatoid arthritis and its relationship to other vascular lesions. *Am. J. Rheumatoid Dis.* **16**:84.
11. Arnoldi, C. C., and Reimann, I. (1979). The pathomechanism of human coxarthrosis. *Acta Orthop. Scand.,* Suppl. **181**.
12. Lund-Olesen, K., and Menander, K. B. (1974). Orgotein: A new anti-inflammatory metalloprotein drug. Preliminary evaluation of clinical efficacy and safety in degenerative joint disease. *Curr. Ther. Res.* **16**:706–717.

13. Huskisson, E. C., and Scott, J. (1981). Orgotein in osteoarthritis of the knee joint. *Eur. J. Rheum. Inflam.* **4**(2):212–218.
14. Beckmann, R., and Flohé, L. (1980). The pathogenic role of O_2^- in inflammation: Efficacy of exogenous superoxide dismutase. *Bull. Eur. Physiopathol. Respir.* **17** (Suppl.):275–286.
15. Goebel, K.-M., Storck, U., and Neurath, F. (1981). Intrasynovial orgotein therapy in rheumatoid arthritis. *Lancet* **1**:1015–1017.
16. Huber, W., and Menander-Huber, K. B. (1980). Orgotein. *Clin. Rheum. Dis.* **6**(3):476.
17. Del Maestro, *et al.,* this volume.
18. Johnson, K. J., Fantone, J. C., Kaplan, J., and Ward, P. A. (1981). In vivo damage of rat lungs by oxygen metabolites. *J. Clin. Invest.* **67**:983–93.
19. Bodansky, M. (1938). "Introduction to Physiological Chemistry" pp. 331–333. Wiley, New York.
20. Crapo, J. D., and Tierney, D. F. (1974). Superoxide dismutase and pulmonary oxygen toxicity. *Am. J. Physiol.* **226**:1401–1407.
21. Stevens, J. B., and Autor, A. P. (1980). A proposed mechanism for neonatal rat tolerance to normobaric hyperoxia. *Fed. Proc., Fed. Am. Soc. Exp. Biol.* **39**:3138–3143.

Chapter 22

Evaluation of Safety of Superoxide Dismutase in the Treatment of Urological Disorders*

JOSEPH D. SCHMIDT AND
THOMAS L. SCHULTE

INTRODUCTION

In this study, superoxide dismutase was administered as orgotein†
(Diagnostic Data, Inc.). Orgotein is the nonproprietary name adopted for
the metalloprotein described in 1971 in the federal "New Drug Names"
list as "water-soluble protein congeners isolatable from red blood cells,
liver, and other tissues" (1). Its activity is thought to reside principally, if
not wholly, in its superoxide dismutase content. Animal and human clinical studies have demonstrated that the preparation has a marked antiinflammatory activity. Investigators at two European medical centers have
reported its efficacy in the treatment of interstitial cystitis and acute radiation damage to the rectum and urinary bladder. To examine the superoxide dismutase preparation specifically for its safety, we studied 53 patients
receiving the protein for various urological disorders at the University of
Iowa.

* The work reported here was conducted with patients in the Department of Urology,
University of Iowa, Iowa City, between the years 1973 and 1977, when one of the authors
(J. D. S.) was a professor in that department. The work was supported in part by the Alex-
ander Medical Foundation.
 † Orgotein is supplied as Ontosein and is available for investigational use only.

MATERIALS AND METHODS

Subject Population

Beginning in 1973, fifty-three patients with various urological disorders at the Department of Urology, University of Iowa, received superoxide dismutase for the evaluation of the toxicity of the preparation. The patients included in the study and their diagnoses are listed in Table I.

Superoxide Dismutase Administration

The copper/zinc-containing superoxide dismutase used in these studies has a molecular weight of about 33,000 with a compact conformation maintained by 4 g atoms of chelated divalent metals. The injectable preparation (orgotein) is currently produced from beef liver in substantially pure form as the copper/zinc enzyme having high enzymatic activity. The dosage forms used in this study included 2 parts sucrose by weight in a freeze-dried solid.

The study was open-labeled, with each dosage unit containing 4 mg of the active ingredient. The duration of administration of the drug ranged from 1 week to more than 3 years, with the drug dose ranging from as little as 4 mg to over 400 mg per patient. The routes of administration varied (Table II).

TABLE I

Diagnoses of 53 Patients Participating in the Safety
Evaluation Study of Superoxide Dismutase

Diagnosis	Number of patients
Benign prostatic hyperplasia	13
Radiation cystitis	9
Chronic cystitis	8
Chronic prostatitis	6
Peyronie's disease	6
Interstitial cystitis	3
Epididymitis	3
Ureteral calculus	1
Penile lymphedema	1
Prostatic cancer	1
Rheumatoid arthritis	2

TABLE II

**Routes of Administration Used in the Study of the
Safety of Superoxide Dismutase Treatment for
Urological Disorders**

Systemic
   Intramuscular
   Subcutaneous
Local
   Intramural (bladder)
   Intralesional (penis)
   Intraprostatic
Topical
   Intravesical

Determination of Toxicity

History, physical examination, complete blood count, biochemical screening profile, prothrombin time, and urinalysis were established as the laboratory parameters that would reflect drug toxicity. These determinations were performed upon each patient's entry into the study and at appropriate intervals thereafter.

Informed Consent

Informed consent was obtained in writing from all patients upon their entry into the study.

RESULTS

Complete hematological and biochemical data indicated no toxicity in any patient receiving either acute or long-term courses of superoxide dismutase (as orgotein). Injections of the drug were pain free; no patient developed signs of systemic toxicity such as skin rash, serum sickness, or fever. The single effect that could be considered adverse occurred in a 39-year-old man with bilateral chronic epididymitis who was receiving 4 mg daily as intramuscular injections. When the route was changed to subcutaneous, he developed erythema and pruritus at the injection site. Subsequent intramuscular injections were well tolerated. Coincidental beneficial effects were noted in several patients; two brief case reports follow.

Case 1

A 47-year-old woman with a 6-year history of interstitial cystitis requiring hydraulic dilations under general anesthesia every 3 months plus antispasmodic drugs and corticosteroids was given superoxide dismutase intramurally (20 mg) injected cystoscopically. A repeat administration via the same route was performed 6 months later. The patient volunteered that this series of injections had given her the best and most lasting relief of symptoms to date.

Case 2

A 49-year-old man with stage C prostatic cancer and a radiation-induced vesicoperineal–cutaneous fistula received 4 mg superoxide dismutase intramuscularly daily for 7 days. An incidental acute thrombophlebitis in an upper extremity resolved completely during the first 48 hr of superoxide dismutase injections. The patient had been receiving no anticoagulant or specific antiinflammatory therapy for his phlebitis.

CONCLUSIONS

The amino acid sequence and crystal structure of superoxide dismutase have been determined (2–4). The protein is a compact globular molecule consisting of two identical subunits tightly but noncovalently bound. It is presumed that the therapeutic effect of this enzyme resides in its antiinflammatory activity. There is no evidence that it is immunosuppressive or that it retards normal wound healing (5). The mechanisms of action of the enzyme are listed in Table III.

The production of the potentially toxic oxygen-derived free radical, superoxide (O_2^-), occurs in biological systems according to the following

TABLE III

Mechanisms of Action of Superoxide Dismutase

Known
   Superoxide anion scavenging
Possible
   Inhibition of platelet aggregation
   Chemotaxis of polymorphonuclear leukocytes
   Stabilization of cell membranes

reaction:

$$O_2 + e^- \xrightarrow[\text{enzymes}]{\text{oxidative}} O_2^- \qquad (1)$$

The protective reaction of dismutation (simultaneous oxidation and reduction) of superoxide catalyzed by superoxide dismutase occurs via the reaction

$$O_2^- + O_2^- + 2H^+ \rightarrow H_2O_2 + O_2 \qquad (2)$$

Formation of the toxic free hydroxyl radical (HO·) from superoxide and hydrogen peroxide has been proposed to occur in the following way:

$$O_2^- + H_2O_2 \xrightarrow[\text{catalyzed}]{\text{iron-}} O_2 + OH^- + HO· \qquad (3)$$

The superoxide radical is produced under various conditions by many sources, including aerobic bacteria, animal and human erythrocytes, polymorphonuclear leukocytes, phagocytes, and macrophages, and also by the reaction to ionizing radiation (6). It then can act as a reactant for the production of HO·.

Investigators from two medical centers in Europe have published reports of the efficacy of superoxide dismutase in the treatment of urological disorders. At Innsbruck, Austria, Marberger and co-workers reported their experience with the administration of superoxide dismutase (as orgotein) in over 50 women with chronic radiation and interstitial cystitis (7,8). Superoxide dismutase therapy via the cystoscopic intramural bladder injection route gave excellent to good results in most patients. Some women required repeat injections for the treatment of clinical relapses.

In Sweden, Edsmyr and associates compared intramuscular superoxide dismutase with placebo on a double-blind basis in a series of 40 bladder cancer patients receiving definitive radiotherapy (9). Orgotein or placebo was administered following each daily radiation treatment. The patients receiving superoxide dismutase showed statistically significant improvement in signs and symptoms related to acute radiation damage to the urinary bladder and rectum. Edsmyr and associates are currently evaluating superoxide dismutase in men receiving radiotherapy for prostatic cancer, and the results to date are encouraging (10).

The results of the current study indicate that superoxide dismutase may be given without toxic effects in a variety of dosages and via several different routes of administration. Our incidental findings of therapeutic benefit in several cases corroborate other evidence that the drug is effective in the treatment of urological disorders. The potential indications for the use of superoxide dismutase in genitourinary diseases are listed in Table IV. If used in conjunction with radiotherapy or cytotoxic chemotherapy,

TABLE IV

**Potential Indications for Superoxide Dismutase
Treatment in Genitourinary Disease**

Radiation therapy
Prostatitis
Benign prostatic hyperplasia
Interstitial cystitis
Urethral syndrome
Herpes progenitalis
Systemic chemotherapy
Peyronie's disease

the effect of superoxide dismutase may be considered analogous to the
rescue via citrovorum factor of toxicity secondary to high-dose methotrexate administration. Further study of the mechanism of action of superoxide dismutase and its efficacy in the treatment of a variety of disorders is warranted.

REFERENCES

1. Anonymous (1971). New drug names: Orgotein. *JAMA, J. Am. Med. Assoc.* **218:**1936.
2. Steinman, H. M., Naik, V. R., Abernethy, J. L., and Hill, R. L. (1974). Bovine erthro-
   cyte superoxide dismutase: Complete amino acid sequence. *J. Biol. Chem.* **249:**7326–
   7338.
3. Richardson, J. S., Thomas, K. A., and Richardson, D. C. (1975). Crystal structure of
   bovine Cu,Zn superoxide dismutase at 3 Å resolution: Chain tracing and metal ligands.
   Proc. Natl. Acad. Sci. U.S.A. **72:**1349–1353.
4. Richardson, J. S., Thomas, K. A., and Richardson, D. C. (1975). Alpha-carbon coordinates for bovine Cu,Zn superoxide dismutase. *Biochem. Biophys. Res. Commun.*
   63:986–992.
5. Huber, W., Schulte, T. L., Carson, S., Goldhamer, R. E., and Vogin, E. E. (1968).
   Some chemical and pharmacologic properties of a novel antiinflammatory protein. *Toxicol. Appl. Pharmacol.* **12:**308.
6. Fridovich, I. (1975). Superoxide dismutase. *Annu. Rev. Biochem.* **44:**147–159.
7. Marberger, H., Huber, W., Bartsch, G., Schulte, T., and Swoboda, P. (1974). Orgotein:
   A new antiinflammatory metalloprotein drug evaluation of clinical efficacy and safety in
   inflammatory conditions of the urinary tract. *Int. Urol. Nephrol.* **6:**61–74.
8. Marberger, H., Bartsch, G., Huber, W., Menander, K. B., and Schulte, T. L. (1975).
   Orgotein: A new drug for the treatment of radiation cystitis. *Curr. Ther. Res.* **18:**466–
   475.
9. Edsmyr, F., Huber, W., and Menander, K. B. (1976). Orgotein efficacy in ameliorating
   side effects due to radiation therapy. I. Double-blind, placebo-controlled trial in patients
   with bladder tumors. *Curr. Ther. Res.* **19:**198–211.
10. Menander, K. B., Edsmyr, F., and Huber, W. (1980). Orgotein efficacy in ameliorating
    side effects due to radiation therapy. *Scand. J. Urol. Nephol., Suppl.* pp. 1–6.

Index

A